Genetic Disorders Sourcebook,
  1st Edition
Genetic Disorders Sourcebook,
  2nd Edition
Head Trauma Sourcebook
Headache Sourcebook
Health Insurance Sourcebook
Health Reference Series Cumulative
  Index 1999
Healthy Aging Sourcebook
Healthy Heart Sourcebook for Women
Heart Diseases & Disorders
  Sourcebook, 2nd Edition
Household Safety Sourcebook
Immune System Disorders Sourcebook
Infant & Toddler Health Sourcebook
Injury & Trauma Sourcebook
Kidney & Urinary Tract Diseases &
  Disorders Sourcebook
Learning Disabilities Sourcebook
Liver Disorders Sourcebook
Lung Disorders Sourcebook
Medical Tests Sourcebook
Men's Health Concerns Sourcebook
Mental Health Disorders Sourcebook,
  1st Edition
Mental Health Disorders Sourcebook,
  2nd Edition
Mental Retardation Sourcebook
Obesity Sourcebook
Ophthalmic Disorders Sourcebook
Oral Health Sourcebook
Osteoporosis Sourcebook
Pain Sourcebook, 1st Edition
Pain Sourcebook, 2nd Edition
Pediatric Cancer Sourcebook
Physical & Mental Issues in Aging
  Sourcebook
Podiatry Sourcebook
Pregnancy & Birth Sourcebook
Prostate Cancer

Public Health Sourcebook
Reconstructive & Cosmetic Surgery
  Sourcebook
Rehabilitation Sourcebook
Respiratory Diseases & Disorders
  Sourcebook
Sexually Transmitted Diseases
  Sourcebook, 1st Edition
Sexually Transmitted Diseases
  Sourcebook, 2nd Edition
Skin Disorders Sourcebook
Sleep Disorders Sourcebook
Sports Injuries Sourcebook
Stress-Related Disorders Sourcebook
Substance Abuse Sourcebook
Surgery Sourcebook
Transplantation Sourcebook
Traveler's Health Sourcebook
Women's Health Concerns Sourcebook
Workplace Health & Safety Sourcebook
Worldwide Health Sourcebook

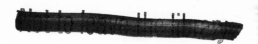

Teen Health Series

Diet Information for Teens
Drug Information for Teens
Mental Health Information
  for Teens
Sexual Health Information
  for Teens

Injury and Trauma
SOURCEBOOK

Health Reference Series

First Edition

Injury and Trauma
SOURCEBOOK

Basic Consumer Health Information about the Impact of Injury, the Diagnosis and Treatment of Common and Traumatic Injuries, Emergency Care, and Specific Injuries Related to Home, Community, Workplace, Transportation, and Recreation

Along with Guidelines for Injury Prevention, a Glossary, and a Directory of Additional Resources

Edited by
Joyce Brennfleck Shannon

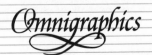

Omnigraphics

615 Griswold Street • Detroit, MI 48226

Bibliographic Note

Because this page cannot legibly accommodate all the copyright notices, the Bibliographic Note portion of the Preface constitutes an extension of the copyright notice.

Edited by Joyce Brennfleck Shannon

Health Reference Series

Karen Bellenir, *Managing Editor*
David A. Cooke, MD, *Medical Consultant*
Elizabeth Barbour, *Permissions Associate*
Dawn Matthews, *Verification Assistant*
Carol Munson, *Permissions Assistant*
Laura Pleva, *Index Editor*
EdIndex, Services for Publishers, *Indexers*

* * *

Omnigraphics, Inc.

Matthew P. Barbour, *Senior Vice President*
Kay Gill, *Vice President—Directories*
Kevin Hayes, *Operations Manager*
David P. Bianco, *Marketing Consultant*

* * *

Peter E. Ruffner, *President and Publisher*

Frederick G. Ruffner, Jr., *Chairman*

Copyright © 2002 Omnigraphics, Inc.

ISBN 0-7808-0421-X

Library of Congress Cataloging-in-Publication Data

Injury and trauma sourcebook : basic consumer health information about the impact of injury, the diagnosis and treatment of common and traumatic injuries, emergency care, and specific injuries related to home, community, workplace, transportation, and recreation; along with guidelines for injury prevention, a glossary, and a directory of additional resources / edited by Joyce Brennfleck Shannon. -- 1st ed.

p. ; cm. -- (Health reference series)
Includes bibliographical references and index.
ISBN 0-7808-0421-X
1. Wounds and injuries--Popular works. I. Shannon, Joyce Brennfleck. II. Health reference series (Unnumbered)
[DNLM: 1. Wounds and Injuries--Popular Works. 2. Wounds and Injuries--Resource Guides. 3. Accident Prevention--Popular Works, 4. Accident Prevention--Resource Guides. WO 39 I56 2002]
RD93 .I55 2002
617.1--dc21

2002022060

Table of Contents

Part III: Trauma Injuries

Part IV: Emergency Care

Part V: Injury Prevention Strategies for the Community and Home

Part VI: Work-Related Injuries

Part VII: Transportation Injuries and Safety

Part VIII: Recreation-Related Injuries and Prevention

Part IX: Additional Help and Information

Preface

About This Book

Injuries are a leading cause of death for Americans of all ages, regardless of gender, race, or economic status. But injury deaths are only part of the picture. Millions of Americans are injured each year and survive. For many of them, the injury causes temporary pain and inconvenience, but for some the injury leads to disability, chronic pain, and a profound change in lifestyle.

Prevention reduces the risk of injury. By following simple safety rules, taking proper precautions, and teaching safety to children, injuries can be avoided. For example, seat belts and motorcycle helmets save thousands of lives each year; smoke detectors halve the risk of dying from fire; and bicycle helmets reduce the risk of head injury in bicycle crashes by 85 percent.

This *Sourcebook* provides health information about common injuries and trauma injuries in the U.S. Readers will learn essential information about injuries that occur at home, in the community, at work, and during transportation and recreation, as well as facts about emergency care. Injury prevention guidelines are included, along with a glossary and a listing of additional resources.

How to Use This Book

This book is divided into parts and chapters. Parts focus on broad areas of interest. Chapters are devoted to single topics within a part.

Part I: The High Toll of Injury in the U.S. provides an overview of injury as a public health issue. Injury visits to hospital emergency departments are documented, and injuries and risk factors specific to children, adolescents, and older adults are also presented.

Part II: Common Injuries reviews bites and stings, burns, cuts and abrasions, and fractures, along with specific injuries to the back, elbow, foot and ankle, growth plate, head and brain, hip, knee, neck, and shoulder.

Part III: Trauma Injuries offers information about firearm injuries, spinal cord and traumatic brain injuries, and abuse and violence that can lead to injury in family, dating, child, and elder relationships. Advice about the psychological effects of trauma is presented with specific information for parents of children who have experienced a trauma injury.

Part IV: Emergency Care describes how to handle severe and life-threatening injuries, what to expect in the emergency room, childcare emergency first aid, and emergency care for severe wounds.

Part V: Injury Prevention Strategies for the Community and Home gives practical advice for creating safe homes and communities. Issues addressed include alcohol-related injury risks, avoiding accidents, preventing falls, and keeping children safe from poison, choking, and playground injuries. Information about the necessity of smoke alarms and home detectors for natural gas and carbon monoxide is also provided.

Part VI: Work-Related Injuries presents the rates of injury associated with specific occupations and workplace factors that lead to musculoskeletal disorders, hearing loss, and risks for adolescent workers. It also includes facts about workplace violence and offers safety guidelines for preventing injury.

Part VII: Transportation Injuries and Safety reviews crash-related statistics associated with motor vehicles, motorcycles, all-terrain vehicles (ATVs), and bicycles. Safety recommendations describe helmet use, pedestrian safety, and the risks of alcohol-impairment.

Part VIII: Recreation-Related Injuries and Prevention examines the risks of injury associated with common leisure activities involving water and winter sports and amusement rides. It also reviews injuries from use of unpowered scooters, fireworks, BB guns, in-line skates, and skateboards.

Part IX: Additional Help and Information includes a glossary of important terms, and directories of on-line resources and organizations that provide additional information.

Bibliographic Note

This volume contains documents and excerpts from publications issued by the following U.S. government agencies: Administration on Aging (AoA); Bureau of Labor Statistics (BLS); Centers for Disease Control and Prevention (CDC); Consumer Product Safety Commission (CPSC); Division of Healthcare Quality Promotion (DHQP); Elder Abuse Center; National Center for Health Statistics (NCHS); National Center for Injury Prevention and Control (NCIPC); National Clearinghouse on Child Abuse and Neglect Information; National Highway Traffic Safety Administration (NHTSA); National Institute on Aging (NIA); National Institute on Alcohol Abuse and Alcoholism (NIAAA); National Institute of Arthritis and Musculoskeletal and Skin Diseases (NIAMS); National Institute of Child Health and Human Development; National Institute of Dental and Craniofacial Research (NIDCR); National Institute of General Medical Sciences (NIGMS); National Institutes of Health Osteoporosis and Related Bone Disorders—National Resource Center; National Institute of Neurological Disorders and Stroke (NINDS); National Institute for Occupational Safety and Health (NIOSH); National Institute on Deafness and Other Communications Disorders (NIDCD); Office of Justice Programs (OJP); SafeKids; SafeUSA; U.S. Coast Guard; U.S. Department of Labor; and U.S. Fire Administration (USFA).

In addition, this volume contains copyrighted documents from the following organizations and individuals: A.D.A.M., Inc.; American Academy of Family Physicians; American Association of Neurological Surgeons/Congress of Neurological Surgeons; American Burn Association; American College of Emergency Physicians; American Psychiatric Association; Brain Injury Association; Dr. Ricky Greenwald; Injury Prevention Research Center (University of Iowa); International Shrine Headquarters; Medical Multimedia Group; MedicineNet.com; National Fire Protection Association; and National Spinal Cord Injury Statistical Center/University of Alabama at Birmingham.

Full citation information is provided on the first page of each chapter. Every effort has been made to secure all necessary rights to reprint the copyrighted material. If any omissions have been made, please contact Omnigraphics to make corrections for future editions.

Acknowledgements

Special thanks to the many organizations, agencies, and individuals who have contributed materials for this *Sourcebook* and to the managing editor Karen Bellenir, medical consultant Dr. David Cooke, permissions specialists Liz Barbour and Carol Munson, verification assistant Dawn Matthews, indexer Edward J. Prucha, and document engineer Bruce Bellenir.

Note from the Editor

This book is part of Omnigraphics' *Health Reference Series*. The series provides basic information about a broad range of medical concerns. It is not intended to serve as a tool for diagnosing illness, in prescribing treatments, or as a substitute for the physician/patient relationship. All persons concerned about medical symptoms or the possibility of disease are encouraged to seek professional care from an appropriate health care provider.

Our Advisory Board

The *Health Reference Series* is reviewed by an Advisory Board comprised of librarians from public, academic, and medical libraries. We would like to thank the following board members for providing guidance to the development of this series:

Dr. Lynda Baker, Associate Professor of Library and Information Science, Wayne State University, Detroit, MI

Nancy Bulgarelli, William Beaumont Hospital Library, Royal Oak, MI

Karen Imarasio, Bloomfield Township Public Library, Bloomfield Township, MI

Karen Morgan, Mardigian Library, University of Michigan-Dearborn, Dearborn, MI

Rosemary Orlando, St. Clair Shores Public Library, St. Clair Shores, MI

Medical Consultant

Medical consultation services are provided to the *Health Reference Series* editors by David A. Cooke, M.D. Dr. Cooke is a graduate of Brandeis University, and he received his M.D. degree from the University of Michigan. He completed residency training at the University of Wisconsin Hospital and Clinics. He is board-certified in Internal Medicine. Dr. Cooke currently works as part of the University of Michigan Health System and practices in Brighton, MI. In his free time, he enjoys writing, science fiction, and spending time with his family.

Health Reference Series *Update Policy*

The inaugural book in the *Health Reference Series* was the first edition of *Cancer Sourcebook* published in 1992. Since then, the *Series* has been enthusiastically received by librarians and in the medical community. In order to maintain the standard of providing high-quality health information for the layperson the editorial staff at Omnigraphics felt it was necessary to implement a policy of updating volumes when warranted.

Medical researchers have been making tremendous strides, and it is the purpose of the *Health Reference Series* to stay current with the most recent advances. Each decision to update a volume will be made on an individual basis. Some of the considerations will include how much new information is available and the feedback we receive from people who use the books. If there is a topic you would like to see added to the update list, or an area of medical concern you feel has not been adequately addressed, please write to:

Editor
Health Reference Series
Omnigraphics, Inc.
615 Griswold Street
Detroit, MI 48226

The commitment to providing on-going coverage of important medical developments has also led to some format changes in the *Health Reference Series*. Each new volume on a topic is individually titled and called a "First Edition." Subsequent updates will carry sequential edition numbers. To help avoid confusion and to provide maximum flexibility in our ability to respond to informational needs, the practice of consecutively numbering each volume has been discontinued.

Part One

The High Toll of Injury in the U.S.

Chapter 1

Working to Prevent and Control Injury

Injuries Affect Everyone

Injuries are a leading cause of death for Americans of all ages, regardless of gender, race, or economic status. But injury deaths are only part of the picture. Millions of Americans are injured each year and survive. For many of them, the injury causes temporary pain and inconvenience, but for some, the injury leads to disability, chronic pain, and a profound change in lifestyle.

An injury affects more than just the person injured—it affects everyone who is involved in the injured person's life. With a fatal injury, family, friends, coworkers, employers, and other members of the injured person's community feel the loss. In addition to experiencing grief, they may experience a loss of income or the loss of a primary caregiver, as well.

With a nonfatal injury, family members are often called upon to care for the injured person, which can result in stress, time away from work, and possibly lost income. They may also experience a change in their relationship with the injured person and with others in the family. For instance, if a wife and mother is seriously injured, her spouse may find himself in the role of primary caregiver—not only for his wife, but also for his children. Friends of the injured person may be called upon to help out and, like family members, may experience a change in their relationship with the injured person. The

Excerpted from "Injury Fact Book 2001-2002," National Center for Injury Prevention and Control, 2001.

injured person's employer may struggle with the temporary or permanent loss of a valued employee. Others in the community—volunteer groups, religious organizations, and neighbors—may also feel the effects of the injury.

Society at large is also profoundly affected by injuries. The financial cost of injuries is estimated at more than $224 billion each year. These costs include direct medical care, rehabilitation, lost wages, and lost productivity. The federal government pays about $12.6 billion each year in injury-related medical costs and about $18.4 billion in death and disability benefits. Insurance companies and other private sources pay about $161 billion.

Table 1.1. Deaths by Age Group Caused by Unintentional Injuries 1998

Age Group	Number of Deaths	Rank*
Under 1 year	754	8
1-4 years	1,935	1
5-9 years	1,544	1
10-14 years	1,710	1
15-24 years	13,349	1
25-34 years	12,045	1
35-44 years	15,127	2
45-54 years	10,946	3
55-64 years	7,340	6
65 years and over	32,975	7
Total	97,835	5

* (1-10 with 1 being the leading cause of death)

Source: National Center for Health Statistics, 2000.

The Public Health Approach to Injury Prevention

To solve public health problems—including injuries—Centers for Disease Control and Prevention (CDC) uses a systematic process called the public health approach. This approach has four steps:

1. define the problem,

2. identify risk and protective factors,

3. develop and test prevention strategies, and

4. assure widespread adoption of injury prevention principles and strategies.

Define the Problem

Before we can tackle an injury problem, we need to know how big the problem is, where it is, and whom it affects. CDC accomplishes this by gathering and analyzing data—often called surveillance. These data can show us how an injury problem changes over time, alert us to troubling trends in a particular type of injury, and let us know what impact prevention programs are having. These data are critical because they help decision-makers allocate programs and resources where they are needed most.

Identify Risk and Protective Factors

It is not enough to simply know that a certain type of injury is affecting a certain group of people in a certain area. We also need to know why. What factors put people at risk for that injury? And conversely, what factors protect people from it? CDC conducts and supports research to answer these important questions. Once the information is gathered, programs can be developed and implemented to eliminate or reduce risk factors for injuries and to capitalize on or increase factors that protect people from being injured.

Develop and Test Prevention Strategies

In this step, knowledge is put into action. Using information gathered in research, CDC develops strategies to prevent particular injury problems. The strategies are implemented in communities that are experiencing the problem. Effects of these strategies are studied to determine whether and how well they're working. This information is used to identify any elements needed to change to eliminate difficulties or increase effectiveness.

Assure Widespread Adoption

What is learned in the developing and testing step has little benefit if the information is kept to ourselves. In this final step of the public health approach, CDC shares the "best practices" or "lessons learned" for a strategy. This information helps communities to replicate successful strategies. CDC may also provide funding or expert consultation to help communities adopt these strategies

The Public Health Approach at Work

CDC has already moved through the first three steps of the public health approach for some injury issues and is ready to encourage widespread adoption. Since the study of injury is a relatively new public health field, however, in several cases CDC is still trying to fully define the problem. Here's how the public health approach works in injury.

Defining the Problem

Violence in America

In the U.S. in 1998, 17,983 people died as a result of homicide and 30,575 died from suicide. While public health officials may know how many people die from violence each year, they don't know much about the circumstances surrounding those deaths. Federal, state, and local agencies all have detailed information that could answer important, fundamental questions about trends and patterns in violence, but the information is fragmented and difficult to access. CDC is working to establish a National Violent Death Reporting System to gather data from states about violent deaths in America. The system would pull together this vital information so it could be shared among states and communities in order to gain an accurate understanding of the problem of violence in America. Such a system would assist policy makers and community leaders in making educated decisions about strategies and programs to prevent violence.

Traumatic Brain Injury among Children

Many injury professionals describe traumatic brain injury (TBI) as the leading cause of disability among children, but evidence to support this assertion is lacking. CDC's Injury Center will fund a study to find out how many children have disabilities related to TBI and how those disabilities affect them and their families. This research will build on recommendations generated by a group of injury researchers, professionals, and advocates convened by CDC in October 2000.

Intimate Partner Violence

An estimated 2.3 million Americans—1.5 million of them women— are raped or physically assaulted by an intimate partner each year.

But inconsistencies in data collection and different ways of describing the problem have fostered a lack of consensus about the magnitude of the problem. Early in Fiscal Year 2000, CDC's Injury Center published a set of definitions designed to improve data collected concerning violence against women by standardizing the terminology used by all parties involved in the problem—the criminal justice system, hospitals, and others. Five states are now establishing tracking systems for intimate partner violence. The states will use the Injury Center's *Uniform Definitions and Recommended Data Elements* in gathering their data. These pilot tests will help CDC assess states' capacity to identify existing data sources that include some or all of these elements, identify opportunities to link data sources, and develop and implement more comprehensive systems.

Identifying Risk and Protective Factors

Suicide

More than 30,000 people took their own lives in 1998, but no one really knows why. Public health officials are still learning what puts people at risk for committing or attempting suicide and what prevents them from doing so. Injury Center staff and CDC-funded researchers have begun studying factors that may increase or decrease a person's risk for suicide. One study in Texas, which interviewed people who experienced nearly lethal suicide attempts, found that many factors—in addition to mental health factors—may influence suicidal behavior, including alcohol use, geographic mobility, exposure to suicidal behavior, hopelessness, help-seeking behavior, impulsiveness, and physical illness. Researchers at Atlanta's Emory University examined suicide risk factors among African Americans ages 18 to 44. They found a strong connection between intimate partner violence and suicidal behavior among African American women.

Assessing Attitudes and Beliefs about Child Maltreatment

CDC is funding an analysis of attitudes, beliefs, and behaviors relating to child maltreatment in various cultural and ethnic populations. The analysis will describe how communities feel about outcomes of abuse, characteristics of abusers, risk, and protective factors for abuse, and efforts to prevent it. This information will help practitioners develop prevention messages that are more meaningful to those groups and can more effectively change behavior.

Developing and Testing Prevention Strategies

Fire Injury Prevention

Through tracking and monitoring injuries and deaths from residential fires, CDC has learned that one of the biggest risk factors is not having a functional smoke alarm in the home. For several years, CDC funded states to distribute smoke alarms and educate citizens most at risk for residential fires (older adults, poor families, and families living in manufactured housing). As part of the program, the Injury Center conducted a long-term evaluation of these efforts and found that only two-thirds of homes receiving smoke alarms through a distribution program had a working alarm three to four years later. The researchers concluded that future programs should distribute alarms that do not require annual battery changes or find ways to ensure that batteries are changed routinely.

Preventing Pressure Ulcers after Spinal Cord Injury

Persons with spinal cord injuries are at risk for pressure ulcers, a condition that can be quite debilitating and costly. Over a one-year period, participants in a CDC-funded intervention experienced a 46% decrease in pressure sore occurrence and a 36% decrease in pressure sore severity. The intervention, part of the Arkansas Spinal Cord Commission's Consumer Action to Prevent Pressure Sores (CAPPS) project, eliminated sores among one-third of the intervention group and saved $660,000 in hospital costs associated with pressure sores.

This project demonstrated that in-home education conducted by public health nurses can prevent new pressure sores and reduce the number and severity of existing sores among a rural, underserved population of persons with spinal cord injury.

Assuring Widespread Adoption

Alcohol and Motor Vehicle Crashes

Epidemiologists from CDC's Injury Center recently found that laws lowering the legal blood alcohol concentration (BAC) for drivers from 0.10% to 0.08% are effective in reducing deaths from alcohol-related motor vehicle crashes. They shared their findings with the Task Force on Community Preventive Services, which strongly recommended that state policy makers consider enacting this type of law. The Task Force's recommendation led the House Appropriations Committee to add language to its appropriations bill requiring states to enact such laws; states that do not will lose federal funding for highway construction. On October 23, 2000, the President signed the transportation appropriations bill containing the 0.08% BAC language, thus creating a new, national standard for the legal BAC for motor vehicle drivers. The new standard does not guarantee that all states will adopt the lower BAC limit, but the funding consequences increase the likelihood.

Preventing Falls among Older Adults

Nearly 10,000 Americans 65 and older die from falls each year. In 2001, the Injury Center published a compendium of selected, community-based programs to prevent falls among older people. *U.S. Fall Prevention Programs for Seniors: Selected Programs Using Home Assessment and Modification* describes 18 fall prevention programs that include education, home assessment, and home modification strategies for fall prevention. Using the detailed program descriptions, as well as sample program materials provided in the appendix, communities can develop similar strategies to protect their older residents from fall-related injuries.

National Poison Control Center Access

CDC and the Health Resources and Services Administration are funding the American Association of Poison Control Centers to implement a single, toll-free, poison control number nationwide. All state poison centers were expected to implement this toll-free number by the end of 2001. One, nationwide number will improve access to poison control services for all Americans, including those in underserved areas. An education program and media campaign will inform Americans about the new number and raise awareness about the services that poison control centers provide.

Chapter 2

Injury Visits to Hospital Emergency Departments

Alcohol, Injuries, and the Emergency Department

Alcohol problems, a known risk factor for a wide range of illnesses and injuries, are prevalent among patients in emergency departments. This fact makes the emergency department a logical setting in which to screen and intervene for alcohol problems. While ED-based screening and intervention has shown promise in ongoing studies, we should continue to explore this strategy for preventing alcohol-related injuries.

- Excessive alcohol consumption is an important factor in more than 100,000 deaths in the United States each year.

- Between 20% and 30% of the patients seen in U.S. hospital emergency departments (ED) have alcohol problems.

- Nearly half of alcohol-related deaths are the result of injuries from motor-vehicle crashes, falls, fires, drowning, homicides, and suicides.

- Emergency departments do not routinely screen patients for alcohol problems.

This chapter includes "Table 84," and excerpts from "Alcohol, Injuries, and the Emergency Department," *Health, United States, 2001,* National Center for Health Statistics, 2001; and "Ambulatory Health Care Data," National Center for Health Statistics, 2001.

- An alcohol-related motor vehicle crash kills someone every 33 minutes and nonfatally injures someone every two minutes. In 1999, 15,786 people died in alcohol-related motor vehicle crashes. That's 38% of the year's total traffic deaths.

- Approximately 1.4 million drivers were arrested in 1998 for driving under the influence of alcohol or narcotics. That's just over 1% of the estimated 120 million or more episodes of impaired driving that occur among U.S. adults each year.

- About 3 in 10 Americans will be involved in an alcohol-related crash in their lifetimes.

- Nearly three-quarters of drivers convicted of driving while impaired are either frequent heavy drinkers (alcohol abusers) or alcoholics (alcohol dependent).

- The National Safety Council estimates that alcohol-related motor vehicle crashes cost the nation $26.9 billion in 1998.

Additional Reading

Burt CW, Overpeck MD. Emergency visits for sports-related injuries. *Ann Emerg Med*. March 2001; 37:301-308.

Table 2.1. Average Annual Injury Visits to Hospital Emergency Departments by Persons between 5 and 24 Years of Age by Type of Activity Performed when Injury Occurred: United States, 1997-98.

Injury	Number of visits in thousands	Percent of visits in thousands	Percent of sports-related injury visits
All injury visits	11,904	100.0	
All sport-related activities[1]	2,616	22.0	100.0
Group sport	1,170	9.8	44.7
Basketball	447	3.8	17.1
Football	271	2.3	10.3
Baseball/softball	245	2.1	9.4
Soccer	95	0.8	3.6
Other group sport[2]	112	0.9	4.3
Individual sport	1,446	12.2	55.3
Pedal cycling	421	3.5	16.1
Ice- or roller skating/boarding	150	1.3	5.7
Gymnastics/cheerleading	146	1.2	5.6
Playground	137	1.2	5.2
Snow sport	111	0.9	4.2
Water sport	100	0.8	3.8
Exercising/track	94	0.8	3.6
Combative	61	0.5	2.3
Recreational	50	0.4	1.9
Other sport[3]	178	1.5	6.8
Nonsport activities[4]	7,947	66.8	
Visits without a specified cause[5]	1,340	11.3	

[1]Includes all visits with a cause indicating an organized or unorganized sport, game, or recreational activity.

[2]Includes other group sports such as volleyball, hockey, and lacrosse.

[3]Includes all other categories such as games, all terrain vehicles, and unspecified sport/recreational activities.

[4]Includes all visits with a specified activity not categorized under sports. This includes transport, household, personal, work, or maintenance activities. It also includes visits for any injuries caused by intentional behavior.

[5]Includes any visits for which no cause was listed or the entry stated unknown causes.

Source: National Hospital Ambulatory Medical Care Survey.

Table 2.2. Injury-Related Visits to Hospital Emergency Departments by Sex, Age, Intent, and Mechanism of Injury: United States, Average Annual 1995-96 and 1998-99. [Data are based on reporting by a sample of hospital emergency departments]

Sex, age, and intent and mechanism of injury[1]	Visits in thousands		Visits per 10,000 persons	
	1995-96	1998-99	1995-96	1998-99
Both sexes				
All ages[2,3]	36,081	37,361	1,360.9	1,378.3
Male				
All ages[2,3]	20,030	20,445	1,530.7	1,535.2
Under 18 years[2]	6,238	6,054	1,720.2	1,644.3
Unintentional injuries	5,478	5,190	1,510.5	1,409.7
Falls	1,402	1,247	386.5	338.7
Struck by or against objects or persons	1,011	1,398	278.9	379.7
Motor vehicle traffic	453	388	125.0	105.5
Cut or pierce	493	505	136.0	137.1
Intentional injuries	290	222	80.0	60.3
18-24 years[2]	2,980	2,948	2,396.9	2,295.1
Unintentional injuries	2,423	2,319	1,948.7	1,805.3
Falls	299	333	240.8	259.5
Struck by or against objects or persons	387	389	311.0	303.1
Motor vehicle traffic	347	412	279.4	320.9
Cut or pierce	304	344	244.8	268.2
Intentional injuries	335	291	269.2	226.5
25-44 years[2]	7,245	7,112	1,767.4	1,751.7
Unintentional injuries	5,757	5,391	1,404.3	1,327.8
Falls	817	847	199.4	208.6
Struck by or against objects or persons	619	819	151.0	201.6
Motor vehicle traffic	912	839	222.6	206.6
Cut or pierce	860	786	209.8	193.7
Intentional injuries	701	473	171.0	116.5

Table 2.2. Injury-Related Visits to Hospital Emergency Departments by Sex, Age, Intent, and Mechanism of Injury: United States, Average Annual 1995-96 and 1998-99. [Data are based on reporting by a sample of hospital emergency departments] (continued)

Sex, age, and intent and mechanism of injury[1]	Visits in thousands		Visits per 10,000 persons	
	1995-96	1998-99	1995-96	1998-99
Male, continued				
45-64 years[2]	2,240	2,822	883.4	1,011.9
Unintentional injuries	1,845	2,213	727.6	793.4
Falls	445	569	175.6	204.0
Struck by or against objects or persons	186	197	73.3	70.6
Motor vehicle traffic	244	322	96.3	115.5
Cut or pierce	203	290	79.9	104.1
Intentional injuries	86	73	33.8	26.2
65 years and over[2]	1,327	1,509	1,000.7	1,100.3
Unintentional injuries	1,009	1,151	760.6	839.3
Falls	505	584	380.9	426.0
Struck by or against objects or persons	*39	101	*29.4	73.3
Motor vehicle traffic	99	113	74.7	82.7
Cut or pierce	*81	85	*61.1	*61.7
Intentional injuries	*	16	*	*
Female				
All ages[2,3]	16,051	16,917	1,186.4	1,217.6
Under 18 years[2]	4,372	4,290	1,263.9	1,220.4
Unintentional injuries	3,760	3,598	1,087.0	1,023.4
Falls	1,040	964	300.7	274.2
Struck by or against objects or persons	477	689	137.9	196.1
Motor vehicle traffic	447	394	129.3	112.1
Cut or pierce	253	258	73.0	73.4
Intentional injuries	220	147	63.6	41.7

15

Table 2.2. Injury-Related Visits to Hospital Emergency Departments by Sex, Age, Intent, and Mechanism of Injury: United States, Average Annual 1995-96 and 1998-99. [Data are based on reporting by a sample of hospital emergency departments] (continued)

Sex, age, and intent and mechanism of injury[1]	Visits in thousands		Visits per 10,000 persons	
	1995-96	1998-99	1995-96	1998-99
Female, continued				
18-24 years[2]	1,900	2,049	1,523.4	1,589.6
Unintentional injuries	1,430	1,464	1,146.7	1,135.8
Falls	268	208	214.5	161.7
Struck by or against objects or persons	134	169	107.4	130.8
Motor vehicle traffic	373	442	298.8	342.7
Cut or pierce	131	122	105.3	94.8
Intentional injuries	239	230	191.7	178.6
25-44 years[2]	5,098	5,257	1,205.8	1,246.7
Unintentional injuries	3,877	3,820	916.8	906.1
Falls	817	908	193.3	215.5
Struck by or against objects or persons	380	405	89.8	95.9
Motor vehicle traffic	872	794	206.2	188.4
Cut or pierce	338	472	79.8	111.9
Intentional injuries	422	422	99.8	100.2
45-64 years[2]	2,369	2,802	873.7	940.4
Unintentional injuries	1,857	2,109	685.2	707.9
Falls	600	706	221.5	237.0
Struck by or against objects or persons	160	193	58.8	64.8
Motor vehicle traffic	343	317	126.5	106.4
Cut or pierce	127	214	46.9	71.8
Intentional injuries	*64	111	*23.5	37.4

Table 2.2. Injury-Related Visits to Hospital Emergency Departments by Sex, Age, Intent, and Mechanism of Injury: United States, Average Annual 1995-96 and 1998-99. [Data are based on reporting by a sample of hospital emergency departments] (concluded)

Sex, age, and intent and mechanism of injury[1]	Visits in thousands		Visits per 10,000 persons	
	1995-96	1998-99	1995-96	1998-99
Female, continued				
65 years and over[2]	2,313	2,518	1,256.1	1,346.8
Unintentional injuries	1,931	2,016	1,049.0	1,078.1
Falls	1,230	1,258	667.9	672.7
Struck by or against objects or persons	82	119	44.8	63.6
Motor vehicle traffic	169	148	91.6	79.3
Cut or pierce	*42	73	*22.7	*39.0
Intentional injuries	*	34	*	*

*Estimates are considered unreliable. Data preceded by an asterisk have a relative standard error of 20-30 percent. Data not shown have a relative standard error greater than 30 percent.

1.Intent and mechanism of injury are based on the first-listed external cause of injury code (E code). Intentional injuries include suicide attempts and assaults.

2. An emergency department visit was considered injury-related if the checkbox for injury was indicated. In addition, injury visits were identified if the physician's diagnosis or the patient's reason for the visit were injury-related. All injury-related visits include visits not shown separately in table including those with intent (about 1 percent in 1998-99); visits with insufficient or no information to code cause of injury (about 12 percent in 1998-99); and visits resulting from effects of medical treatment (about 4 percent in 1998-99). Unintentional injury-related visits include visits with mechanism of injury not shown in table.

3. Rates are age adjusted to year 2000 standard using six age groups: Under 18 years of age, 18-24 years, 25-44 years, 45-64 years, 65-74 years, and 75 years and over.

Note: Some data for 1998-99 have been revised and differ from previous editions of *Health, United States*. Rates are based on the civilian non-institutionalized population adjusted for net under enumeration using the 1990 National Population Adjustment Matrix from Bureau of the Census.

17

Chapter 3

Childhood Injuries

Chapter Contents

Section 3.1

How Frequently Are Children Injured?

"Childhood Injury Fact Sheet," National Center for Injury
Prevention and Control, July 2, 1999; and "Major Causes of Early
Childhood Death from Injury Identified," News Releases, National
Institute of Child Health & Human Development (NICHD),
May 3, 1999.

Each year between 20%-25% of all children sustain an injury sufficiently severe to require medical attention, missed school, and/or bed
rest.

- For every childhood death caused by injury, there are approximately 34 hospitalizations, 1,000 emergency department
  visits, many more visits to private physicians and school
  nurses, and an even larger number of injuries treated at
  home.

- Deaths: Unintentional injuries are the leading cause of death
  in children from 1-21 years of age. However, deaths are still a
  rare event. Even so, they are relatively easy to count accurately,
  given the sophisticated vital statistics surveillance system in
  the United States. These records are maintained by the National Center for Health Statistics, CDC

- Nonfatal: These are much less rare, but are more difficult to
  count accurately, since injured children are treated at so
  many types of sites by so many types of health care professionals. Very few national surveillance systems exist for such
  data. The Department of Transportation (National Highway
  Traffic Safety Administration) maintains the Fatal Accident
  Reporting System for fatal traffic-related events, and its com-
  panion General Estimates System to estimate the number of
  nonfatal traffic-related events. The U.S. Consumer Product
  Safety Commission maintains the National Electronic Injury
  Surveillance System to monitor hospital emergency department visits for product-related injuries.

Who Is At-Risk?

Each type of injury has a particular demographic pattern, which is determined by:

- Developmental level of the child: physical, mental, emotional

- Prevalence of the threat in that community (e.g., all-terrain vehicles, backyard swimming pools, firearms, kerosene heaters, etc.)

- Access to and use of environmental countermeasures (e.g., bike helmets, smoke detectors)

- Importance of supervision in avoiding the threat, relative to the degree provided (e.g., toddler living in a low-income apartment complex with an in-ground swimming pool that lacks protective fencing, with a 5-year-old supervising the toddler)

- Several demographic features are common to most types of injuries. The injury rates are greatest in those with:
    - Low socioeconomic status, especially urban African-American children and American Indians/Alaska Natives
    - Males

The principal exception to this is young motor vehicle occupants before adolescence, in whom the male to female ration is nearly even.

What Are the Leading Causes of Fatal Injuries

Overall, motor vehicles, fires/burns, drowning, falls, and poisoning are the leading causes of fatal injuries.

What Determines What Body Site(s) Are Injured?

Injury-specific. For example:

- Motor vehicle—blunt thoracoabdominal trauma, head injuries
- Sports—extremity fractures, sprains, and strains
- House fires—body burns, inhalation injuries
- Near-drowning—coma, brain damage
- Falls—head injuries, fractures, blunt trauma
- Poisoning—coma, kidney failure, etc.

Was the child a projectile?

- Head injury quite likely
- Bicycle-motor vehicle collision, falling forward over the handlebars
- Unrestrained occupant in a motor vehicle collision, thrown forward through the windshield or ejected from vehicle unto roadway

Where Do Injuries Occur most Commonly?

Locations and conditions associated with possible danger are:

- In the home:
    - Water—kitchen, bathroom, backyard swimming pool
    - Intense heat or flames—kitchen, backyard barbecue pit
    - Toxic agents—under the kitchen sink, bathroom medicine chest, mother's purse, garage
    - High potential energy—stairwells, loaded firearms

- At school:
    - Related to sports activities (especially in the absence of proper gear)
    - Carrying of weapons
    - Industrial arts classes

- After school on the job:
    - Hostile relationships in work environment
    - Use of machinery

- After school during transport:
    - Motor vehicle crashes (especially if unrestrained or if driver has been drinking alcohol)
    - Bicycle crashes
    - Pedestrian injuries

What Criteria Determine the Priority Level for Each Type of Childhood Injury?

- High mortality rate or hospitalization rate
- High long-term disability rate, especially mechanisms likely to result in head and spinal cord injuries
- Existence of effective countermeasure

In other words, the highest priorities are assigned to those types of injuries which are common, severe, and readily preventable. Often, however, the only difference between a nonfatal and fatal event is only a few feet (e.g., pedestrian injury which results in fracture rather than massive trauma), a few inches (gunshot wound to the arm instead of the head), or a few seconds (as in the survivor of a near-drowning event). Therefore, each nonfatal event that involves a great mismatch of momentum must be taken very seriously. Surveillance of nonfatal injuries would be appropriate to help determine risk factors and possible interventions, as a proxy for fatal events.

Major Causes of Early Childhood Death from Injury

Homicide, accidental suffocation, motor vehicle accidents, fire, drowning, and choking were the major causes of injury-related death for children less than a year of age, according to a study by researchers at the National Institute of Child Health and Human Development (NICHD). "This important study examines some major causes of death for small children," said NICHD Director Duane Alexander, MD. "The study provides vital information for planning interventions that can help prevent this needless, tragic loss of life."

The investigators were led by Ruth Brenner, MD, MPH, of NICHD as Division of Epidemiology, Statistics, and Prevention Research. They began by analyzing a set of linked infant birth and death certificates, compiled by the National Center for Health Statistics, for the years 1983 through 1991. Homicides claimed the greatest number of lives. A listing of deaths by all categories follows.

- Homicide: 2,345 (22.6 percent)
- Suffocation: 1,839 (17.7 percent)
- Motor vehicle accident: 1,580 (15.2 percent)
- Fire: 990 (9.5 percent)
- Drowning: 745 (7.2 percent)
- Choking on food: 734 (7.1 percent)
- Choking on objects: 609 (5.9 percent)
- Other unintentional injuries: 1,097 (10.6 percent)
- Injuries of undetermined intent: 431 (4.2 percent)

The study found that infants were more likely to die from injuries if their mothers were young, unmarried, had lower levels of education, had more older children, had received prenatal care either late or not at all, or were Native American or African American. Infants who died from an injury were more likely to be of low birth weight, premature, and male. In addition, the researchers found that specific injuries corresponded with specific risk factors. For example, children born to mothers who were younger or had given birth previously were at twice the risk for suffocation. Infants born to Native American mothers were at greatest risk for motor vehicle-related deaths and drownings, while the rate of death from choking was highest among low birth weight infants.

Dr. Brenner cautioned that the study was limited to information that was listed consistently on birth and death certificates, such as birth weight on birth certificates, and cause of death on death certificates. This limitation prevented the researchers from examining the influence of paternal characteristics and other important factors, such as household income.

Dr. Brenner added that efforts to prevent childhood injuries and injury-related deaths should continue to focus on such general strategies as the use of car safety seats for infants and visiting home nurse programs for young, unmarried mothers. She pointed out, however, that there is also a need to develop specific intervention strategies for children at particularly high risk of death.

"Our study identified groups of infants at increased risk of death due to injury," she said. "This will help in the design of more focused interventions to prevent injuries in high risk groups of children.

Section 3.2

Hidden Hazards—Why Kids Are at Risk

"Hidden Hazards, Why Kids Are at Risk," National SAFE KIDS Campaign, 2000; and "Shopping Cart Injuries: Victims 5 Years Old and Younger," Consumer Product Safety Commission (CPSC).

Children are at risk from hidden hazards due to their curiosity, tendency to put things in their mouths, and their size. Lack of supervision increases the risk for some of these hazards. Some result from activity that comes naturally to children. Others result from products that just don't mix with kids. Some of the most common hidden hazards:

- **Shopping cart injury**—In 1999, nearly 23,600 children were treated in hospital emergency rooms for injuries associated with shopping carts. Children ages 4 and under accounted for the majority of these injuries. Children can suffer cuts, bruises, fractures, concussions, and even internal injuries when they jump or fall from a shopping cart, the cart overturns, they get pinched in the folding mechanism, or they fall against or are hit by a cart.

  - An annual average of 21,600 children 5 years old and younger were treated in U.S. hospital emergency rooms for shopping cart injuries during the years 1985-1996.

  - There has been a significant increase in the estimated number of these injuries between 1985 and 1996.

  - In 1996 there were 22,200 injuries versus 16,900 in 1985.

  - An annual average of 12,800 of these children were treated for falls from the carts.

  - There has been a significant increase in the number of fall injuries between 1985 and 1996.

  - There has been a decline in other hazard patterns over these years.

- In 1996 there were over 16,000 injuries from falls versus 7,800 in 1985.

- A detailed analysis of the incidents during 1995 and 1996 showed that 66 percent of the fall victims were treated for head injuries (11,000 per year).

- This analysis of data from 1995 and 1996 also showed that 54 percent of the head injury victims suffered severe injuries such as concussions and fractures (5940 per year).

- A special investigation study in 1994 showed that 51 percent of the fall victims fell from the seat and 49 percent fell from the basket.

- **Trunk entrapment**—At least 20 children have died from unintentional trunk entrapment since July 1987. All children involved were 6 years old or younger. Unintentional entrapments typically occur during children's games or exploration, or while retrieving items from the trunk. Heat stroke is the most common cause of death associated with unintentional trunk entrapment.

- **Automobile heat-related deaths**—When the outside temperature is 93 degrees Fahrenheit, even with a window cracked, the temperature inside a car can reach 125 degrees in just 20 minutes. In these extreme conditions, children can die or suffer permanent disability quickly. Heat-related deaths often occur when parents leave children alone in a vehicle, or when playing children climb into unlocked cars and cannot get out.

- **Fireworks**—Fireworks displays hosted by professionals are a safe and festive way to celebrate a holiday. However, more than 3,000 children ages 14 and under are treated in hospital emergency rooms each year for injuries from family firework activities. And illegal fireworks aren't the only culprits: firecrackers, rockets, and sparklers, legal in many states, cause the bulk of emergency room-treated injuries.

- **Bunk beds**—In 1999, more than 36,600 children ages 14 and under were treated in hospital emergency rooms for injuries related to bunk beds. Children are injured due to falls (greatest risk), entrapment in guardrails, and suffocation due to falling mattresses or foundations. It is estimated that 10 children die each year after becoming trapped in bunk beds.

- **Sledding**—More than 14,000 children ages 5 to 14 were treated in emergency rooms in 1999 for injuries related to sledding. Children are especially at risk when not sledding on open terrain or when equipment is not inspected for wear or breakage.

- **Pool Drains**—Spending time in a whirlpool, spa, or hot tub can be great fun for kids. However, the strong suction caused by pool drains can cause serious injury or death when hair or body parts become entrapped. Since 1978, at least 67 incidents have been recorded, including 18 deaths.

- **Wired Glass**—Wired glass is commonly used in windows and doors of schools and recreation centers where fire-rated glass is required. While wired glass protects against fire, it is only about half as strong as ordinary glass, and can be extremely dangerous upon impact. Many children have suffered serious injuries from the shattered glass and exposed wires, including permanent nerve damage and amputations.

- **Other hidden hazards**:
  - Clothing with drawstrings
  - Window-covering cords
  - Five-gallon buckets and other water hazards
  - Latex balloons
  - Open window falls
  - Used cribs

Section 3.3

Trauma Season—The Seasonality of Unintentional Childhood Injury

"Trauma Season: A National Study of the Seasonality of Unintentional Childhood Injury," by B.E. Kane, A.D. Mickalide, H.A. Paul, National SAFE KIDS Campaign, May 2001.

This study is the first one to look at seasonal trends in national injury mortality among children, confirming that a "trauma season" does exist. Public health and medical professionals have long assumed that childhood unintentional injuries follow a seasonal pattern. During the summer months, when children are out of school, lack adequate supervision, and spend more time outdoors, the risks are heightened.

Current research indicates that unintentional injury remains the number one killer of children ages 14 and under and that motor vehicle occupant injury, drowning, falls, pedestrian injury, and bike-related injury are among the leading risks to children. To determine the seasonality of injury, SAFE KIDS researched the following questions: How much more dangerous are these risks during warm weather months—May through August? Which risks are more prevalent during specific months? Are children of certain ages more at risk than others? Are particular summer months or particular regions of the country inherently more dangerous for children than others?

Methodology

SAFE KIDS studied national data on mortality among children ages 14 and under between 1991 and 1996. This data, obtained from the National Center for Health Statistics, was based on death certificates documenting external causes of injury (e-codes). SAFE KIDS specifically analyzed e-codes for drowning, fall-related injury, pedestrian-related injury, bicycle-related injury, and motor vehicle occupant injury.

Data were examined by month, and the number of injuries that occurred between May and August was compared with the number

28

of injuries that would be expected to occur during that four-month period if the injury rate was constant throughout the year. Data were also examined by age group (under 1 year, 1-4 years, 5-9 years, and 10-14 years old) and geographic location based on the state where the injury occurred. A total of 40,240 death records of children who died from unintentional injury were analyzed from the six-year period.

SAFE KIDS also analyzed national morbidity data obtained from the National Center for Health Statistics. This data included estimates of U.S. hospital emergency department visits by children ages 14 and under who suffered from an unintentional injury between 1993 and 1998. To examine variations in injury trends around the country, local morbidity data were gathered from seven different cities (Hartford, CT; Anderson, SC; Wichita, KS; Twin Falls, ID; Phoenix, AZ; Sacramento, CA; and Washington, DC). SAFE KIDS analyzed data from multiple years of pediatric unintentional injuries treated in hospital emergency rooms to see if there were peaks in the occurrence of injury between May and August.

Fatal Unintentional Injury among Children Ages 14 and Under during Summer Months

- Nearly half (42 percent) of all unintentional injury-related deaths occurred during the summer months.

- July was the deadliest month for unintentional childhood injury, with 12 percent of deaths occurring in this month alone.

- Deaths among children ages 10-14 increased most dramatically—45 percent occurred in the summer months. Deaths among children ages 5-9 also increased substantially.

- Mountain states and West North Central states experienced the greatest summer increases (greater than 30 percent) in unintentional childhood injury deaths.

Fatal Unintentional Injury

- From 1991 to 1996, 40,240 children ages 14 and under died as a result of unintentional injuries. Of these deaths, 16,966 (42.2 percent) occurred May through August, a 25 percent increase above average. The majority (two-thirds) of these deaths were a result of bike, pedestrian, motor vehicle occupant injury, falls, and drowning.

Fatal Drowning

- From 1991-1996, 6,237 children ages 14 and under died as a result of unintentional drowning. Of these deaths, 4,124 (66.1 percent) occurred May through August, a 96.1 percent increase above average.

Fatal Bicycle-Related Injury

- From 1991 to 1996, 1,547 children ages 14 and under died as a result of unintentional bicycle-related injury. Of these deaths, 827 (52.5 percent) occurred May through August, a 55.8 percent increase above average.

Fatal Fall-Related Injury

- From 1991 to 1996, 801 children ages 14 and under died as a result of unintentional fall-related injury. Of these deaths, 394 (49.2 percent) occurred May through August, a 46.0 percent increase above average.

Fatal Pedestrian-Related Injury

- From 1991 to 1996, 6,018 children ages 14 and under died as a result of unintentional pedestrian-related injury. Of these deaths, 2,458 (40.8 percent) occurred May through August, a 21.1 percent increase above average.

Fatal Motor Vehicle Occupant Injury

- From 1991 to 1996, 8,263 children ages 14 and under died as a result of motor vehicle occupant injury. Of these deaths, 3,331 (40.3 percent) occurred May through August, a 19.6 percent increase above average.

Conclusions

This report confirms the assumption that the summer months pose a heightened risk for childhood injury. More specifically:

- July is the deadliest time of the year for childhood unintentional injury.
- Drowning occurs more often during July than any other month. The increase in deaths may be attributed to the number of

children out of school during July, as well as the likelihood of warm, long days.

- Motor vehicle-related injuries also hit their peak during July. The increases may be attributed to the number of families who travel by car during this month in addition to the number of children out of school during July.

- Older children experience the greatest increase in unintentional injury-related death during the summer months. This is primarily because children ages 10-14 tend to engage in more risky behavior and are presumably given more freedom from their parents.

- Young school-age children ages 5-9 are also at high risk because they lack the skills to make clear judgments necessary to bike, walk, swim, and play safely without adult supervision. Many parents of children this age also fail to restrain them properly in booster seats in motor vehicles, which can lead to severe injuries or even death in the event of a car crash.

- Summer injury peaks are less pronounced in mild-weather regions of the country. Temperate climates enable children to spend more time outdoors; therefore injuries in these regions tend to be distributed more evenly throughout the entire year.

Call to Action

The National SAFE KIDS Campaign urges others to join its more than 300 coalitions in all 50 states, the District of Columbia, and Puerto Rico, in a multifaceted approach to reducing unintentional injury during the summer months. Specifically, communities need to:

- Spread the word to parents, caregivers, and older children about summer risks through television, radio and print media, and community events.

- Provide safety devices, including bike helmets, child safety seats, window guards, and life jackets to parents in need through community networks.

- Create safer roads by building bike paths, sidewalks, and speed-reduction measures into communities where children live, targeting high-risk areas.

- Increase the number of pools with four-sided isolation fencing.

- Pass and enforce child safety laws, including bike helmet, personal flotation device, and child occupant protection laws.

- Advocate for affordable childcare options for parents to ensure adequate supervision during the summer months.

Additional Information

National SAFE KIDS Campaign
1301 Pennsylvania Avenue, NW
Suite 1000
Washington, DC 20004
Tel: 202-662-0600
Fax: 202-393-2072
Website: www.safekids.org

Chapter 4

Adolescent Injury Statistics

How Big Is the Problem of Injuries for U.S. Adolescents?

- At least one adolescent (10-19 years old) dies of an injury every hour of every day; about 15,000 die each year.[1]

- Injuries kill more adolescents than all diseases combined.[2]

- For every injury death, there are about 41 injury hospitalizations and 1,100 cases treated in emergency departments.[2]

- Unintentional injury accounts for around 60% of adolescent injury deaths, while violence (homicide and suicide) accounts for the remaining 40%.[1]

Who Is Most at Risk for Injury Death?

- In general, males are more likely than females to die of any type on injury.

- The most pronounced differences between sexes in injury death rates occur within the older adolescent group (15-19 years). In this group, males are about 2.5 times more likely to die of any

"Fact Sheet on Adolescent Injury," National Center for Injury Prevention and Control, reviewed July 1999; and excerpts from "Adolescent Health Chartbook," Health, United States, 2000, National Center for Health Statistics, DHHS Publication No. (PHS) 2000-1232-1, July 2000.

unintentional injury and 5 times more likely to die of homicide or suicide. The gender difference is most pronounced in drowning, where males are 10.6 times more likely to die than females of the same age.

- Among adolescents 15-19 years old, one in every four deaths is caused by a firearm. For this age group, the risk of dying from a firearm injury has increased by 77% since 1985.[3]

What Are the Most Common Types of Injuries among Adolescents?

- The largest proportion of adolescent injuries are due to motor vehicle crashes.

- Adolescents are far less likely to use seat belts than any other age group.[2]

- Adolescents are especially vulnerable to fatal crashes at night; they do 20% of their driving at night, but they have more than 50% of their fatalities at night.[2]

- When adolescents drive after drinking alcohol, they are more likely than adults to be in a crash, even when drinking less alcohol than adults.[2]

- Adolescents also cause a disproportionate number of deaths among non-adolescent drivers, passengers, and pedestrians.[2]

Does Alcohol Contribute to Adolescent Injuries?

- Alcohol is involved in about 35% of adolescent (15-20 years) driver fatalities.

- Alcohol is involved in about 40% of all adolescent drownings.[2]

References

1. Runyan CW, Gerken EA. Epidemiology and prevention of adolescent injury: a review and research agenda. *JAMA* 1989;262:16:2273-2278.

2. Centers for Disease Control and Prevention. *Injury mortality: national summary of injury mortality data 1984-1990*. Atlanta, GA: Centers for Disease Control and Prevention, 1993.

3. Fingerhut LA. *Firearm mortality among children, youth, and young adults 1-34 years of age, tends and current status: U.S., 1985-90.* Advance Data No. 231. Hyattsville, MD: National Center for Health Statistics, Centers for Disease Control and Prevention, 1993.

Suicide Ideation and Attempts

In 1997 suicide was the third leading cause of injury death among adolescents 13-19 years of age. However, many teens seriously consider suicide without attempting, or attempt without completing suicide. Among those adolescents seriously considering suicide, factors influencing suicidal thoughts may include depression, feelings of hopelessness or worthlessness, and a preoccupation with death, but may not be related to risk factors associated with actually attempting suicide.[1] Factors which may contribute to attempting suicide among adolescents include impulsive, aggressive, and antisocial behavior; family influences, including a history of violence and family disruption; severe stress in school or social life; and rapid sociocultural change.[2] Substance abuse or dependence can be an important contributor in the escalation from suicidal thoughts to suicide attempts.[3]

- In 1999 one-fifth of all high school students reported having seriously considered or attempted suicide during the previous 12 months. Less than one-half of students who seriously considered suicide actually attempted suicide (8 percent of all students). Less than 3 percent of all students reported having an injurious attempt, that is, a suicide attempt that resulted in an injury, poisoning, or overdose that had been treated by a doctor.

- Female students were substantially more likely to consider suicide than male students. This difference was identified for all racial/ethnic and grade level subgroups.

- Although a substantial decrease in suicide attempts was apparent between 9th and 12th grade among female students, a decrease by grade level among male students was not significant. Suicide attempts among non-Hispanic white and Hispanic female students were significantly higher than among their male counterparts; among non-Hispanic black students there was no difference by gender. In contrast, the rate of completed suicides is higher among male adolescents than female adolescents.

- *Healthy People 2010* identifies a reduction in the rate of suicide attempts by adolescents as a critical adolescent objective.[4]

References

1. Behrman RE, Kliegman RM, Arvin AM, eds. *Nelson Textbook of Pediatrics.* 15th ed. Philadelphia: W.B. Saunders Company. 1996.

2. Goodwin FK, Brown GL. Risk factors for youth suicide. In: *Alcohol, Drug Abuse, and Mental Health Administration. Report of the Secretary's Task Force on Youth Suicide.* Vol 2. Washington: U.S. Department of Health and Human Services, Public Health Service, Alcohol, Drug Abuse, and Mental Health Administration; DHHS publication no. (ADM)89-1622. 1989.

3. Gould MS, King R, Greenwald S, et al. Psychopathology associated with suicidal ideation and attempts among children and adolescents. *J Am Acad Child Adolesc Psychiatry* 37(9):915-23. 1998.

4. U.S. Department of Health and Human Services. *Healthy People 2010* (Conference Edition, in Two Volumes). Washington: January 2000.

Emergency Department Visits

Use of the emergency department may be influenced by underlying health status, the severity of the current illness or injury, access to other sources of health care, and health insurance status.

- In general, adolescents 10-19 years of age visit the emergency department less often than younger children, young adults 20-24 years, and the elderly 65 years and older. Adolescents visit the emergency department about as often as adults 25-64 years. Adolescents and young adults 20-24 are more likely than others to use the emergency department for reasons related to an injury.

- In 1995-97 visits to emergency departments for injuries comprised about one-half of all visits for adolescents 10-19 years, with higher proportions for males than for females (63 percent compared with 41 percent). This is related to the higher visit rates among males for injuries associated with being struck or cut.

- Injury-related emergency department visit rates among male adolescents were consistently higher than noninjury visit rates. In contrast, noninjury visit rates among female adolescents exceeded injury-related visit rates by ages 14-15 and the gap widened with age.

- Emergency department visit rates for injury increased with age. The injury-related visit rates for adolescent females and males 18-19 years of age were 1.5 and 1.6 times the rates for their respective counterparts 10-11 years of age.

Injury-Related Visits to Emergency Departments

Injuries are a major cause of emergency department visits. The morbidity associated with injuries is costly on an individual and a societal level.[1,2] A greater understanding of the epidemiology of injuries should lead to improved injury prevention strategies and decreases in the incidence of injuries.

- Four external causes of injury—being struck by or against an object or person, falls, motor vehicle traffic-related injuries, and being cut by a sharp object—accounted for nearly 60 percent of all injury-related visits to emergency departments among adolescents in 1995-97. Of these four causes, only motor vehicle traffic-related injuries are a significant source of mortality among adolescents.

- One in five injury-related emergency department visits among adolescents resulted from "being struck by or against an object or a person." Sports-related injuries made up 41 percent of the injuries in this category. At each age, the "struck by.." rate for males was about twice the rate for females. Rates for male adolescents 14-19 years of age were higher than for younger males.

- Visit rates for falls (16 percent of all injury-related visits) generally decreased with age. Rates in this category were similar for males and females across ages 10-19 years.

- Injury visit rates associated with motor vehicle traffic injuries (14 percent of all injury-related visits) were similar for males and females at each age, with large relative increases at 14-15 years and at 16-17 years for both sexes. In contrast to nonfatal motor vehicle injuries, motor vehicle traffic-related death rates for males were higher than for females at each age from 10-19 years.

- Visits for injuries from being cut (9 percent of all injury-related visits) also increased with age, especially from ages 12-13 years to 16-19 years.

References

1. Rice DP, Mackenzie EJ, Associates. *Cost of injury in the United States: A report to Congress.* San Francisco, California: Institute for Health and Aging, University of California and Injury Prevention Center. The Johns Hopkins University. 1989.

2. Burt CW, Fingerhut LA. Injury visits to hospital emergency departments: United States, 1992-95. National Center for Health Statistics. *Vital Health Stat* 13(131). 1998.

Open Wounds, Fractures, Sprains and Strains, and Contusions

In 1995-97 open wounds, fractures, sprains and strains, and contusions were the four most common injury diagnoses for emergency department visits among adolescents 10-19 years of age. These four injury diagnoses accounted for 80 percent of all first-listed injury diagnoses for adolescents. Open wound injuries were the most often reported diagnoses for male adolescents and sprains, strains, and contusions were the most often reported for female adolescents.

- The emergency department visit rate for open wounds for male adolescents 18-19 years of age was nearly twice that for adolescents 12-15 years of age. Open wound injury visit rates for female adolescents 10-19 years of age were about one-half the rates for males at each age. These injuries are caused primarily by knives and other instruments for cutting or piercing.

- Emergency department visit rates for fractures among male adolescents did not vary by age. The rates for female adolescents declined with age; the visit rate for fractures at 18-19 years was less than one-half the rate at 10-11 years. Among males 14-19 years of age, age-specific visit rates for fractures were about 3 times those for females. Upper extremity fracture was the most common fracture site reported for males and females. Injuries resulting from falls and being struck were the primary causes of these fractures.

- Sprains, strains, and contusions were the most commonly reported diagnoses in emergency department visits for female adolescents 10-19 years, accounting for one-half of all first-listed injury diagnoses. There were no significant gender differences by age for visits for sprains and strains or contusions. Among the leading external causes of these injuries were motor vehicle traffic crashes, falls, being struck, and overexertion.

Violent Crime Victimization

Adolescents are the victims of violent acts in the home, at school, and in the community. Violent crime includes rape or sexual assault, aggravated and simple assaults, and robbery.

- During the period 1992-97 an average of approximately 3.4 million adolescents 12-19 years of age were reported to be victims of violent crime each year. Sixty-five percent of the crimes were classified as simple assaults, 21 percent as aggravated assaults, 10 percent as robbery, and 4 percent as rape and sexual assault. The proportions for aggravated assault and for robbery were somewhat higher for male adolescents than for female adolescents; there were more female than male victims (10 percent) of rape and sexual assault.

- The 1992-97 overall rate of violent assault for male adolescents was 50 percent higher than for female adolescents. Among the youngest adolescents, male victimization rates were nearly twice those for females; however, the disparity narrowed with increasing age. Among males there was no variation in the rates by age; among females adolescents 18-19 years of age were more likely to be victims of violence than those 12-13 years.

- Among female adolescents 12-19 years of age the rates for rape and sexual assault increased with age (data not shown). The reported rates for older adolescents were about twice those for younger adolescents. Overall, female adolescents and young adult women are four times as likely to be victims of sexual assault as women in all other age groups.[1]

- From 1992 to 1997 the rate of violent crime victimization for adolescents 12-15 years and 16-19 years decreased. Declines were noted for each of the major categories of victimization.

Reference

1.   Rickert VI, et al. Date rape among adolescents and young adults. *J Pediatr Adolesc Gynecol* 11(4):167-75. 1998.

Death Rates

*   Injuries cause more deaths among adolescents than do natural causes. ("Natural" is a term similar to "noninjury" that is used to categorize causes of death.) For the period 1996-97, nearly 14,000 adolescents died annually from injuries compared with about 5,000 adolescents who died from natural causes; that is, 73 percent of all deaths among adolescents 10-19 years of age were caused by an injury. The proportion of all deaths that were injuries increases with age from 47 percent at age 10 years to 81 percent at age 18 years.

*   Among male adolescents injury death rates exceeded natural cause death rates at each age 11-19 years (the rates were similar at 10 years of age), and the difference increased with age. Among male adolescents 19 years of age, the injury death rate was 12 times the rate of those 10 years of age. Compared with death rates for injuries, death rates for natural causes increased more slowly with age. Among male adolescents 19 years of age, the natural cause death rate was twice that of males 10 years of age.

*   Among female adolescents 10-12 years, death rates for natural causes exceeded those for injuries; the rates were similar at age 13 years, and for those 14-19 years of age injury death rates were higher than natural cause death rates. Injury death rates for female adolescents did not increase as consistently with age as did the rates for male adolescents.

*   The injury death rate for males 10-19 years of age was 2.7 times that for females, while for natural causes the death rate for males was 1.3 times the rate for females.

*   Among adolescents unintentional injuries comprised the majority of injury deaths, 57 percent among males and 74 percent among females. For both sexes, the proportion of unintended injury deaths declined with age, as homicide and suicide deaths increased with age.

- The unintentional injury death rates increased with age, with a particularly large relative increase, 73 percent for males and 79 percent for females, between ages 15 and 16 years. Suicide and homicide rates for males also increased with age, more sharply for ages 10-15 years than for ages 16-19 years. Unlike the pattern for males, suicide rates for females 15-19 years did not increase.

- Race and ethnicity specific death rates also increased with age. In 1996-97 injury death rates were higher for black and American Indian adolescents than for non-Hispanic white, Hispanic, and Asian and Pacific Islander adolescents. The higher rates for black adolescents were due to higher homicide rates at each age; striking disparities exist in homicide rates for black adolescents compared with other race and ethnic groups. Higher rates for American Indian adolescents were due to higher unintentional injury mortality as well as higher suicide rates especially among those 15 years of age and over. Death rates for natural causes were consistently higher for black adolescents and lower for Asian and Pacific Islander adolescents than for non-Hispanic and Hispanic adolescents.

- *Healthy People 2010* has identified reduction of adolescent mortality as a critical adolescent objective. The objectives call for a reduction of death rates to 16.8 per 100,000 for adolescents 10-14 years of age and 43.2 per 100,000 for adolescents 15-19 years of age.[1] *Healthy People 2010* has specifically targeted the reduction of suicide and homicide rates as critical adolescent objectives.

Reference

1. U.S. Department of Health and Human Services. *Healthy People 2010* (Conference Edition, in Two Volumes). Washington: 2000.

Motor Vehicle and Firearm-Related Deaths

- Motor vehicle traffic-related injuries and firearm-related injuries are the two leading causes of death among adolescents 10-19 years of age. For the period 1996-97, motor vehicle traffic injuries were the leading cause of injury death for adolescents 10-19 years of age (averaging 6,260 deaths per year), followed by injuries from firearms (averaging 4,250 per year). Together these two causes accounted for 55 percent of all deaths and for 75 percent of all injury deaths for adolescents. By comparison, malignant neoplasms, the leading natural cause of death for this age group, accounted for 6 percent of all deaths.

• For motor vehicle traffic injury deaths, rates increased markedly with age for male and female adolescents. Notably, between ages 15 and 16 years the rates for males and females doubled. A similar increase at these ages was noted in the emergency department visit rates for motor vehicle traffic-related injuries. Motor vehicle death rates for males 10-17 years were 1.3-1.7 times those for females; by ages 18 and 19 years, the death rates for males were 2.1-2.5 times those for females.

• Disparities by race and ethnicity were apparent in the rates of death from motor vehicle injuries for male and female adolescents, although the differences for males were more pronounced. Among males and females motor vehicle injury rates were highest among American Indian or Alaska Native adolescents and lowest among Asian or Pacific Islander adolescents. Rates among non-Hispanic white teens were higher than those of non-Hispanic black and Hispanic teens.

• The high rates of death from motor vehicle injuries are partially attributable to risk behavior among adolescents. In 1999, 33 percent of high school students reported that in the previous 30 days they rode in a car with a driver who had been drinking alcohol, and 13 percent reported that they drove after drinking alcohol.[1] Sixteen percent of students surveyed had rarely or never worn seat belts when riding in a car or truck driven by someone else. Overall, male students (21 percent) were significantly more likely than female students (12 percent) to have rarely or never worn seat belts.[1]

• *Healthy People 2010* has identified reduction of deaths caused by motor vehicle crashes and the reduction of deaths and injuries caused by alcohol- and drug-related motor vehicle crashes as critical adolescent objectives.[2] The objectives also call for increased use of safety belts and a reduction in the proportion of adolescents who report that they rode, during the previous 30 days, with a driver who had been drinking alcohol.

- Firearm death rates also increase substantially with age; the rate for males 19 years of age was 28 times the rate for those 11 years of age. In contrast, the firearm death rates for 19 year old females was 10 times the rate for 11 year old females. The disparity between male and female firearm-related death rates increased from threefold for the youngest adolescents (10-11) to ninefold for older adolescents (18-19 years).

- Differences exist in firearm-related death rates by race and ethnicity for male and female adolescents. Rates were strikingly higher among black adolescents than among other race and ethnic groups. Firearm death rates were lowest among non-Hispanic white and Asian or Pacific Islander adolescents. Firearm deaths include deaths that were classified as unintentional, suicide, homicide, legal intervention, or undetermined intent. Among adolescents 10-19 years of age, 60 percent of all firearm deaths were homicides, 31 percent were suicides, 6 percent were unintentional and 2 percent were of undetermined intent.

References

1. Centers for Disease Control and Prevention. *Youth Risk Behavior Survey*. 1999.

2. U.S. Department of Health and Human Services. *Healthy People 2010* (Conference Edition, in Two Volumes). Washington: January 2000.

Motor Vehicle and Firearm-Related Deaths and Residence

Where adolescents reside, whether in urban, suburban, or more rural settings, has been shown to influence mortality risks.[1-3] Teenagers living in the most densely populated metropolitan counties have higher death rates associated with interpersonal violence, while those in more rural counties have higher rates of motor vehicle fatalities. In general, motor vehicle death rates are higher in less densely populated settings and firearm homicide is higher in more densely populated settings.[1]

- In 1996-97 motor vehicle traffic death rates in non-metropolitan counties were 2-3 times the rates in the core metropolitan (counties with large central cities) counties, while rates in the non-core but still metropolitan counties were in between.

- In all urbanization categories, the motor vehicle traffic death rates increased with age, with most of the increase occurring by age 17 years. Motor vehicle traffic death rates for adolescents 16 years of age (when many adolescents can begin to drive) were approximately twice those for adolescents 15 years of age in all three county groups. Between ages 18 and 19 years the rate declined by 5-7 percent in each of the three county groups.

- Age and urbanization patterns for firearm mortality differ from those for motor vehicle mortality. Most notably, the increases in firearm death rates by age were steeper. Between ages 11 and 13 years, firearm death rates more than doubled and were higher in non-metropolitan counties than in either of the two metropolitan groups. With increasing age, the pattern changed and rates in the core counties were higher than those in non-core metropolitan and non-metropolitan counties. With each single year of age between 13 and 16 years, firearm death rates in the core counties doubled or nearly doubled. Between 16 and 19 years, the rate came close to doubling again. Core county firearm death rates for 15-19 year olds were more than twice the rates in the other two county groups.

- The manner or intent of firearm deaths, that is, whether deaths were ruled unintentional, a suicide, or a homicide, differs significantly by urbanization category. For example, the higher firearm death rates among younger adolescents in the non-metropolitan areas resulted from higher unintentional and suicide rates. Among older adolescents, the majority of firearm deaths in the core counties were homicides while among adolescent who resided in the non-metropolitan counties, suicide was the mostly likely manner of firearm death.

References

1. Fingerhut LA, Ingram DD, Feldman JJ. Firearm and nonfirearm homicide among persons 15-19 years of age: Differences by level of urbanization, United States, 1979-1989. *JAMA*, 267;3048-3053. 1992.

2. Fingerhut LA, Ingram DD and Feldman JJ. Homicide rates among U.S. teenagers and young adults—differences by

mechanism, level of urbanization, race and sex, 1987-1995. *JAMA* 280(5):423-7. 1998.

3. Cubbin C, Pickle LW, Fingerhut, LA. Social context and the geographic patterns of homicide in black and white males in the United States. *AJPH* 90:579-87. 2000.

Table 4.1. Emergency Department Visit Rates for Selected External Causes of Injury among Adolescents 10-19 Years of Age (Visits per 10,000 adolescents)

Age and external cause	Female		Male	
	Rate	SE	Rate	SE
Struck by or against				
10-11 years	164.9	30.2	282.4	45.2
12-13 years	150.8	31.9	294.1	37.7
14-15 years	237.1	38.2	452.3	51.9
16-17 years	229.4	39.7	588.4	68.9
18-19 years	247.5	38.9	483.1	59.7
Cut or pierce				
10-11 years	94.1	21.3	168.5	28.3
12-13 years	71.7	17.2	103.7	20.5
14-15 years	67.9	18.0	124.2	24.2
16-17 years	91.5	25.0	238.2	33.9
18-19 years	89.0	34.4	226.9	36.1
Fall				
10-11 years	288.1	39.7	310.4	47.0
12-13 years	314.6	51.5	275.1	41.5
14-15 years	220.1	39.0	268.7	46.5
16-17 years	194.4	30.6	246.3	45.3
18-19 years	197.4	32.2	202.1	33.4
Motor vehicle traffic				
10-11 years	81.7	28.7	90.1	25.4
12-13 years	105.1	25.2	94.3	23.7
14-15 years	221.1	38.2	161.6	33.4
16-17 years	385.3	50.4	311.9	49.1
18-19 years	416.6	48.4	349.2	50.3

SE Standard error.

Table 4.2. Emergency Department Visit Rates for Selected Injury Diagnoses among Adolescents 10-19 Years of Age (Visits per 10,000 adolescents)

Age and injury diagnosis	Female Rate	SE	Male Rate	SE
Fractures				
10-11 years	179.1	32.8	250.7	38.7
12-13 years	156.2	34.0	253.2	30.9
14-15 years	103.7	22.4	330.9	44.1
16-17 years	103.8	27.3	257.7	41.9
18-19 years	83.0	21.2	225.7	40.8
Sprains and strains				
10-11 years	189.0	39.1	175.9	31.9
12-13 years	319.1	46.7	277.9	39.9
14-15 years	362.3	46.9	325.2	42.3
16-17 years	398.3	50.3	334.1	44.1
18-19 years	286.9	43.1	348.8	43.2
Open wounds				
10-11 years	212.4	31.0	396.7	51.9
12-13 years	198.0	41.3	318.0	40.6
14-15 years	203.5	33.6	319.5	33.7
16-17 years	214.7	30.6	488.0	52.4
18-19 years	338.2	57.4	616.2	76.4
Contusions				
10-11 years	223.9	37.4	235.9	37.6
12-13 years	194.8	34.9	244.0	36.2
14-15 years	267.6	40.4	318.5	41.6
16-17 years	313.3	48.3	382.7	54.0
18-19 years	282.2	34.6	313.6	40.4

SE Standard error.

Table 4.3. Violent Crime Victimization Rates among Adolescents 12-19 Years of Age (Victimizations per 1,000 adolescents)

Age	Female		Male	
	Rate	SE	Rate	SE
12-13 years	82.0	4.8	137.0	6.0
14-15 years	92.4	5.1	137.5	6.1
16-17 years	90.6	5.1	129.8	5.9
18-19 years	98.6	5.4	129.9	6.1

Year	12-15 years of age		16-19 years of age	
	Rate	SE	Rate	SE
1992	118.3	7.9	112.6	7.8
1993	132.1	6.3	122.1	6.2
1994	123.9	5.4	127.6	5.6
1995	111.3	5.1	113.7	4.8
1996	96.8	4.9	98.9	5.1
1997	95.9	5.2	102.2	5.4

SE Standard error.

Table 4.4. Death Rates for Motor Vehicle Traffic-Related and Firearm-Related Injuries among Adolescents 10-19 Years of Age (Deaths per 100,000 adolescents)

| | Motor vehicle deaths | | | | Firearm-related deaths | | | |
| | Female | | Male | | Female | | Male | |
Age	Rate	SE	Rate	SE	Rate	SE	Rate	SE
10 years	3.1	0.3	4.8	0.3	*	*	1.0	0.2
11 years	3.3	0.3	4.4	0.3	0.5	0.1	1.8	0.2
12 years	4.4	0.3	5.9	0.4	0.6	0.1	2.8	0.3
13 years	4.5	0.3	7.3	0.4	1.2	0.2	4.6	0.3
14 years	7.5	0.4	10.0	0.5	2.5	0.3	9.4	0.5
15 years	11.3	0.6	15.5	0.6	3.6	0.3	15.9	0.6
16 years	21.7	0.8	33.0	0.9	4.9	0.4	25.6	0.8
17 years	22.6	0.8	37.3	1.0	4.7	0.4	34.5	0.9
18 years	22.2	0.8	46.7	1.1	5.5	0.4	46.7	1.1
19 years	18.4	0.7	45.5	1.1	5.2	0.4	49.8	1.1

SE Standard error.

* Number in this category is too small to calculate reliable rates; fewer than 20 deaths.

Chapter 5

Older Adult Injuries

The Cost of Fall Injuries among Older Adults

- Falls are a serious public health problem among older adults. In the United States, one of every three people 65 years and older falls each year.[1,2]

- Older adults are hospitalized for fall-related injuries five times more often than they are for injuries from other causes.[3]

- Of those who fall, 20%-30% suffer moderate to severe injuries that reduce mobility and independence, and increase the risk of premature death.[3]

Calculating Cost Estimates

- The cost of fall-related injuries is usually expressed in terms of direct costs.

  - Direct costs include out-of-pocket expenses and charges paid by insurance companies for the treatment of fall-related injuries. These include costs and fees associated

This chapter includes "The Costs of Fall Injuries Among Older Adults," National Center for Injury Prevention and Control, 2000; "Indicator 24—Criminal Victimization," *Older Americans 2000: Key Indicators of Well-Being*, Federal Interagency Forum on Aging-Related Statistics, 2000; and "Older Adult Drivers," *Injury Fact Book 2001-2002*, National Center for Injury Prevention and Control (NCIPC), 2001.

with hospital and nursing home care, physician and other professional services, rehabilitation, community-based services, the use of medical equipment, prescription drugs, local rehabilitation, home modifications, and insurance administration.[4]

- Direct costs do not account for the long term consequences of these injuries, such as disability, decreased productivity, or quality of life.

The Costs of Fall-Related Injuries

- In 1994, the average direct cost for a fall injury was $1,400 for a person over the age of 65.[4]

- The total direct cost of all fall injuries for people age 65 and older in 1994 was $20.2 billion.[4]

- By 2020, the cost of fall injuries is expected to reach $32.4 billion.[4]

Fall-Related Fractures

- The most common fall-related injuries are osteoporotic fractures. These are fractures of the hip, spine, or forearm.

- In the United States in 1986, the direct medical costs for osteoporotic fractures were $5.15 billion. By 1989, these costs exceeded $6 billion.[5]

- Over the next 10 years, total direct medical costs for osteoporotic fractures among postmenopausal women will be more than $45.2 billion.[6]

Hip Fractures

- Of all fall-related fractures, hip fractures are the most serious and lead to the greatest number of health problems and deaths.

- In the United States, hospitalization accounts for 44% of direct health care costs for hip fracture patients.[7]

- In 1991, Medicare costs for this injury were estimated to be $2.9 billion.[5]

- Hospital admissions for hip fractures among people over age 65 have steadily increased, from 230,000 admissions in 1988 to 340,000 admissions in 1996.[8] The number of hip fractures is expected to exceed 500,000 by the year 2040.[9,10]

- The cost of a hip fracture, including direct medical care, formal non-medical care, and informal care provided by family and friends, was between $16,300 and $18,700 during the first year following the injury.[10]

- Assuming 5% inflation and the growing number of hip fractures, the total annual cost of these injuries may reach $240 billion by the year 2040.[11]

References

1. Tinetti ME, Speechley M, Ginter SF. Risk factors for falls among elderly persons living in the community. *New England Journal of Medicine* 1988;319(26):1701-7.

2. Sattin RW. Falls among older persons: A public health perspective. *Annual Review of Public Health* 1992;13:489-508.

3. Alexander BH, Rivara FP, Wolf ME. The cost and frequency of hospitalization for fall-related injuries in older adults. *American Journal of Public Health* 1992;82(7):1020-3.

4. Englander F, Hodson TJ, Terregrossa RA. Economic dimensions of slip and fall injuries. *Journal of Forensic Science* 1996;41(5):733-46.

5. CDC. Incidence and costs to Medicare of fractures among Medicare beneficiaries aged >65 years—United States, July 1991-June 1992. *MMWR* 1996;45(41):877-83.

6. Chrischilles E, Shireman T, Wallace R. Costs and health effects of osteoporotic fractures. *Bone* 1994;15(4):377-86.

7. Barrett-Connor, Elizabeth. The economic and human costs of osteoporotic fracture. *American Journal of Medicine* 1995;98 (suppl 2A):2A-3S to 2A-8S.

8. Graves EJ, Owings MF. 1996 summary: *National hospital discharge survey. Advance data from vital and health statistics;*

no. 301. Hyattsville, MD: National Center for Health Statistics, 1998.

9. Cooper C, Campion G, Melton LJ III. Hip fractures in the elderly; a world-wide projection. *Osteoporosis International* 1992;2:285-9.

10. Brainsky GA, Lydick E, Epstein R, Fox KM, Hawkes W, Kashner TM, Zimmerman SI, Magaziner J. The economic cost of hip fractures in community-dwelling older adults: A prospective study. *Journal of the American Geriatrics Society* 1997;45:281-7.

11. Schneider EL, Guralnick JM. The aging of America: Impact on health care costs. *Journal of the American Medical Association* 1990;263(17):2335-40.

Older Adult Drivers

In 1999, more than 7,000 Americans 65 and older died and another 246,000 suffered nonfatal injuries in motor vehicle crashes.

- Drivers 65 and older have higher crash death rates per mile driven than all but teen drivers.

- Rates for motor vehicle-related injury are twice as high for older men as for older women.

- Motor vehicle-related deaths and injuries among older adults are rising. During 1990-1997, the number of deaths rose 14% and the number of nonfatal injuries climbed 19%.

- The over-65 age group is the fastest growing segment of the population. It is estimated that more than 40 million older adults will be licensed drivers by 2020.

Why Older Adults Stop Driving

Scientists at CDC's Injury Center worked with the University of California, San Diego, to survey older drivers living in community settings to find out why they stop driving. Medical conditions and poor vision were the most common reasons for stopping. This research provides useful insight into why older drivers decide that they are no longer fit to drive, which can help inform development of programs to reduce motor vehicle-related injuries among this population.

Older Drivers Less Likely Than Younger Drivers to Kill Others in a Crash.

Injury Center researchers analyzed fatality data to determine whether older drivers were more likely than younger drivers to be involved in crashes that killed someone else. They found that, in fact, older drivers were involved in fewer of these crashes than were drivers 16 to 34 years old. This study helps dispel the myth that older drivers present a threat to others on the road.

Violent Crime and Older Adults

The fear of crime is an important concern among persons of all ages. Although older persons may be more fearful of violent crime, they are more likely to be victims of property crime.

- Violent crime rates against persons age 65 or older declined from 9 per 1,000 older persons in 1973 to 3 per 1,000 in 1998.

- In 1998, persons age 65 or older were much less likely to be victims of violent crimes (3 per 1,000) than were persons ages 12 to 64 (45 per 1,000).

- Among persons in all age groups, most measured crime was property crime. Property crime rates have fallen in recent decades. Among households headed by older persons, 88 per 1,000 were victims of property crimes in 1998, down from 205 per 1,000 households in 1973.

- Households headed by persons age 65 or older were much less likely to be victims of property crime than were households headed by persons under age 65 (88 per 1,000 for older households, compared with 249 per 1,000 for younger households in 1998).

Part Two

Common Injuries

Chapter 6

Back Injuries

[Editor's Note: Spinal Cord Injuries are addressed in Chapter 24 under Part III: Trauma Injuries.]

Sprain and Strain

Lumbar, low back sprain/strain occurs with a sudden stressful injury to the low back region, causing stretching or tearing of the muscle/tendons/ligaments of the low back region. The muscles are large in this area and when a strain occurs, severe low back pain is the result. However, a sprain or strain may be misdiagnosed when an underlying disc injury has not yet made itself evident.

The erector spinae muscles are the firm prominent muscles that you can feel in the lower part of your back, on either side of the midline. These muscles can be painful when they get tensed and cramped up in spasms. When strains are imposed on the psoas muscle, tremendous forces are exerted on the lumbar spine. These forces can be very irritating to the low back.

Typical Pain and Findings

The low back pain from a sprain or muscle strain is in a broad area of the back and may be on either side, with consequent painful muscle

"Sprain and Strain," © 2000 American Association of Neurological Surgeons/Congress of Neurological Surgeons, reprinted with permission from Neurosurgery://ON-CALL ® at www.neurosurgery.org; "A Patient's Guide to Low Back Pain," © Medical Multimedia Group, reprinted with permission; and CDC Media Relations: Press Release, December 5, 2000.

spasms occurring with activity, or at night during sleep. The pain is worsened by activities and bed rest is an absolute necessity for a short period of time—one to three days.

The pain is typically limited to five to ten days and does not involve either leg. There is no weakness in the legs. There is marked restriction and painful limitation in range of motion. Patients are typically bent over and unable to straighten up or maintain a normal posture. Any particular activity is impossible, including sitting, standing, walking, driving, etc.

What Diagnostic Tests Are Used for Evaluations

No diagnostic testing is indicated, except in a case of unremitting sprain or strain which has been present for several weeks and is not improving as expected. At this point, x-rays of the lumbar spine will be needed to rule out underlying spinal injury or disease. If symptoms persist, an MRI is indicated to diagnoses underlying disc injury such as ruptured or degenerated disc, not evident or suspected at the initial examination.

Treatment

Treatment initially should involve nonsteroidal anti-inflammatory medications such as Nuprin, Motrin, Voltaren, Naprosyn, Tolectin, Lodine, Dolobid, Clinoril, or Feldene. A rehabilitation program involving physical therapy is prescribed. Physical therapy with ultrasound, heat and ice applied to the low back region allows the muscle spasms to relax. Exercises to stretch out painfully contracted muscles which are in spasm, followed by muscle strengthening exercises to build up the muscles to prevent further sprain and strain injuries completes a physical therapy program.

Prognosis

The prognosis is excellent for a complete recovery of a lumbar sprain or strain injury. The muscle typically recovers nearly 100% with some minimal scar tissue, if there was tearing of the muscle. Recurrent episodes of sprain and strain injury to the lumbar spine may be prevented by a conscientious daily exercise program to stretch and strengthen the lumbar spine muscles. This will avoid muscles that are weak and chronically underused or in a state of "chronic deconditioning."

Recommendations

An active strengthening and stretching program for the lumbar spine. This program should be done daily to build up strength and muscle mass, as well as maintain their normal length by simultaneous stretching program. This will definitely decrease the frequency and severity of episodes of sprain and strain injuries when the back is subjected to an abnormal force.

If overweight, get down to your ideal body weight. Reducing one's weight decreases force on the spine. Weight which hangs out in front on the spine causes chronic spasms in the low back region. When the back muscles contract to hold the belly up, abnormal forces on the spine result in disc degeneration and arthritis in the spine. Heat and ice treatment are indicated on an "as needed" basis at home to treat sudden flare-ups of low back pain, along with anti-inflammatory medications, as stated above. The cornerstone of treatment, however, is prevention, which is accomplished through an active exercise program.

A Patient's Guide to Low Back Pain—Understanding Spinal Rehabilitation

Back pain is a serious subject. As you recover from a back injury, it is important that you begin to learn how to safely strengthen your back to help prevent injuries to your back later. Your physical therapist can teach you specific exercises that will help reduce your back pain now—and help you begin a new set of habits that will help keep your back healthy.

This section will help you understand what each part of your back rehabilitation program is meant to do. It will also teach you how your back works and how to reduce or prevent further injury while your back heals. There are many different exercises that are recommended for the rehabilitation of the lumbar spine. This section won't try to teach you what to do—but rather why you'll be doing the exercises.

Understanding the Neutral Spine Position

Management and prevention of back pain begins by understanding the neutral spine position. Three natural curves are present in a healthy spine. The neck, or the cervical spine, curves slightly inward. The mid-back, or the thoracic spine, is curved outward. The low back, or the lumbar spine, curves inward again. The neutral alignment is important in helping to cushion the spine from too much stress and strain. Learning how to maintain a neutral spine position also helps you move safely during activities like sitting, walking, and lifting.

The natural curves of the spine are the result of the muscles, ligaments, and tendons that attach to the vertebrae of the spine. Without these supporting structures, the spine would collapse. They support the spine—much like guide wires support the mast of a ship. This guide wire system is made up mainly of the abdominal and back muscles. The abdominal muscles provide support by attaching to the ribs, pelvis, and indirectly, the lumbar spine. The muscles of the back are arranged in layers (deep layer, the intermediate layer, and the superficial layer), with each layer playing an important role in balancing the spine. By using these muscles together, we are able to balance the spine.

Controlling pelvic tilt is one way to begin helping to balance the spine. As certain muscles of the back and abdomen contract, the pelvis rotates. As the pelvis rotates forward, the curve of the low back increases. As the pelvis rotates backward, the curve of the low back straightens. Rotation of the pelvis is like a wheel centered at the hip joint. The muscles of the upper thighs also attach to the pelvis and contraction of these muscles can also be used to change the curve of the spine.

The abdominal muscles work alone, or with the hamstring muscles to produce a backward rotation of the pelvis. This causes the slight inward curve of the low back to straighten. If these muscles cause the curve of the low back to straighten too much, this may produce an unhealthy slouching posture.

In the other direction, as the hip flexors contract and back extensors contract, the pelvis is rotated forward—increasing the curvature of the lower back. If this curve is increased too much another unhealthy posture may result. This condition is called lordosis in medical terminology, or swayback in common terms.

A balance of strength and flexibility is the key to maintaining the neutral spine position. This balance is the basis for good muscle function. Like an automobile or any other piece of machinery, an imbalance may lead to wear and tear, eventually damaging the parts of the machine.

Muscle imbalances that affect the spine have many causes. One common cause of muscle imbalance is weak abdominal muscles, the muscles in the belly. As the abdominal muscles sag the hip flexors become tight, causing an increase in the curve of the low back. Leading to the swayback posture mentioned above. Another common problem results from tight hamstring muscles. As the hamstring muscles become tight the pelvis is rotated backwards. This produces an abnormal slouching posture.

Putting Safe Posture into Practice

Understanding body mechanics means understanding how we use our body. Proper body mechanics result when we put the neutral spine posture into action. To use proper body mechanics we need to learn how the spine should work during activities like:

• rising from a chair,
• walking, and
• lifting.

Sitting

Healthy sitting posture is based on the neutral spine position. Positioning your hips and knees at 90 degrees can help you keep a neutral sitting posture. Remember this position is balanced between the extremes of lumbar movement. Remember to choose a properly designed chair to help support the lumbar spine. The neutral spine position is also important when getting up from a chair. Holding the spine safely in neutral, the pelvic wheel turns forward, placing the "nose over the toes." With the feet placed shoulder width apart, stand upright. Use the buttock and thigh muscles to push yourself up. Don't twist or bend too far over at the waist and put too much strain on the lumbar spine.

Walking

Proper body mechanics are also important while walking—try to maintain the neutral spine position while walking. In the neutral position, the legs and arms swing naturally during forward motion. Conditions which alter the normal way of walking, and cause a limp, can severely stress the spine. While walking, always try to maintain your spine in the neutral position.

Lifting

Lifting is one of the most dangerous activities for the spine. The neutral position must be used to reduce the risk of injury. With the spine held in the neutral position, the movement occurs as the pelvic wheel turns. The hip joint is the center of the axis of pelvic rotation—not the back! The back loses the neutral position when the pelvis does not rotate forward. This posture can put too much of the force on the back muscles during a lift. Lifting in a neutral position allows the larger and more powerful leg muscles to do the lifting.

When lifting—first find the neutral position. Bend at the hips by rotating the pelvic wheel at the hip joint axis. Keep the safe posture, hold the object securely, and use the large leg muscles to generate power. Tighten the abdominal muscles during the lift to create a stabilizing corset around the trunk.

The Rules of Lifting

Many back injuries occur during lifting. The risks of injury can be reduced by making a complete checklist for safe lifting.

- First, plan and prepare for the lift. It only takes a moment to insure safety. The consequences of a back injury can be long lasting! Insure a safe and clear path. Before beginning to actually lift and move something, think through the lift.

- Obtain good footing with a wide base of support, by placing the feet a minimum of shoulder width apart. This lowers the center of gravity and increases stability.

- Keep the load close! Keeping the load close to the body can reduce stress on the spine and back muscles. Think of how a lever and fulcrum works. The back muscles, the spine, and the arms are the parts that form this lever system. The force needed to lift an object is lower if the load is nearer the fulcrum point. If the load is too far away from the body, the muscles of the spine have to work harder to help with the lift. This can lead to too much stress on the muscles or the spine, leading to injury.

- Maintain the neutral spine position! By moving the pelvic wheel around its axis, the upper body hinges forward, but the spine stays in neutral. Remember the neutral spine position at all times!

- Remember to lift with the large muscles of the legs!

- Avoid twisting and bending of the lower back at the same time! This is one the most damaging movements to the spine. To avoid twisting, pivot the feet to complete the lift.

- Get help if necessary! If the load is too bulky or heavy, don't hesitate to get help or use a handtruck! Don't be too tough or too busy to get help. A strong will does not take the place of a reasonably safe lift.

The Importance of Exercise

Exercise is important during all stages of recovery from a back injury. Different types of exercises will be used by your physical therapist as you progress. In the early stages, when your back is still quite painful, you may be taught specific exercises that are used to reduce your pain. These exercises are helpful in easing pain through relaxation. You also may be taught positioning exercises that will place the spine at a resting position. These exercises can give relief to sore muscles and joints.

Back pain can physically and emotionally draining. Relaxation exercises may not correct your problem, but they can help control pain and its accompanying stress. Movement is also important, even when the back is still painful. Careful movements may be suggested by your therapist that can safely ease pain by providing nutrition and lubrication to injured areas. Movement of joints and muscles also signals the nervous system to block incoming pain.

As your back becomes less painful, the exercises will be changed to focus on improving the overall health of your back. These changes will focus on:

- flexibility
- strength
- coordination
- aerobic conditioning

Exercises that increase flexibility help by reducing pain and making it easier to keep the spine in the neutral position. Tight muscles can cause an imbalance in spinal movements.

This can make the risk of injury to these structures more likely. Flexibility exercises for the trunk and lower limbs are helpful in establishing a pattern of safe movement. A slow progression of stretching exercises can increase the flexibility in the muscles and ligaments of the back and reduce the chance of re-injury.

The next stage of exercise focuses on the strength of the muscles that support the spine. These muscles help bring the spine into the neutral position—and keep it there. Well-trained abdominal, back, and hip muscles can help hold the back in a neutral position almost forming a natural corset. Strength training is simple to do at home and doesn't require any expensive equipment.

Posture exercises help train the muscles in the right movements between the pelvis and low back. Learning how to find and hold the neutral position of the spine is the key for a safe and healthy posture. Remember that the position of the pelvis determines the curve in the low back. Forward rotation increases the curve. Backward rotation straightens the curve. By practicing these exercises, you will become more comfortable in using the neutral spine position in your daily activities.

Strong muscles need to be coordinated. As the strength of the spinal muscles increases, it becomes important to train those muscles to work together.

Learning any physical activity takes practice. Muscles must be trained so that the physical activity is under control. Muscles trained to control safe movement of the spine reduce the chance of injury. You will be taught exercises that will help you train your back muscles to work together to protect the spine.

Finally, attention will be directed to increasing your overall fitness. Muscles can get the energy they need to work in one of two ways—by using oxygen to burn calories from the bloodstream or by burning sugars in the bloodstream quickly without using oxygen. By using oxygen as they work, muscles are better able to move continuously, rather than in spurts. The word aerobic means with oxygen. Fitness training, or aerobic training, conditions the muscles to become better able to obtain the nutrients and oxygen that they need from the blood. If muscles are more used to working in fits and spurts they are more likely to burn sugars without using oxygen. This is called anaerobic metabolism, and it doesn't work nearly as well as aerobic metabolism. As the muscles use up the nutrients and oxygen, they switch to anaerobic metabolism and chemical waste products are created that can cause pain in the muscles. Aerobic training increases the muscles ability to get rid of these waste products.

Exercise has other benefits as well. Exercise can cause chemicals called endorphins to be released into the blood. These chemical hormones act as natural pain relievers in reducing your pain. So, exercise can actually make you feel better and help control your pain through the body's natural pain medication! It will be important that you pick an aerobic activity you can enjoy and stick with it!

No Evidence That Back Belts Reduce Injury Seen in Landmark Study of Retail Users

In the largest study of its kind ever conducted, the Centers for Disease Control and Prevention's (CDC)'s National Institute for Occupational Safety and Health (NIOSH) found no evidence that back belts reduce back injury or back pain for retail workers who lift or move merchandise, according to results published in the *Journal of the American Medical Association* (JAMA) December 6, 2000 issue.

The study, conducted over a two-year period, found no statistically significant difference between the incidence rate of workers' compensation claims for job-related back injuries among employees who reported using back belts usually every day, and the incidence rate of such claims among employees who reported never using back belts or using them no more than once or twice a month.

Similarly, no statistically significant difference was found in comparing the incidence of self-reported back pain among workers who reported using back belts every day, with the incidence among workers who reported never using back belts or using them no more than once or twice a month. Neither did the study find a statistically significant difference between the rate of back injury claims among employees in stores that required the use of back belts, and the rate of such claims in stores where back belt use was voluntary.

Back belts, also called back supports or abdominal belts, resemble corsets. In recent years, they have been widely used in numerous industries to prevent worker injury during lifting. There are more than 70 types of industrial back belts, including the lightweight, stretchable nylon style used by workers in this study. Approximately four million back belts were purchased for workplace use in 1995, the most recent year for which data were available. The results of the new study are consistent with NIOSH's previous finding, reported in 1994, that there is insufficient scientific evidence that wearing back belts protects workers from the risk of job-related back injury.

"Work-related musculoskeletal disorders cost the economy an estimated $13 billion every year, and a substantial proportion of these are back injuries," said CDC Director Jeffrey P. Koplan, M.D., M.P.H. "By taking action to reduce exposures, employers can go a long way toward keeping workers safe and reducing the costs of work-related back injury."

This study was the largest prospective study ever conducted on use of back belts. From April 1996 to April 1998, NIOSH interviewed 9,377 employees at 160 newly opened stores owned by a national retail chain. The employees were identified by store management as involved in materials handling tasks (lifting or moving merchandise). Through interviews, data was gathered on detailed information on workers' back-belt wearing habits, work history, lifestyle habits, job activities, demographic characteristics, and job satisfaction. The study also examined workers' compensation claims for back injuries among employees at the stores over the two-year period.

In a prospective study, researchers identify a cohort or group of workers for evaluation, and then collect current information on that group as the study progresses. In this study, NIOSH determined workers' habits in wearing back belts in advance of any injuries, and collected data as workers filed back injury claims.

Findings from this study included:

- There was no statistically significant difference between the rates of back injuries among workers who wore back belts every day (3.38 cases per 100 full time equivalent workers or FTEs) and back injury rates among workers who never wore back belts or wore them no more than once or twice a month (2.76 cases per 100 FTEs).

- There was no statistically significant difference between the incidence of self-reported back pain among workers who wore back belts usually every day (17.1 percent) and the incidence of self-reported back pain among workers who never wore back belts or wore them no more than once or twice a month (17.5 percent).

- There was no statistically significant difference between the rate of back injury claims in stores requiring the use of back belts (2.98 cases per every 100 FTEs) and the rate in stores where back belt use was voluntary (3.08 cases per 100 FTEs).

- A history of back injury was the strongest risk factor for predicting either a back injury claim or reported back pain among employees, regardless of back belt use. The rate of back injury among those with a previous history of back pain (5.14 cases per 100 FTEs) nearly twice as high as the rate among workers without a previous history of back pain (2.68 per 100 FTEs).

- Even for employees in the most strenuous types of jobs, comparisons of back injury claims and self-reported back pain failed to show any differences in rates or incidence associated with back belt use.

Chapter 7

Bites and Stings

Cat and Dog Bites

How Should I Take Care of a Bite from a Cat or a Dog?

Here are some things you should do to take care of a wound caused by a cat or dog bite:

- Wash the wound gently with soap and water.
- Apply pressure with a clean towel to the injured part to stop the bleeding.
- Apply a sterile bandage to the wound.
- Keep the injury elevated above the level of the heart to slow swelling and prevent infection.
- Report the incident to the proper authority in your community (for example, police or animal control).
- Apply antibiotic ointment to the area 2 times every day until it heals.

Should I Call My Doctor if I've Been Bitten by a Cat or a Dog?

Call your doctor in any of these situations:

"Cat and Dog Bites," Reprinted with permission from http://www.familydoctor. org/handouts/203.html; Revised April 2000. Copyright © American Academy of Family Physicians. All Rights Reserved. And, "First Aid for Bee and Insect Stings," by Dawna L. Cyr and Steven B. Johnson, Ph.D., National Ag Safety Database (NASD).

- You have a cat bite. Cat bites are very prone to infection. You don't need to call your doctor for a cat scratch, unless you think the wound is infected.

- You have a dog bite on your hand, foot, or head, or you have a bite that is deep or gaping.

- You have diabetes, liver or lung disease, cancer, acquired immunodeficiency syndrome (AIDS), or other conditions that weaken your ability to fight infection.

- You have any signs of infection, such as redness, swelling, warmth, increased tenderness, oozing of pus from the wound, or fever.

- You have bleeding that doesn't stop after 15 minutes of pressure or you think you may have a broken bone, nerve damage, or other serious injury.

- Your last tetanus shot was more than 5 years ago. (If so, you may need a booster shot.)

What Will My Doctor Do?

Here are some things your doctor may do to treat a cat or dog bite:

- Examine the wound for possible nerve or tendon damage, or bone injury. He or she will also check for signs of infection.

- Clean the wound with a special solution and remove any damaged tissue.

- May use stitches to close a bite wound, but often the wound is left open to heal, so the risk of infection is lowered.

- May prescribe an antibiotic to prevent infection.

- May give you a tetanus shot if you had your last shot more than 5 years ago.

- May ask you to schedule an office visit to check your wound again in 1 to 2 days.

- If your injury is severe, or if the infection has not gotten better even though you're taking antibiotics, your doctor may suggest that you see a specialist and/or go to the hospital, where you can get special medicine given directly in your veins (intravenous antibiotics) and further treatment if necessary.

How Can I Prevent Cat and Dog Bites?

Here are some things you can do to prevent bites:

- Never leave a young child alone with a pet.
- Do not try to separate fighting animals.
- Avoid strange and sick animals.
- Leave animals alone while they're eating.
- Keep pets on a leash when in public.
- Select your family pet carefully.

First Aid for Bee and Insect Stings

Most bees and insects will not attack if left alone. If provoked, a bee will sting in defense of its nest or itself. Thousands of people are stung each year and as many as 40 to 50 people in the United States die each year as a result of allergic reactions.

What to Do If a Person Is Stung

- Have someone stay with the victim to be sure that they do not have an allergic reaction.
- Wash the site with soap and water.
- The stinger can be removed using a 4 x 4 inch gauze wiped over the area or by scraping a fingernail over the area. Never squeeze the stinger or use tweezers. It will cause more venom to go into the skin and injure the muscle.
- Apply ice to reduce the swelling.
- Do not scratch the sting. This will cause the site to swell and itch more, and increase the chance of infection.
- Persons with severe allergic reactions to insect stings should consider wearing a medical ID bracelet and carrying an insect allergy kit where appropriate.

Allergic Reactions to Bee Stings

Allergic reactions to bee stings can be deadly. People with known allergies to insect stings should always carry an insect sting allergy kit and wear a medical ID bracelet or necklace stating their allergy. See a physician about getting either of these.

There are several signs of an allergic reaction to bee stings. Look for swelling that moves to other parts of the body, especially the face or neck. Check for difficulty in breathing, wheezing, dizziness, or a drop in blood pressure. Get the person immediate medical care if any of these signs are present. It is normal for the area that has been stung to hurt, have a hard swollen lump, get red, and itch. There are kits available to reduce the pain of an insect sting. They are a valuable addition to a first aid kit.

Reducing the Risk of Being Stung

1. Wear light-colored, smooth-finished clothing.

2. Avoid perfumed soaps, shampoos, and deodorants. Don't wear cologne or perfume. Avoid bananas and banana-scented toiletries.

3. Wear clean clothing and bathe daily. Sweat angers bees.

4. Cover the body as much as possible with clothing.

5. Avoid flowering plants.

6. Check for new nests during the warmer hours of the day during July, August, and September. Bees are very active then.

7. Keep areas clean. Social wasps thrive in places where humans discard food, so clean up picnic tables, grills, and other outdoor eating areas.

8. If a single stinging insect is flying around, remain still or lie face down on the ground. The face is the most likely place for a bee or wasp to sting. Swinging or swatting at an insect may cause it to sting.

9. If you are attacked by several stinging insects at the same time, run to get away from them. Bees release a chemical when they sting. This alerts other bees to the intruder. More bees often follow. Go indoors or jump into water. Outdoors, a shaded area is better than an open area to get away from the insects.

10. If a bee comes inside your vehicle, stop the car slowly, and open all the windows.

11. For information on safely removing known nests, contact the Extension Office in your area.

Chapter 8

Cuts and Abrasions

While most minor injuries can be tended at home, there are some that require more specialized medical attention. This chapter is intended to help you to recognize and manage such injuries until professional medical care is available. It will also review the kinds of treatment that may be provided by physicians.

Major Trauma and Life Threatening Wounds

Serious Bleeding

Steady or heavy bleeding is an urgent situation, especially after major trauma. While the wound itself may not be severe, large amounts of blood loss can be life threatening.

When is bleeding "serious?" Most healthy adults can tolerate the loss of one to two pints of blood without much consequence. Losses in excess of this, especially in weak or ill individuals, can cause serious harm. Similarly, rapid bleeding (steadily flowing blood or bleeding that soaks through gauze dressings quickly) can lead to large blood losses in a short period of time.

As a lay person helping an injured person, it is not necessary for you to make accurate measurements or estimates of blood loss. It is essential that you summon professional medical attention, and do what you can to prevent further blood loss.

"Cuts and Abrasions: When a Band-Aid Won't Do," David A. Cooke, MD, © 2001, Omnigraphics, Inc.

Before attempting to help a victim, send for an ambulance, or call for one yourself if no other help is available. The measures you take will not cure the victim, but only buy time for the Emergency Medical System to arrive.

Stopping Bleeding

- Virtually all bleeding can be stopped quickly and easily, with no special tools or training required. Direct pressure and elevation are the keys to stopping bleeding.

- Direct pressure is exactly that. Using your fingers, or for a larger wound, the heel of your hand, press firmly around the edges, but not into, the wound. The pressure you exert will compress blood vessels and capillaries, slowing the rate of bleeding. Often, this will slow bleeding enough that blood can clot, sealing the injured vessels.

- If the wound is in an extremity, elevate it if possible. This uses gravity to your advantage, slowing the rate at which new blood flows into the wound.

- Pressure may need to be held for several minutes, or possibly even much longer periods of time for serious wounds. For this reason, it is essential to make sure that help has been summoned before you attempt to stop the bleeding.

- If you have gauze pads available, use them. In a pinch, a strip of cloth from clothing will do. Lay them over the wound, and exert pressure through them. This will help protect the wound, as well as help with clot formation. If blood soaks through the dressing, do not remove it. Instead, place a new dressing on top of the old one, and resume holding pressure. Removing old dressings will disrupt clots, and may make matters worse.

- Tourniquets should be used only as *a last resort*! As stated above, it is very rare that bleeding cannot be stopped with direct pressure and elevation. A tourniquet should only be considered when a wound on a limb continues to bleed heavily despite direct pressure and elevation, and professional medical rescuers are not expected to arrive quickly. Use of a tourniquet is likely to result in permanent loss of the limb, so it is truly an option of last resort.

- A tourniquet may *only* be used on an arm or a leg. If it must be used, select a wide band or strap, the wider the better. A belt will often do. Put it around the limb between the wound and the rest of the body. It should be as close to the wound as possible, without actually covering the wound. Once in place, tighten it until the bleeding slows, then tie it. Once placed, a tourniquet should never be loosened or removed except by medical personnel. Note the time it was placed, and write this down. If you have a pen or marker available, write on the victim's forehead "TK" and the time it was placed. This will be very important for future care of the patient.

Open Fractures

Occasionally, a broken bone will protrude through the skin. This is known as an open, or compound, fracture. These fractures are quite serious, as infection is likely to ensue.

An ambulance should be summoned immediately. If bleeding is heavy, use the direct pressure and elevation techniques described above until help arrives. If clean, dry gauze is available, lightly cover the wound with it. *Do not attempt to push the bone back into the skin.*

Amputations

An amputation is the term for the loss of a limb, or an appendage such as an ear. Such wounds require immediate medical attention for two reasons. First, bleeding may be heavy after an amputation. Second, in some circumstances, it may be possible to reattach the severed tissue, but only if it is done quickly.

In the event of an amputation, summon help and control bleeding as above. If possible, try to find the missing tissue. Try to keep it cool, but do not freeze it. Send it with the patient to the medical facility when Emergency Medical Services arrive.

Minor Trauma: No Ambulance Required

Open Wounds

Most open wounds are referred to as lacerations, which usually have irregular edges. While not life-threatening, they can be problematic because they can lead to infection. Additionally, if they are not properly cared for, a large scar may develop, which can be unsightly, and sometimes even interfere with normal function of the affected body part.

When does an open wound need professional medical attention? Generally speaking, any wound more than 1 inch long and more than 1/4 inch deep should be evaluated by a physician. Any wound that clearly extends through all the skin layers should also be checked.

Time is of the essence in care of open wounds. In order to be properly repaired, the wound should be treated before eight to twelve hours from the time of injury have passed. Longer delays sharply increase the risk of infection, and it may not be possible to repair them if more than twelve hours have passed.

Kinds of Wound Repair

There are several ways in which a laceration may be repaired. Which method is used depends on the size and location of the wound, degree of contamination with infectious material, the materials available to the physician, and the treating physician's clinical judgement.

Suturing (stitches): This is probably the oldest form of wound repair. Thread is used to draw the wound edges together and hold them there. This speeds healing, and generally results in a smaller, neater, stronger scar. This technique is especially good for clean, relatively straight wounds, as well as wounds in body areas subject to high skin tension, such as skin overlying a joint. It may not be suitable for "dirty" wounds.

Once the wound has been cleansed, the skin surrounding the wound is numbed using a local anesthetic. A needle and thread pushed through the surrounding skin and wound, pulling the edges together, much like repairing a tear in a piece of cloth. There are a large variety of specific suturing techniques, depending on the wound type. The thread (suture) is pulled taut to bring the edges together, and knots are tied to hold it in place.

While some kinds of suture material are available which slowly dissolve in place, most sutures need to be removed one to two weeks after they are placed. The absorbable type are usually not suitable for use on exposed skin because they become infected more easily. Removing sutures is usually a simple and painless procedure, simply cutting the threads and pulling out the ends.

Wound Adhesive (glue): In the past ten years, several kinds of adhesives have become available for closing wounds. These are essentially forms of "glue" which stick wound edges together. They differ from ordinary glues in that they are safe for use in tissue, and slowly dissolve away as the wound heals. They are good for irregular wounds, as well as in body locations where there is little skin tension, such as on the scalp or back.

Once the wound has been cleansed, the wound adhesive is squeezed from a tube into the wound, and the edges are pushed together. The wound is allowed to sit for a period of time while the glue hardens. Once the glue has hardened, the repair is generally durable. The skin edges will grow together, dissolving the glue as it does so. This usually results in a very cosmetically acceptable scar.

Wound adhesives have the advantage of being quick, easy, and relatively painless treatment for open wounds. However, the repair is generally not as strong as with suturing, so it may not be suitable for large wounds or wounds near joints. It is also relatively expensive. Not all emergency departments or physicians' offices stock the adhesives, so availability may also govern its use.

Secondary Intention: In certain cases, it is not possible or advisable to close an open wound by either of the above techniques. A wound that is already infected should not be closed, because this tends to lead to abscess formation. Similarly, a "dirty" wound usually will not be closed, because the risk of infection is high, even after aggressive cleaning. In these cases, the wound is allowed to close by secondary intention.

Secondary intention is the body's natural healing process. Generally, the wound will heal from the inside out as scar tissue grows in. This produces an effective repair. However, healing tends to take much longer than with other methods. Additionally, the resulting scar is often large and bulky, and typically unsightly.

When it is necessary to allow a wound to close by secondary intention, packing material will often be used to aid in healing. Gauze strips will be pushed into the wound, keeping the edges apart. This forces the bottom of the wound to heal before the top. Packing is changed regularly, and over time, less and less is placed until the wound cavity is finally completely closed by scar tissue.

Abrasions

Abrasions are wounds where the upper layers of skin are removed, while the deeper layers remain intact. This usually occurs from friction or shearing type forces. It is frequently seen after sliding on rough ground or pavement. Usually, these wounds are less serious than lacerations. However, because abrasions may be quite large, they still may require extra care.

Abrasions are most often "dirty" wounds by nature of the injuries that cause them. Careful cleansing of the wound as soon as possible is very important. This is preferably done with warm water, soap, and alcohol or hydrogen peroxide. If embedded material remains after cleansing, the wound should be evaluated by a physician. Abrasions should usually be covered with a dry, plastic-lined gauze dressing to prevent the dressing from sticking to the wound. Within a few days, a hard crust or scab will appear covering the wound. Once this has occurred, the wound can be left open to the air. Most abrasions heal well, usually without scarring.

Wound Healing and Infections

Infection is always a concern with a healing wound. A major function of skin is to provide a barrier against entry of bacteria into the body. When skin is disrupted, this barrier fails. Even with very careful cleansing, it is rarely possible to completely sterilize a wound. Usually, the immune system is adequate to handle what bacteria enter the wound, but this is not always the case.

Normal Healing

Some degree of swelling and redness surrounding a healing wound is normal. Swelling is usually most prominent in the first three days following the injury, and generally decreases afterwards. Clear to yellow fluid drainage may also be seen in the first few days. Moderate pink or red coloration at the wound edges is also common. As healing becomes more advanced, a pink or red rim will often form around the wound. This typically extends less than one half inch from the wound edge. As the wound heals further, it will shrink and contract, until it disappears entirely.

Signs of Infection

An infected wound usually will have multiple indications of a problem. Most frequently seen is spreading redness surrounding the wound. As stated above, a red rim is not unusual in normal healing. However, the redness may extend for one or more inches around an infected wound. This will also typically be bright red and hot to the touch.

Infected wounds may also drain fluid. In contrast to normal wound healing, an infected wound will often drain large amounts of fluid. The fluid is often thick and opaque, and may be yellow to green in color. It may also be quite foul-smelling. Pus may be obvious.

Pain is also often present with an infected wound. A wound that suddenly becomes increasingly painful is suspicious for infection, since pain usually decreases as healing progresses.

In the event of any signs of infection, obtain medical care immediately. Depending on the degree and severity, it may be necessary to reopen the wound, start antibiotic therapy, or both.

Chapter 9

Elbow Injuries

How Is the Elbow Designed, and What Is Its Function?

The elbow is the joint where three long bones meet in the middle portion of the arm. The bone of the upper arm (humerus) meets the inner bone of the forearm (ulna) and the outer bone of the forearm (radius) to form a hinge joint. The radius and ulna also meet in the elbow to allow for rotation of the forearm. The elbow functions to move the arm like a hinge (forward and backward) and in rotation (twisting outwards and inwards). The biceps muscle is the major muscle that flexes the elbow hinge. The triceps muscle is the major muscle that extends the elbow hinge. The outer bone of the elbow is referred to as the lateral epicondyle and is a part of the humerus bone. Tendons are attached to this area which can be injured, causing inflammation or tendinitis (lateral epicondylitis, or "tennis elbow"). The inner portion of the elbow is a bony prominence called the medial epicondyle. Additional tendons from the muscles attach here and can be injured, causing medial epicondylitis, "golfer's elbow." A fluid-filled sac (bursa), which serves to reduce friction, overlies the tip of the elbow (olecranon bursa). The elbow can be affected by inflammation of the tendons or the bursae (plural for bursa), or conditions which affect the bones and joints, such as fractures, arthritis, or nerve irritation.

Reprinted with permission "Elbow Pain," reviewed 5/3/01, © MedicineNet.com; and "Bursitis," by William C. Shiel Jr., MD, FACP, FACR, reviewed 8/20/01, © MedicineNet.com., reprinted with permission.

What Injuries Can Cause Elbow Pain?

Tendinitis

- **Lateral Epicondylitis (Tennis Elbow)** The lateral epicondyle is the outside bony portion of the elbow where large tendons attach to the elbow from the muscles of the forearm. These tendons can be injured, especially with repetitive motions of the forearm, such as using a manual screwdriver, washing windows, or hitting a backhand in tennis play. Tennis elbow results in pain over the outside of the elbow, occasionally with warmth and swelling, but always with local tenderness. The elbow maintains its full range of motion, as the inner joint is not affected, and the pain can be particularly noticed toward the end of the day. Repeated twisting motions or activities which strain the tendon typically elicit increased pain. X-rays are usually normal, but can reveal calcium deposits in the tendon or reveal other unforeseen abnormalities of the elbow joint.

  The treatment of lateral epicondylitis includes ice packs, resting the involved elbow, and antiinflammatory medications. Antiinflammatory medications typically used include aspirin and other nonsteroidal antiinflammatory drugs (NSAIDs) such as naproxen (Naprosyn ®), diclofenac (Voltaren ®), and ibuprofen (Motrin ®). Bracing the elbow can help. Local cortisone injections are given for persistent pain. Activity involving the elbow is resumed gradually. Ice application after activity can reduce or prevent recurrent inflammation. Occasionally, supportive straps can prevent reinjury. In severe cases, an orthopedic surgical repair is performed.

- **Medial Epicondylitis (Golfer's Elbow)** Medial epicondylitis is inflammation at the point where the tendons of the forearm attach to the bony prominence of the inner elbow. As an example, this tendon can become strained in a golf swing, but many other repetitive motions can injure the tendon. Golfer's elbow is characterized by local pain and tenderness over the inner elbow. The range of motion of the elbow is preserved because the inner joint of the elbow is not affected. Those activities which require twisting or straining the forearm tendon can elicit pain and worsen the condition. X-rays for epicondylitis are usually normal but can indicate calcifications of the tendons if the tendinitis has persisted for extended periods of time.

Olecranon Bursitis

Bursitis is inflammation of a bursa. A bursa is a tiny fluid-filled sac that functions as a gliding surface to reduce friction between tissues of the body. The major bursae are located adjacent to the tendons near the large joints, such as the shoulders, elbows, hips, and knees.

A bursa can become inflamed from injury, infection (rare in the shoulder), or underlying rheumatic condition. Examples include injury as subtle as lifting a bag of groceries into the car to inflame the shoulder bursa (shoulder bursitis), infection of the bursa in front of the knee from a knee scraping on asphalt (septic prepatellar bursitis), and inflammation of the elbow bursa from gout crystals (gouty olecranon bursitis).

The treatment of any form of bursitis depends on whether or not it involves infection. Bursitis that is not infected (from injury or underlying rheumatic disease) can be treated with ice compresses, rest, and antiinflammatory and pain medications. Occasionally, it requires aspiration of the bursa fluid. This procedure involves removal of the fluid with a needle and syringe under sterile conditions. It can be performed in the doctor's office. Sometimes the fluid is sent to the laboratory for further analysis. Noninfectious shoulder bursitis can also be treated with an injection of cortisone medication into the swollen bursa. This is sometimes done at the same time as the aspiration procedure.

Infectious (septic) bursitis requires even further evaluation and treatment. This is unusual in the shoulder bursa, but does occur. The bursal fluid can be examined in the laboratory for the microbes causing the infection. Septic bursitis requires antibiotic therapy, often intravenously. Repeated aspiration of the inflamed fluid may be required. Surgical drainage and removal of the infected bursa sac (bursectomy) may also be necessary. Generally, the elbow functions normally after the surgical wound heals.

Fractures

The bones of the elbow can break (fracture) into the elbow joint or adjacent to the elbow joint. Fractures generally require immobilization and casts and can require orthopedic pinning or open joint surgery.

Arthritis of the Elbow

Inflammation of the elbow joint (arthritis) can occur as a result of many systemic forms of arthritis, including rheumatoid arthritis, gouty arthritis, psoriatic arthritis, ankylosing spondylitis, and reactive arthritis (formerly called Reiter's disease). Generally, they are associated with signs of inflammation of the elbow joint, including heat, warmth, swelling, pain, tenderness, and decreased range of motion. Range of motion of the elbow is decreased with arthritis of the elbow because the swollen joint impedes the range of motion.

Information on elbow pain is provided for informational purposes only and is not a substitute for professional medical advice. You should not use this information for diagnosing or treating a medical or health condition. You should carefully read all product packaging. If you have or suspect you have a medical problem, promptly contact your professional healthcare provider. Statements and information regarding dietary supplements have not been evaluated or approved by the Food and Drug Administration. Please consult your healthcare provider before beginning any course of supplementation or treatment.

Chapter 10

Foot and Ankle Injuries

Immediate Treatment

Foot and ankle emergencies happen every day. Broken bones, dislocations, sprains, contusions, infections, and other serious injuries can occur at any time. Early attention is vitally important. Whenever you sustain a foot or ankle injury, you should seek immediate treatment from a podiatric physician.

That advice is universal, even though there are lots of myths about foot and ankle injuries. Some of them follow.

Myths

1. **"It can't be broken, because I can move it."** False, this widespread idea has kept many fractures from receiving proper treatment. The truth is that often you can walk with certain kinds of fractures. Some common examples: breaks of the thinner of the two leg bones; small "chip" fractures of either foot or ankle bones; and the frequently neglected fracture of a toe.

2. **"If you break a toe, immediate care isn't necessary."** False, a toe fracture needs prompt attention. If x-rays reveal it to be a simple, displaced fracture, care by your podiatrist

usually can produce rapid relief. However, x-rays might identify a displaced or angulated break. In such cases, prompt realignment of the fracture by your podiatric physician will help prevent improper or incomplete healing. Many patients develop post-fracture deformity of a toe, which in turn results in formation of a painfully deformed toe with a most painful corn. A good general rule is to seek prompt treatment for injury to foot bones.

3. **"If you have a foot or ankle injury, soak it in hot water immediately."** False, don't use heat or hot water if you suspect a fracture, sprain, or dislocation. Heat promotes blood flow, causing greater swelling. More swelling means greater pressure on the nerves, which causes more pain. An ice bag wrapped in a towel has a contracting effect on blood vessels, produces a numbing effect, and prevents swelling and pain. After seeing a podiatric physician, warm compresses, and soaks may be used.

4. **"Applying an elastic bandage to a severely sprained ankle is adequate treatment".** False, ankle sprains often mean torn or severely overstretched ligaments, and they should receive immediate care. X-ray examination, immobilization by casting or splinting, and physiotherapy to insure a normal recovery all may be indicated. Surgery may even be necessary.

5. **"The terms 'fracture,' 'break,' and 'crack' are all different".** False, all of those words are proper in describing a broken bone.

Before Seeing the Podiatrist

If an injury or accident does occur, the steps you can take to help yourself until you can reach your podiatric physician are easy to remember if you can recall the word "rice."

1. **Rest.** Cut back on your activity, and get off your feet if you can.

2. **Ice.** Gently place a plastic bag of ice, or ice wrapped in a towel, on the injured area in a 20-minute-on, 40-minute-off cycle.

3. **Compression.** Lightly wrap an Ace bandage around the area, taking care not to pull it too tight.

4. **Elevation.** Sit in a position that you can elevate the foot higher than the waist, to reduce swelling and pain.

5. Switch to a soft shoe or slipper, preferably one that your podiatrist can cut up in the office if it needs to be altered to accommodate a bulky dressing.

6. For bleeding cuts, cleanse well, apply pressure with gauze or a towel, and cover with a clean dressing. It's best not to use any medication on the cut before you see the doctor.

7. Leave blisters unopened if they are not painful or swollen.

8. Foreign materials in the skin, such as slivers, splinters, and sand, can be removed carefully with a sterile instrument. A deep foreign object, such as broken glass or a needle, must be removed professionally.

9. Treatment for an abrasion is similar to that of a burn, since raw skin is exposed to the air and can easily become infected. Cleansing is important to remove all foreign particles. Sterile bandages should be applied, along with an antibiotic cream or ointment.

Prevention

1. Wear the correct shoes for any event. Good walking shoes provide more comfort and better balance.

2. Wear hiking shoes or boots in rough terrain.

3. Different sports activities call for specific footwear to protect feet and ankles. Use the correct shoes for each sport. Don't wear any sports shoe beyond its useful life.

4. Wear safety shoes if you're in an occupation which threatens foot safety. There are specific safety shoes for a variety of on-the-job conditions. Be certain they are fitted properly.

5. Always wear hard-top shoes when operating a lawn mower or other grass-cutting equipment.

6. Don't walk barefoot on paved streets or sidewalks.

7.   Watch out for slippery floors at home and at work. Clean up obviously dangerous spills immediately.

8.   If you get up during the night, turn on a light. Many fractured toes and other foot injuries occur while attempting to find your way in the dark.

Additional Information

American Podiatric Medical Association
9312 Old Georgetown Road
Bethesda, MD 20814
Tel: 301-571-9200
Fax: 301-530-2725
Website: www.apma.org
E-mail: aaskapma@apma.org

The APMA produces a series of pamphlets that discuss several foot health conditions and concerns, including diabetes, arthritis, high blood pressure, athlete's foot, occupational foot health, warts, foot orthoses, aging, children's feet, surgery, Medicare coverage, heel pain, nail problems, walking, women's feet, footwear, and others. The pamphlets are available from many podiatrist members of APMA.

Chapter 11

Fractures

Fracture of Bone

A fracture is a break in the bone or cartilage. It usually is a result of trauma. It can, however, be a result of disease of the bone that leads to weakening, such as osteoporosis, or abnormal formation of the bone from congenital diseases at birth, such as osteogenesis imperfecta.

How Are Fractures Classified?

Fractures are classified by their character and location. Examples of classification include:

- *Spiral Fracture*: A fracture that goes around the axis of the bone.

- *Greenstick Fracture*: A fracture that does not go all the way through the bone.

- *Transverse (Linear) Fracture*: A "clean" or straight break of the bone without jagged edges.

- *Oblique Fracture*: A fracture which goes at an angle to the axis.

"Facture of Bone," © 1996-2001 MedicineNet, Inc., reprinted with permission; excerpts from "Falls and Related Fractures," Osteoporosis and Related Bone Diseases National Resource Center (ORBD~NRC), revised 4/2000; and "Fast Facts on Osteoporosis," Osteoporosis and Related Bone Diseases National Resource Center (ORBD~NRC), revised 10/2000.

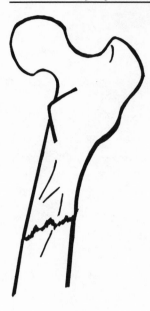

Figure 11.1. Spiral Fracture of the Femur (illustration by William A. Shannon; © 2002 Omnigraphics, Inc.)

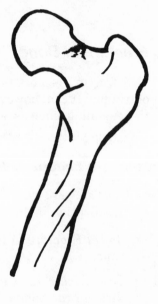

Figure 11.2. Greenstick Fracture of the Femur (illustration by William A. Shannon; © 2002 Omnigraphics, Inc.)

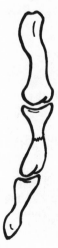

Figure 11.3. Transverse (Linear) Fracture of the Second Phalanx of the Thumb (illustration by William A. Shannon; © 2002 Omnigraphics, Inc.)

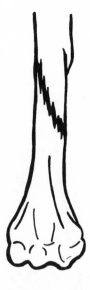

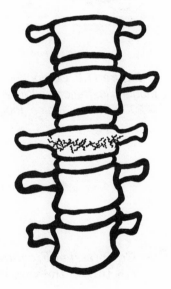

Figure 11.4. Oblique Fracture of the Humerus (illustration by William A. Shannon; © 2002 Omnigraphics, Inc.)

Figure 11.5. Compression Fracture of a Lumbar Vertebrae (illustration by William A. Shannon; © 2002 Omnigraphics, Inc.)

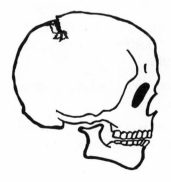

Figure 11.6. Depressed Fracture of the Cranium (illustration by William A. Shannon; © 2002 Omnigraphics, Inc.)

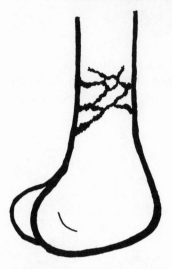

Figure 11.7. Comminuted Fracture of the Femur (illustration by William A. Shannon; © 2002 Omnigraphics, Inc.)

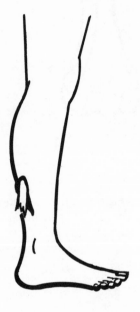

Figure 11.8. Compound Fracture of the Fibula (illustration by William A. Shannon; © 2002 Omnigraphics, Inc.)

- *Compression Fracture of a Lumbar Vertebrae*: In a compression fracture of the vertebrae, the bone tissue of the vertebral body collapses.

- *Depressed Fracture of the Cranium*: A depressed skull fracture is a break in a cranial bone (or "crushed" portion of skull) with depression of the bone in toward the brain.

- *Comminuted Fracture*: A comminuted fracture is where a bone is broken into a number of pieces

- *Compound Fracture*: A compound fracture is a fracture in which there is an associated open wound of the skin which leads directly to the broken bone.

Fractures are also named by the trauma event that caused the bone breakage. Examples include: "boxer's fracture" of the metacarpal bone of the hand, "blowout fracture" of the bones behind the eye, and "stress fracture" of the bones of tibia. Some fractures are also named by conditions associated with the bone breakage.

How Are Fractures Treated?

The treatment of a fracture depends on the type of fracture, its severity, and location, as well as the underlying condition of the patient. Fractures are treated with resting, non-weight bearing, splints, casting, and surgical procedures.

Falls and Related Fractures

The Risk of Undiagnosed Osteoporosis

Falls are serious at any age, and breaking a bone after a fall becomes more likely as a person ages. Everyone knows someone who has fallen and broken or fractured a bone. While healing, the fracture limited activities and sometimes required surgery, and, often, the person wore a heavy cast to support the broken bone and needed physical therapy to resume normal activities. People are unaware that there is often a link between the broken bone and osteoporosis, a silent disease in which there is a gradual loss of bone tissue or bone density that makes bones so fragile they break under the slightest strain. Because osteoporosis progresses without symptoms, falls are especially dangerous for people who are unaware that they have low bone density. If the patient and the physician fail to connect the broken bone to osteoporosis, the chance to make a diagnosis with a bone density test and begin a prevention or treatment program is lost. Bone loss continues until another bone breaks. Even though bones do not break after every fall, the person who has fallen and broken a bone almost always becomes fearful of falling again. As a result, she or he may limit activities for the sake of "safety." Among Americans age 65 and older, fall-related injuries are the leading cause of death due to unintentional injuries.[1]

Did You Know?

- More than 90% of hip fractures are associated with osteoporosis?

- Nine out of ten hip fractures in older Americans are the result of a fall?[2]

- Individuals who have a hip fracture are 5-20% more likely to die in the first year following that injury than others in this age group?[3]

- For those living independently before a hip fracture, 15%-25% will still be in long-term care institutions a year after their fracture?[3]

- Most falls happen to women in their homes in the afternoon?[4]

If one of these factors is modified, the chances of breaking a bone are greatly reduced.

The Force and Direction of a Fall

The force of a fall (how hard a person lands) plays a major role in determining whether a person will fracture or not. For example, the greater the distance of the hip bone to the floor, the greater the risk of fracturing a hip so tall people seem to have an increased risk of fractures when they fall. The angle at which a person falls also is important. Falling sideways or straight down is more risky than falling backwards, for example.

- Being tall increases your risk of a hip fracture

- How you land increases fracture risk

- Catching yourself so you land on your hands or grabbing onto an object as you fall can prevent a hip fracture

Protective responses, such as reflexes and changes in posture that break the fall, can reduce the risk of fracturing a bone as a result of a fall. Individuals who land on their hands or grab an object on their descent are less likely to fracture their hip, but they may fracture their wrist or arm. While these fractures are painful and interfere with daily activities, they do not carry the same risks that are associated with a fractured hip. The type of surface on which one lands can also affect whether a bone breaks or not. Landing on a soft surface is less likely to cause a broken bone than landing on a hard surface.

Bone Fragility

While most serious falls happen when people are older, steps to prevent and/or treat bone loss and falls can never begin too early. Many people begin adulthood with less than optimal bone mass, so the fact that bone mass or density is lost slowly over time puts them at increased risk for fractures. Bones that once were strong become so fragile and thin that they easily break. Activities that once were done without a second thought are now avoided for fear they will lead to breaking another bone.

Steps to Prevent Fragile Bones

- Take in adequate amounts of calcium and vitamin D
- Exercise several times a week
- Ask your doctor about a Bone Density Test
- Ask about medications to slow bone loss and reduce fracture risk

References

1. National Safety Council, *Accident Facts*, National Safety Council, Chicago, 1992.

2. Riggs B & Melton L (Eds) (1995) *Osteoporosis: Etiology, diagnosis, and management* (2nd ed) New York: Raven Press, p 239.

3. Riggs B & Melton L (1995 Nov.) The worldwide problem of osteoporosis: Insights afforded by epidemiology. *Bone,* 17 (5) Supp. 505S-511S.

4. Seeley DG, Browner WS, Nevitt MC, Genant HK, Scott JC, Cummings SR for the SOF Research Group. Which fractures are associated with low appendicular bone mass in elderly women? *Annals of Internal Medicine.* (1991). 115:837-842.

5. Tinetti M et al. *Reducing the risk of falls among older adults in the community.* Yale FICSIT (1994).

Fast Facts on Osteoporosis

Osteoporosis, or porous bone, is a disease characterized by low bone mass and structural deterioration of bone tissue, leading to bone fragility and an increased susceptibility to fractures of the hip, spine, and wrist. Osteoporosis is a major public health threat for more than 28 million Americans, 80 percent of whom are women. In the U.S. today, 10 million individuals already have the disease and 18 million more have low bone mass, placing them at increased risk for osteoporosis.

- 80% of those affected by osteoporosis are women.

- 8 million American women and 2 million men have osteoporosis, and millions more have low bone density.

- One out of two women and one in eight men over age 50 will have an osteoporosis-related fracture in their lifetime.

- 10% of African-American women over age 50 have osteoporosis; an additional 30% have low bone density that puts them at risk of developing osteoporosis.

- Significant risk has been reported in people of all ethnic backgrounds.

- While osteoporosis is often thought of as an older person's disease, it can strike at any age.

- Osteoporosis is responsible for more than 1.5 million fractures annually, including:
  - 300,000 hip fractures; and approximately
  - 700,000 vertebral fractures,
  - 250,000 wrist fractures, and
  - 300,000 fractures at other sites.

Cost

The estimated national direct expenditures (hospitals and nursing homes) for osteoporotic and associated fractures is $13.8 billion ($38 million each day) and the cost is rising.

Symptoms

Osteoporosis is often called the "silent disease" because bone loss occurs without symptoms. People may not know that they have osteoporosis until their bones become so weak that a sudden strain, bump, or fall causes a fracture, or a vertebra to collapse. Collapsed vertebrae may initially be felt or seen in the form of severe back pain, loss of height, or spinal deformities such as kyphosis, or stooped posture.

Risk Factors

Certain people are more likely to develop osteoporosis than others. Factors that increase the likelihood of developing osteoporosis are called "risk factors." The following risk factors have been identified:

- Being female
- Thin and/or small frame
- Advanced age
- A family history of osteoporosis
- Postmenopause, including early or surgically induced menopause
- Abnormal absence of menstrual periods (amenorrhea)
- Anorexia nervosa or bulimia
- A diet low in calcium
- Use of certain medications, such as corticosteroids and anticonvulsants
- Low testosterone levels in men
- An inactive lifestyle
- Cigarette smoking
- Excessive use of alcohol
- Being Caucasian or Asian, although African Americans and Hispanic Americans are at significant risk as well

Women can lose up to 20% of their bone mass in the 5-7 years following menopause, making them more susceptible to osteoporosis.

Detection

Specialized tests called bone density tests can measure bone density in various sites of the body. A bone density test can:

- Detect osteoporosis before a fracture occurs
- Predict your chances of fracturing in the future
- Determine your rate of bone loss and/or monitor the effects of treatment if the test is conducted at intervals of a year or more

Prevention

By about age 20, the average woman has acquired 98% of her skeletal mass. Building strong bones during childhood and adolescence can be the best defense against developing osteoporosis later. There are four steps to prevent osteoporosis. No one step alone is enough to prevent osteoporosis but all four may. They are:

- A balanced diet rich in calcium and vitamin D
- Weight-bearing exercise
- A healthy lifestyle with no smoking and limited alcohol intake, and
- Bone density testing and medication, when appropriate

Fractures

- The most typical sites of fractures related to osteoporosis are the hip, spine, wrist, and ribs, although the disease can affect any bone in the body.
- The rate of hip fractures is two to three times higher in women than men; however the one year mortality following a hip fracture is nearly twice as high for men as for women.
- A woman's risk of hip fracture is equal to her combined risk of breast, uterine, and ovarian cancer.
- In 1991, about 300,000 Americans age 45 and over were admitted to hospitals with hip fractures. Osteoporosis was the underlying cause of most of these injuries.
- An average of 24% of hip fracture patients age 50 and over die in the year following their fracture.
- One-fourth of those who were ambulatory before their hip fracture require long-term care afterward.
- White women 65 or older have twice the incidence of fractures as African-American women.

Medications

Although there is no cure for osteoporosis, the following medications are approved by the FDA for postmenopausal women to prevent and/or treat osteoporosis:

- Estrogens (brand names such as Premarin®, Ogen®, Estrace®, Estraderm®, Estratab®, Prempro® and others)

- Alendronate (brand name Fosamax®) is also approved as a treatment for men.

- Calcitonin (brand name Miacalcin®)

- Raloxifene (brand name Evista®)

- Risedronate (brand name Actonel®)

- Alendronate is approved for treatment of glucocorticoid-induced osteoporosis in men and women. Risedronate is approved for prevention and treatment of glucocorticoid-induced osteoporosis in men and women.

- Treatments under investigation include sodium fluoride, vitamin D metabolites, parathyroid hormone, and other bisphosphonates and SERMs.

Medical experts agree that osteoporosis is highly preventable. However, if the toll of osteoporosis is to be reduced, the commitment to osteoporosis research must be significantly increased. It is reasonable to project that with increased research, the future for definitive treatment and prevention of osteoporosis is very bright.

Additional Information

Osteoporosis and Related Bone Diseases National Resource Center
1232 22nd Street, N.W.
Washington DC 20037-1292
Toll-Free: 800-624-2663
Tel: 202-223-0344
TTY: 202-466-4315
Fax: 202-293-2356
Website: www.osteo.org
E-mail: orbdnrc@nof.org

Chapter 12

Growth Plate Injuries

This chapter contains general information about growth plate injuries. It describes what the growth plate is, how injuries occur, and how they are treated. At the end is a list of additional resources. If you have further questions after reading this chapter, you may wish to discuss them with your doctor.

What Is the Growth Plate?

The growth plate, also known as the physis, is the area of developing tissue near the end of the long bones in children and adolescents. Each long bone has at least two growth plates: one at each end. The growth plate determines the future length and shape of the mature bone. When growth is complete—sometime during adolescence—the growth plates are replaced by solid bone.

Who Gets Growth Plate Injuries?

These injuries occur in children and adolescents. The growth plate is the weakest area of the growing skeleton, weaker than the nearby ligaments and tendons that connect bones to other bones and muscles. In a growing child, a serious injury to a joint is more likely to damage a growth plate than the ligaments that stabilize the joint. An injury that

"Questions and Answers about Growth Plate Injuries," National Institute of Arthritis and Musculoskeletal and Skin Diseases (NIAMS), March 1999.

would cause a sprain in an adult can be a potentially serious growth plate injury in a young child.

Most injuries to the growth plate are fractures. Growth plate fractures comprise 15 to 30 percent of all childhood fractures. They occur twice as often in boys as in girls, with the greatest incidence among 14 year-old boys and 11-12 year-old girls. Older girls experience these fractures less often because their bodies mature at an earlier age than boys. As a result, their bones finish growing sooner, and growth plates are replaced by stronger, solid bone.

Growth plate fractures occur most often in the long bones of the fingers (phalanges), followed by the outer bone of the forearm (radius) at the wrist. These injuries also occur frequently in the lower bones of the leg: the tibia and fibula. They can also occur in the upper leg bone (femur) or in the ankle, foot, or hip bone.

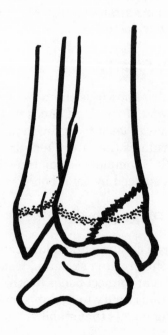

Figure 12.1. *Fracture Across the Growth Plate of the Tibia (illustration by William A. Shannon; © 2002 Omnigraphics, Inc.)*

What Causes Growth Plate Injuries?

While growth plate injuries can be caused by an acute event, such as a fall or a blow to the body, they can also result from overuse. For example, a gymnast who practices for hours on the uneven bars, a long-distance runner, or a baseball pitcher perfecting his curve ball can all have growth plate injuries.

In one large study of growth plate injuries in children, the majority resulted from a fall, usually while running or playing on furniture or playground equipment. Competitive sports, such as football, basketball, softball, track and field, and gymnastics, accounted for one-third of all injuries. Recreational activities, such as biking, sledding, skiing, and skateboarding, accounted for one-fifth of all growth plate fractures, while car, motorcycle, and all-terrain-vehicle accidents accounted for only a small percentage of fractures.

Whether an injury is acute or due to overuse, a child who has pain that persists or affects athletic performance or the ability to move or put pressure on a limb should be examined by a doctor. A child should never be allowed or expected to "work through the pain."

Children who participate in athletic activity often experience some discomfort as their bones and muscles grow and they practice new movements. Some aches and pains can be expected, but a child's complaints always deserve careful attention. Some injuries, if left untreated, can cause permanent damage and interfere with proper physical growth.

Although many growth plate injuries are caused by accidents that occur during play or athletic activity, growth plates are also susceptible to other types of injury, infection, and diseases that can alter their normal growth and development.

Additional Reasons for Growth Plate Injuries

- Child abuse can result in skeletal injuries. These more often occur in very young children, who still have years of bone growth ahead of them. One study reported that half of all fractures due to child abuse were found in children younger than age 1, whereas only 2 percent of accidental fractures occurred in this age group.

- Injury from cold or frostbite can also damage the growth plate in children and result in short, stubby fingers or premature degenerative arthritis.

- Radiation, which is used to treat certain cancers in children, can damage the growth plate. Moreover, a recent study has suggested that chemotherapy given for childhood cancers may also negatively affect bone growth.

- Children with certain neurological disorders that result in sensory deficit, muscular imbalance, or looseness in the ligaments are prone to growth plate fractures, especially at the ankle and knee. Similar types of injury are seen in children who are born with insensitivity to pain.

- The growth plates are the site of many inherited disorders that affect the musculoskeletal system. Scientists are just beginning to understand the genes involved in skeletal formation, growth, and development. This new information is raising hopes for improving treatment of children who are born with poorly formed or improperly functioning growth plates.

How Are Growth Plate Fractures Diagnosed?

After learning how the injury occurred and examining the child, the doctor will probably use x-rays to determine the type of fracture and decide on a treatment plan. Because growth plates have not yet hardened into solid bone, they don't show on x-rays. Instead, they appear as gaps between the shaft of a long bone, called the metaphysis, and the end of the bone, called the epiphysis. Because injuries to the growth plate may be hard to see on x-ray, an x-ray of the noninjured side of the body may be taken so the two sides can be compared. In some cases, other diagnostic tests, such as magnetic resonance imaging (MRI), computed tomography (CT), or ultrasound, will be used. Since the 1960s, the Salter-Harris classification, which divides most growth plate fractures into five categories based on the type of damage, has been the standard. The categories are as follows:

Type I

The epiphysis is completely separated from the end of the bone, or the metaphysis. The vital portions of the growth plate remain attached to the epiphysis. Only rarely will the doctor have to put the fracture back into place, but all type I injuries generally require a cast to keep the fracture in place as it heals. Unless there is damage to the blood supply, the likelihood that the bone will grow normally is excellent.

Type II

This is the most common type of growth plate fracture. The epiphysis, together with the growth plate, is partially separated from the metaphysis, which is cracked. Unlike type I fractures, type II fractures typically have to be put back into place and immobilized for normal growth to continue. Because these fractures usually return to their normal shape during growth, sometimes the doctor does not have to manipulate this fracture back into position.

Type III

This fracture occurs only rarely, usually at the lower end of the tibia, one of the long bones of the lower leg. It happens when a fracture runs completely through the epiphysis and separates part of the epiphysis and growth plate from the metaphysis. Surgery is sometimes necessary to restore the joint surface to normal. The outlook or prognosis for growth is good if the blood supply to the separated portion of the epiphysis is still intact, if the fracture is not displaced, and if a bridge of new bone has not formed at the site of the fracture.

Type IV

This fracture runs through the epiphysis, across the growth plate, and into the metaphysis. Surgery is needed to restore the joint surface to normal and to perfectly align the growth plate. Unless perfect alignment is achieved and maintained during healing, prognosis for growth is poor. This injury occurs most commonly at the end of the humerus (the upper arm bone) near the elbow.

Type V

This uncommon injury occurs when the end of the bone is crushed and the growth plate is compressed. It is most likely to occur at the knee or ankle. Prognosis is poor, since premature stunting of growth is almost inevitable.

A newer classification, called the Peterson classification, adds a type VI fracture, in which a portion of the epiphysis, growth plate, and metaphysis is missing. This usually occurs with an open wound or compound fracture, often involving lawnmowers, farm machinery, snowmobiles, or gunshot wounds. All type VI fractures require surgery, and most will require later reconstructive or corrective surgery. Bone growth is almost always stunted.

What Kind of Doctor Treats Growth Plate Injuries?

For all but the simplest injuries, the doctor may recommend that the injury be treated by an orthopaedic surgeon, a doctor who specializes in bone and joint problems in children and adults. Some problems may require the services of a pediatric orthopaedic surgeon, who specializes in injuries and musculoskeletal disorders in children.

How Are Growth Plate Injuries Treated?

As indicated in the previous section, treatment depends on the type of fracture. Treatment, which should be started as soon as possible after injury, generally involves a mix of the following:

Immobilization

The affected limb is often put in a cast or splint, and the child is told to limit any activity that puts pressure on the injured area. The doctor may also suggest that ice be applied to the area.

Manipulation or Surgery

In about 1 out of 10 cases, the doctor will have to put the bones or joints back in their correct positions, either by using his or her hands (called manipulation) or by performing surgery. After the procedure, the bone will be set in place so it can heal without moving. This is usually done with a cast that encloses the injured growth plate and the joints on both sides of it. The cast is left in place until the injury heals, which can take anywhere from a few weeks to several months for serious injuries. The need for manipulation or surgery depends on the location and extent of the injury, its effect on nearby nerves and blood vessels, and the child's age.

Strengthening and Range-of-Motion Exercises

These treatments may also be recommended after the fracture is healed.

Long-Term Follow-Up

Long-term follow-up is usually necessary to monitor the child's recuperation and growth. Evaluation may include x-rays of matching limbs at 3- to 6-month intervals for at least 2 years. Some fractures require periodic evaluations until the child's bones have finished growing. Sometimes a growth arrest line may appear as a marker of the injury. Continued bone growth away from that line may mean that there will not be a long-term problem, and the doctor may decide to stop following the patient.

What Is the Prognosis for a Child with a Growth Plate Injury?

Most growth plate fractures heal without any lasting harm. Whether long-term damage occurs depends on the following factors, in descending order of importance:

- **Severity of the injury**. If the injury causes the blood supply to the epiphysis to be cut off, growth can be stunted. If the growth plate is shifted, shattered, or crushed, a bony bridge is more likely to form and the risk of growth retardation is higher. An open injury in which the skin is broken carries the risk of infection, which could destroy the growth plate.

- **Age of the child.** In a younger child, the bones have a great deal of growing to do; therefore, growth arrest can be more serious, and closer surveillance is needed.

- **Which growth plate is injured.** Some growth plates are more responsible for extensive bone growth than others.

- **Type of growth plate fracture.** The five fracture types are described in the section, "How Are Growth Plate Fractures Diagnosed?"

The treatment depends on the above factors and also bears on the prognosis.

The most frequent complication of a growth plate fracture is premature arrest of bone growth. The affected bone grows less than it would have without the injury, and the resulting limb could be shorter than the opposite, uninjured limb. If only part of the growth plate is injured, growth may be lopsided and the limb may be crooked.

Growth plate injuries at the knee are at greatest risk of complications. Nerve and blood vessel damage occurs most frequently there. Injuries to the knee have a much higher incidence of premature growth arrest and crooked growth.

105

What Are Researchers Trying to Learn about Growth Plate Injuries?

Researchers continue to develop methods to optimize the diagnosis and treatment of growth plate injuries and to improve patient outcomes. Examples of such work include:

- Removal of a growth-blocking "bridge" or bar of bone that can form across a growth plate following a fracture. After the bridge is removed, fat, cartilage, or other materials are inserted in its place to prevent the bridge from forming again.

- Use of distraction osteogenesis, a procedure in which a bone that is prematurely shortened is surgically cut and gradually lengthened.

- Development of methods to regenerate musculoskeletal tissue by using principles of tissue engineering.

Additional Information

American Academy of Orthopaedic Surgeons
6300 North River Road
Rosemont, IL 60018-4262
Toll-Free: 800-346-AAOS
Tel: 847-823-7186
Fax: 847-823-8125
Fax on Demand: 800-999-2939
Website: www.aaos.org

The academy provides education and practice management services for orthopaedic surgeons and allied health professionals. It also serves as an advocate for improved patient care and informs the public about the science of orthopaedics. The orthopaedist's scope of practice includes disorders of the body's bones, joints, ligaments, muscles, and tendons.

American Academy of Pediatrics
141 Northwest Point Boulevard
Elk Grove Village, IL 60007-1098
Tel: 847-434-4000
Fax: 847-434-8000
Website: www.aap.org
E-mail: kidsdocs@aap.org

The American Academy of Pediatrics (AAP) and its member pediatricians dedicate their efforts and resources to the health, safety, and well-being of infants, children, adolescents, and young adults. Activities of the AAP include advocacy for children and youth, public education, research, professional education, and membership service and advocacy for pediatricians.

American Orthopaedic Society for Sports Medicine
6300 N. River Road, Suite 200
Rosemont, IL 60018
Tel: 847-292-4900
Fax: 847-292-4905
Website: www.sportsmed.org

The society is an organization of orthopaedic surgeons and allied health professionals dedicated to educating health care professionals and the general public about sports medicine. It promotes and supports educational and research programs in sports medicine, including those concerned with fitness, as well as programs designed to advance our knowledge of the recognition, treatment, rehabilitation, and prevention of athletic injuries.

National Arthritis and Musculoskeletal and Skin Diseases Information Clearinghouse (NAMSIC)
National Institutes of Health
1 AMS Circle
Bethesda, MD 20892-3675
Toll-Free: 877-22-NIAMS
Tel: 301-495-4484
Fax: 301-718-6366
TTY: 301-565-2966
Website: www.niams.nih.gov
E-mail: niamsinfo@mail.nih.gov

This clearinghouse, a public service sponsored by the NIAMS, provides information on arthritis and musculoskeletal and skin diseases. The clearinghouse distributes patient and professional education materials and also refers people to other sources of information.

Chapter 13

Head and Brain Injuries

A blow or jolt to the head can disrupt the normal function of the brain. Doctors often call this type of brain injury a "concussion" or a "closed head injury." Doctors may describe these injuries as "mild" because concussions are usually not life threatening. Even so, the effects of a concussion can be serious.

After a concussion, some people lose consciousness or are "knocked out" for a short time, but not always—you can have a brain injury without losing consciousness. Some people are simply dazed or confused. Sometimes whiplash can cause a concussion.

Because the brain is very complex, every brain injury is different. Some symptoms may appear right away, while others may not show up for days or weeks after the concussion. Sometimes the injury makes it hard for people to recognize or to admit that they are having problems.

The signs of concussion can be subtle. Early on, problems may be missed by patients, family members, and doctors. People may look fine even though they're acting or feeling differently.

Because all brain injuries are different, so is recovery. Most people with mild injuries recover fully, but it can take time. Some symptoms can last for days, weeks, or longer.

"Facts about Concussion and Brain Injury, Version 2," National Center for Injury Prevention and Control (NCIPC); and "New Study Links Head Injury, Severity of Injury, with Alzheimer's Disease," Press Release: October 23, 2000, National Institute on Aging (NIA).

In general, recovery is slower in older persons. Also, persons who have had a concussion in the past may find that it takes longer to recover from their current injury.

This chapter explains what can happen after a concussion, how to get better, and where to go for more information and help when needed.

Medical Help

People with a concussion need to be seen by a doctor. Most people with concussions are treated in an emergency department or a doctor's office. Some people must stay in the hospital overnight for further treatment.

Sometimes the doctors may do a CT scan of the brain or do other tests to help diagnose your injuries. Even if the brain injury doesn't show up on these tests, you may still have a concussion.

Your doctor will send you home with important instructions to follow. For example, your doctor may ask someone to wake you up every few hours during the first night and day after your injury. Be sure to carefully follow all your doctor's instructions. If you are already taking any medicines—prescription, over-the-counter, or "natural remedies"—or if you are drinking alcohol or taking illicit drugs, tell your doctor. Also, talk with your doctor if you are taking "blood thinners" (anticoagulant drugs) or aspirin, because these drugs may increase your chances of complications. If it's all right with your doctor, you may take acetaminophen (for example, Tylenol® or Panadol®) for headache or neck pain. Use of trade names is for identification only and does not imply endorsement by the U.S. Department of Health and Human Services.

Danger Signs—Adults

In rare cases, along with a concussion, a dangerous blood clot may form on the brain and crowd the brain against the skull. Contact your doctor or emergency department right away if, after a blow or jolt to the head, you have any of these danger signs:

- Headaches that get worse
- Weakness, numbness, or decreased coordination
- Repeated vomiting

The people checking on you should take you to an emergency department right away if you:

- Cannot be awakened
- Have one pupil—the black part in the middle of the eye—larger than the other
- Have convulsions or seizures
- Have slurred speech
- Are getting more and more confused, restless, or agitated

Danger Signs—Children

Take your child to the emergency department right away if the child has received a blow or jolt to the head and:

- Has any of the danger signs listed for adults
- Won't stop crying
- Can't be consoled
- Won't nurse or eat

Although you should contact your child's doctor if your child vomits more than once or twice, vomiting is more common in younger children and is less likely to be an urgent sign of danger than it is in an adult.

Symptoms of Brain Injury

Persons of All Ages

"I just don't feel like myself."

The type of brain injury called a concussion has many symptoms. These symptoms are usually temporary, but may last for days, weeks, or even longer. Generally, if you feel that "something is not quite right," or if you're "feeling foggy," you should talk with your doctor. Here are some of the symptoms of a concussion:

- Low-grade headaches that won't go away
- Having more trouble than usual:
  - Remembering things
  - Paying attention or concentrating
  - Organizing daily tasks
  - Making decisions and solving problems

- Slowness in thinking, acting, speaking, or reading
- Getting lost or easily confused
- Neck pain
- Feeling tired all the time, lack of energy
- Change in sleeping pattern:
  - Sleeping for much longer periods of time than before
  - Trouble sleeping or insomnia
- Loss of balance, feeling light-headed or dizzy
- Increased sensitivity to:
  - Sounds
  - Lights
  - Distractions
- Blurred vision or eyes that tire easily
- Loss of sense of taste or smell
- Ringing in the ears
- Change in sexual drive
- Mood changes:
  - Feeling sad, anxious, or listless
  - Becoming easily irritated or angry for little or no reason
  - Lack of motivation

Young Children

Although children can have the same symptoms of brain injury as adults, it is harder for young children to let others know how they are feeling. Call your child's doctor if your child seems to be getting worse or if you notice any of the following:

- Listlessness, tiring easily
- Irritability, crankiness
- Change in eating or sleeping patterns
- Change in the way they play
- Change in the way they perform or act at school
- Lack of interest in favorite toys

- Loss of new skills, such as toilet training
- Loss of balance, unsteady walking

Older Adults

Older adults with a brain injury may have a higher risk of serious complications such as a blood clot on the brain. Headaches that get worse or an increase in confusion are signs of this complication. If these signs occur, see a doctor right away.

Getting Better

"Sometimes the best thing you can do is just rest and then try again later."

How fast people recover from brain injury varies from person to person. Although most people have a good recovery, how quickly they improve depends on many factors. These factors include how severe their concussion was, what part of the brain was injured, their age, and how healthy they were before the concussion.

Rest is very important after a concussion because it helps the brain to heal. You'll need to be patient because healing takes time. Return to your daily activities, such as work or school, at your own pace. As the days go by, you can expect to gradually feel better.

If you already had a medical problem at the time of your concussion, it may take longer for you to recover from your brain injury. Anxiety and depression may also make it harder to adjust to the symptoms of brain injury.

While you are healing, you should be very careful to avoid doing anything that could cause a blow or jolt to your head. On rare occasions, receiving another concussion before a brain injury has healed can be fatal.

Even after your brain injury has healed, you should protect yourself from having another concussion. People who have had repeated brain injuries, such as boxers or football players, may have serious problems later in life. These problems include difficulty with concentration and memory and sometimes with physical coordination.

Tips for Healing—Adults

Here are a few tips to help you get better:

- Get plenty of sleep at night, and rest during the day.

- Return to your normal activities gradually, not all at once.

- Avoid activities that could lead to a second brain injury, such as contact or recreational sports, until your doctor says you are well enough to take part in these activities.

- Ask your doctor when you can drive a car, ride a bike, or operate heavy equipment because your ability to react may be slower after a brain injury.

- Talk with your doctor about when you can return to work or school. Ask your doctor about ways to help your employer or teacher understand what has happened to you.

- Consider talking with your employer about returning to work gradually and changing your work activities until you recover.

- Take only those drugs that your doctor has approved.

- Don't drink alcoholic beverages until your doctor says you are well enough to do so. Alcohol and certain other drugs may slow your recovery and can put you at risk of further injury.

- If it's harder than usual to remember things, write them down.

- If you're easily distracted, try to do one thing at a time. For example, don't try to watch TV while fixing dinner.

- Consult with family members or close friends when making important decisions.

- Don't neglect your basic needs such as eating well and getting enough rest.

Tips for Healing—Children

Parents and caretakers of children who have had a concussion can help them heal by:

- Having the child get plenty of rest.

- Making sure the child avoids activities that could result in a second blow or jolt to the head—such as riding a bicycle, playing sports, or climbing playground equipment—until the doctor says the child is well enough to take part in these activities.

- Giving the child only those drugs that the doctor has approved.

114

- Talking with the doctor about when the child should return to school and other activities and how to deal with the challenges the child may face.

- Sharing information about concussion with teachers, counselors, babysitters, coaches, and others who interact with the child so they can understand what has happened and help meet the child's needs.

Help for People with Brain Injuries

"It was the first time in my life that I couldn't depend on myself."

There are many people who can help you and your family as you recover from your brain injury. You don't have to do it alone.

Show this information to your doctor or health care provider and talk with them about your concerns. Ask your doctor whether you need specialized treatment and about the availability of rehabilitation programs.

Your doctor may be able to help you find a health care provider who has special training in the treatment of concussion. Early treatment of symptoms by professionals who specialize in brain injury may speed recovery. Your doctor may refer you to a neurologist, neuropsychologist, neurosurgeon, or specialist in rehabilitation.

Keep talking with your doctor, family members, and loved ones about how you are feeling, both physically and emotionally. If you do not think you are getting better, tell your doctor.

Help for Families and Caregivers

"My husband used to be so calm. But after his injury, he started to explode over the littlest things. He didn't even know that he had changed."

When someone close to you has a brain injury, it can be hard to know how best to help. They may say that they are "fine" but you can tell from how they are acting that something has changed.

If you notice that your family member or friend has symptoms of brain injury that are getting worse or are not getting better, talk to them and their doctor about getting help. They may also need help if you can answer "yes" to any of the following questions:

- Has their personality changed?

- Do they get angry for no reason?
- Do they get lost or easily confused?
- Do they have more trouble than usual making decisions?

You might also want to talk with people who have experienced what you are going through. The Brain Injury Association can put you in contact with people who can help.

New Study Links Head Injury, Severity of Injury, with Alzheimer's Disease

A new analysis of head injuries among World War II veterans links serious head injury in early adulthood with Alzheimer's disease (AD) in later life. The study, by researchers at Duke University and the National Institute on Aging (NIA), also suggests that the more severe the head injury, the greater the risk of developing AD.

For some time, scientists have been examining the association between head injury and AD. Studies in recent years have gone back and forth, some finding a relationship and others not. This new finding, by Brenda L. Plassman, Ph.D., of Duke University, Richard J. Havlik, M.D., M.P.H., of NIA, and colleagues is of great interest not only for its conclusions, but also for how the research was conducted. By looking at documented evidence of head injury from medical records of the veterans, scientists were able to move away from information solely based on a participant's or family member's recall about injuries that may have occurred decades—in this case 50 years—earlier.

The study appeared in the Oct. 24, 2000, issue of the journal *Neurology*. The work by Plassman and colleagues at Duke and Johns Hopkins University was supported by NIA. Dr. Havlik heads the NIA's Epidemiology, Demography, and Biometry program.

Havlik cautions that the new findings do not demonstrate a direct cause-and-effect relationship between head injury in early life and the development of dementia, but rather show an association between the two that needs to be studied further. "This study made a great effort to address some of the limitations of previous epidemiologic research in this area. We now need to hone in on what's behind these findings, especially what may be happening biologically," says Havlik. "While we may not fully understand what's going on, as a practical matter, it may be one more reason to wear that bike helmet instead of keeping it in a closet," Havlik adds. Havlik cautions, however, that the findings from the veterans study may not be applied to today's common exposures to head injury, such as in sports, where helmets are used or where injuries may not be as serious as those examined among veterans who were hospitalized for head trauma.

The researchers began the study by looking at military medical records of male Navy and Marine World War II veterans who were hospitalized during their period of service with a diagnosis of head injury or an unrelated condition. The use of records instead of recall, the scientists said, allowed them to avoid the problem of "recall error," with which, they estimated, probably fewer than 70 percent of people with a true head injury in prior studies would have recalled their injuries many years later.

A specially trained team evaluated the records according to agreed-upon criteria for defining head injury and its severity. (Mild injury involved loss of consciousness or post-traumatic amnesia for less than 30 minutes with no skull fracture, moderate involved loss of consciousness or post-traumatic amnesia for more than 30 minutes but less than 24 hours, and/or a skull fracture, and severe injury was loss of consciousness or post-traumatic amnesia for 24 or more hours.) Veterans were located in 1996-1997 and most contacted agreed to participate in the study. Eventually, 548 veterans who had suffered a head injury and 1,228 veterans without a history of head injury, who comprised the control group for the study, took part.

Using a three-stage screening and assessment process, including home visits in some cases, the scientists then identified the aged veterans with dementia. They also determined whether the veterans had Alzheimer's disease specifically or another type of dementia.

The researchers then compared the number of veterans with AD or other dementias in the group who had suffered a head injury to those in the group with no head injury. The risk of AD and dementia was increased about two-fold among all those with moderate head injury. And risk increased with the severity of the injury. Those with head injuries categorized as severe—who had been hospitalized and who remained unconscious or amnesic for 24 hours or more—had a four-fold greater risk.

Why head injury may be involved in AD and dementia is still unknown. The researchers, in one attempt to help address that question, also looked for a possible interaction effect between head injury and genetic factors associated with AD. Among study participants, they looked at apolipoprotein E, or APOE, an important gene in AD. APOE has various forms, or alleles, and its e4 allele has been associated with increased risk of AD. The scientists wanted to see if increased risk of AD associated with head injury was only present in those men with an APOE e4 allele. The analysis did not find a statistically significant interaction.

The analyses also looked at other factors that possibly could influence the development of dementia among the veterans, including education, positive family history of dementia, and a history of alcohol or tobacco use, but none was involved in the association between head injury and dementia found in this study.

Plassman and her colleagues note more generally that the findings are consistent with current thinking on the etiology, or course, of AD. The increased risk of dementia, some 50 years after the head injuries had occurred, is one more indication that AD is a chronic disease that unfolds over many decades, she points out. "Understanding how head injury and other AD risk factors begin their destructive work early in life may ultimately lead to finding ways to interrupt the disease process early on," says Plassman.

An estimated 1.5 to 2 million individuals per year suffer a significant head injury in the U.S. It is estimated that up to 4 million Americans currently have AD.

The NIA leads the federal effort supporting and conducting basic and clinical research on Alzheimer's disease and on its caregiving aspects. The Institute, a component of the National Institutes of Health, operates the Alzheimer's Disease Education & Referral Center (ADEAR), which provides information to health professionals and the public on AD and memory impairment.

Resources for Getting Help

Several groups help people with brain injury and their families. They provide information and put people in touch with local resources, such as support groups, rehabilitation services, and a variety of health care professionals.

Among these groups, the Brain Injury Association (BIA) has a national office that gathers scientific and educational information and works on a national level to help people with brain injury. In addition, 44 affiliated state Brain Injury Associations provide help locally.

Brain Injury Association (BIA)
105 North Alfred Street
Alexandria, VA 22314
Toll-Free: 800-444-6443
Tel: 703-236-6000

Fax: 703-236-6001
Website: www.biausa.org
E-mail: familyhelpline@biausa.org

Centers for Disease Control and Prevention (CDC)
4770 Buford Highway, NE
Atlanta, GA 30341-3724
Tel: 770-488-4031
Fax: 770-488-4338
Website: www.cdc.gov/ncipc/tbi.
E-mail: DARDINFO@cdc.gov

Alzheimer's Disease Education & Referral Center (ADEAR)
P.O. Box 8250
Silver Spring, MD 20907
Toll-Free: 800-438-4380
Website: www.alzheimers.org
E-mail: adear@alzheimers.org

Chapter 14

Hip Fractures

What Is the Impact of Hip Fractures?

- Of all fractures from falls, hip fractures cause the greatest number of deaths and lead to the most severe health problems.[1]

- In 1996, there were approximately 340,000 hospital admissions for hip fractures in the United States.[2]

- Women sustain 75%-80% of all hip fractures.[3]

- People who are 85 years or older are 10-15 times more likely to experience hip fractures than are people between the ages of 60 and 65.[4]

- Most patients with hip fractures are hospitalized for about 2 weeks.[5]

- Half of all older adults hospitalized for hip fractures cannot return home or live independently after their injuries.[3,4]

- In 1991, Medicare costs for hip fractures were estimated to be $2.9 billion.[6]

Excerpt from "Falls and Hip Fractures among Older Adults," National Center for Injury Prevention and Control (NCIPC); and "Hip Fracture Study Calls for Assessing Patients' Risks of Both Functional Impairment and Death," Press Release, Agency for Healthcare Research and Quality, June 5, 2001.

- Because the U.S. population is aging, the problem of hip fractures will likely increase substantially over the next four decades. By the year 2040, the number of hip fractures is expected to exceed 500,000.[7]

Hip Fracture Study Calls for Assessing Patient's Risks of Both Functional Impairment and Death

A study sponsored by the U.S. Agency for Healthcare Research and Quality (AHRQ) could help acute and post-acute care medical staff improve the outcomes of the approximately 350,000 hip fractures that occur annually in the United States by focusing efforts on reducing the risks that often leave patients unable to walk or lead to death from complications.

Currently, four of every 10 patients are unable to walk without total assistance by six months after the fracture occurs and a quarter of patients die within a year. In addition to its human toll, hip fracture and its consequences have a large economic impact, with hospital charges alone totaling roughly $6 billion a year. The challenge has been to identify characteristics that put patients at higher risk for these adverse outcomes.

The study's analysis of data on hip fracture patients in four New York City hospitals between August 1997 and August 1998, found that when patients required moderate to total assistance for walking or stair climbing prior to admission, there was a higher likelihood of poor post-fracture functional ability, while limited pre-fracture locomotion combined with the presence of chronic medical conditions were risk factors that made death more likely.

Of the 571 elderly patients studied, nearly 2 percent died in the hospitals and roughly equal percentages—about 13 percent—either died within six months or needed total assistance to walk or use a wheelchair.

The researchers, who were led by Albert L. Siu, M.D., of Mount Sinai School of Medicine, identified risk factors that accurately predicted the loss of locomotion and/or death. While previous studies have identified patient factors related to either the recovery of hip fracture patients or to death, most looked at function or mortality independently, and none reported on how risk-adjusted outcomes could be obtained to assess the effectiveness or quality of care in a hospital or post-acute care setting.

AHRQ's director, John M. Eisenberg, M.D., said, "Hip fracture care is increasingly fragmented among acute care providers, and those in rehabilitation units, nursing homes, and home health agencies. The message of this study is that all providers, regardless of where they work, should assess these risks of disability and death, and take action to prevent adverse outcomes in patients with hip fracture."

Hip fracture patients, most of whom are elderly, are first admitted to acute care hospitals where rehabilitative services generally exist to improve functional mobility and where there are nursing services for preventing or treating common postoperative complications, such as thrombophlebitis, surgical site infection, and delirium. Following discharge, the typical hip fracture patient receives post-acute rehabilitative services in a skilled nursing facility, acute rehabilitative unit, home health program, or a combination of these.

Dr. Siu, a professor of medicine at Mount Sinai, said, "Currently, each group involved in the care of a hip fracture patient views only their small section of the overall condition. This means that aspects of care that need to be followed often slip through the cracks." Dr. Siu added that "Close scrutiny and observation is critical to developing effective means of managing the care of hip fracture patients."

Further details of the study are in "Mortality and Locomotion Six Months after Hospitalization for Hip Fracture: Risk Factors and Risk-Adjusted Hospital Outcomes," in the June 6, 2001 issue of the *Journal of the American Medical Association.*

References

1. Barancik JI, Chatterjee BF, Greene YC et al. Northeastern Ohio Trauma Study: I. Magnitude of the problem. *American Journal of Public Health* 1983;73:746-51.

2. Graves EJ, Owings MF. 1996 *Summary: National Hospital Discharge Survey. Advance data from vital and health statistics*; no. 301. Hyattsville, Maryland: National Center for Health Statistics, 1998.

3. Melton LJ III, Riggs BL. *Epidemiology of age-related fractures*, in Avioli LV (ed): The Osteoporotic Syndrome. New York, Grune & Stratton, 1983, pp 45-72.

4. Scott JC. *Osteoporosis and hip fractures*. Rheumatic Diseases Clinics of North America 1990;16(3):717-40.

5. Graves, EJ. 1988 Survey: *National Hospital Discharge Survey. Advance Data from vital and health statistics*; no. 185:1-12. Hyattsville, Maryland: National Center for Health Statistics, 1990.

6. CDC. Incidence and costs to Medicare of fractures among Medicare beneficiaries aged >65 years—United States, July 1991-June 1992. *MMWR* 1996;45(41):877-83.

7. Cummings SR, Rubin SM, Black D. The future of hip fractures in the United States. Numbers, costs, and potential effects of postmenopausal estrogen. *Clinical Orthopaedics and Related Research* 1990;252:163-66.

Chapter 15

Knee Injuries

Knee problems commonly occur in young people and adults. This chapter contains general information about several knee problems. It includes descriptions and a diagram of the different parts of the knee. Individual sections of the chapter describe the symptoms, diagnosis, and treatment of specific types of knee injuries and conditions. Information on how to prevent these problems is also provided.

What Do the Knees Do? How Do They Work?

The knees provide stable support for the body and allow the legs to bend and straighten. Both flexibility and stability are needed for standing and for motions like walking, running, crouching, jumping, and turning.

Several kinds of supporting and moving parts, including bones, cartilage, muscles, ligaments, and tendons, help the knees do their job. Any of these parts can be involved in pain or dysfunction.

What Causes Knee Problems?

There are two general kinds of knee problems: mechanical and inflammatory.

"Questions and Answers about Knee Problems," National Institute of Arthritis and Musculoskeletal and Skin Diseases (NIAMS), NIH Publication No. 01-4912, May 2001. Updated in October 2001 by Dr. David A. Cooke, MD, Diplomate, American Board of Internal Medicine.

Mechanical Knee Problems

Some knee problems result from injury, such as a direct blow or sudden movements that strain the knee beyond its normal range of movement. Other problems, such as osteoarthritis in the knee, result from wear and tear on its parts.

Inflammatory Knee Problems

Inflammation that occurs in certain rheumatic diseases, such as rheumatoid arthritis and systemic lupus erythematosus, can damage the knee.

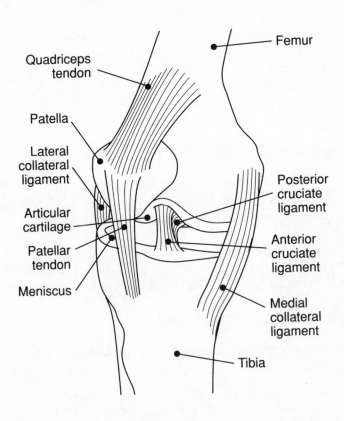

Figure 15.1. *Lateral View of the Knee*

Joint Basics

The point at which two or more bones are connected is called a joint. In all joints, the bones are kept from grinding against each other by padding called cartilage. Bones are joined to bones by strong, elastic bands of tissue called ligaments. Tendons are tough cords of tissue that connect muscle to bone. Muscles work in opposing pairs to bend and straighten joints. While muscles are not technically part of a joint, they're important because strong muscles help support and protect joints.

What Are the Parts of the Knee?

Like any joint, the knee is composed of bones and cartilage, ligaments, tendons, and muscles.

Bones and Cartilage

The knee joint is the junction of three bones: the femur (thigh bone or upper leg bone), the tibia (shin bone or larger bone of the lower leg), and the patella (knee cap). The patella is 2 to 3 inches wide and 3 to 4 inches long. It sits over the other bones at the front of the knee joint and slides when the leg moves. It protects the knee and gives leverage to muscles.

The ends of the three bones in the knee joint are covered with articular cartilage, a tough, elastic material that helps absorb shock and allows the knee joint to move smoothly. Separating the bones of the knee are pads of connective tissue. One pad is called a meniscus (muh-NISS-kus). The plural is menisci (muh-NISS-sky). The menisci are divided into two crescent-shaped discs positioned between the tibia and femur on the outer and inner sides of each knee. The two menisci in each knee act as shock absorbers, cushioning the lower part of the leg from the weight of the rest of the body as well as enhancing stability.

Muscles

There are two groups of muscles at the knee. The quadriceps muscle comprises four muscles on the front of the thigh that work to straighten the leg from a bent position. The hamstring muscles, which bend the leg at the knee, run along the back of the thigh from the hip to just below the knee. Keeping these muscles strong with exercises such as walking up stairs or riding a stationary bicycle helps support and protect the knee.

127

Tendons and Ligaments

The quadriceps tendon connects the quadriceps muscle to the patella and provides the power to extend the leg. Four ligaments connect the femur and tibia and give the joint strength and stability:

- The medial collateral ligament (MCL) provides stability to the inner (medial) part of the knee.

- The lateral collateral ligament (LCL) provides stability to the outer (lateral) part of the knee.

- The anterior cruciate ligament (ACL), in the center of the knee, limits rotation and the forward movement of the tibia.

- The posterior cruciate ligament (PCL), also in the center of the knee, limits backward movement of the tibia.

Other ligaments are part of the knee capsule, which is a protective, fiber-like structure that wraps around the knee joint. Inside the capsule, the joint is lined with a thin, soft tissue called synovium.

How Are Knee Problems Diagnosed?

Doctors use several methods to diagnose knee problems.

Medical history—The patient tells the doctor details about symptoms and about any injury, condition, or general health problem that might be causing the pain.

Physical examination—The doctor bends, straightens, rotates (turns), or presses on the knee to feel for injury and discover the limits of movement and the location of pain. The patient may be asked to stand, walk, or squat to help the doctor assess the knee's function.

Diagnostic tests—The doctor uses one or more tests to determine the nature of a knee problem.

- **X-ray** (radiography)—An x-ray beam is passed through the knee to produce a two-dimensional picture of the bones.

- **Computerized axial tomography** (CAT) scan—X-rays lasting a fraction of a second are passed through the knee at different angles, detected by a scanner, and analyzed by a computer. This produces a series of clear cross-sectional images ("slices") of the knee tissues on a computer screen. CAT scan images show soft tissues such as ligaments or muscles more clearly than conventional x-rays. The computer can combine individual images to give a three-dimensional view of the knee.

- **Bone scan** (radionuclide scanning)—A very small amount of radioactive material is injected into the patient's bloodstream and detected by a scanner. This test detects blood flow to the bone and cell activity within the bone and can show abnormalities in these processes that may aid diagnosis.

- **Magnetic resonance imaging** (MRI)—Energy from a powerful magnet (rather than x-rays) stimulates knee tissue to produce signals that are detected by a scanner and analyzed by a computer. This creates a series of cross-sectional images of a specific part of the knee. An MRI is particularly useful for detecting soft tissue damage or disease. Like a CAT scan, a computer is used to produce three-dimensional views of the knee during MRI.

- **Arthroscopy**—The doctor manipulates a small, lighted optic tube (arthroscope) that has been inserted into the joint through a small incision in the knee. Images of the inside of the knee joint are projected onto a television screen. While the arthroscope is inside the knee joint, removal of loose pieces of bone or cartilage or the repair of torn ligaments and menisci is also possible.

- **Biopsy**—The doctor removes tissue to examine under a microscope.

Knee Injuries and Problems

Arthritis

Arthritis of the knee is most often osteoarthritis. In this disease, the cartilage in the joint gradually wears away. In rheumatoid arthritis, which can also affect the knees, the joint becomes inflamed and cartilage may be destroyed. Arthritis not only affects joints; it can also affect supporting structures such as muscles, tendons, and ligaments.

Osteoarthritis may be caused by excess stress on the joint from deformity, repeated injury, or excess weight. It most often affects middle-aged and older people. A young person who develops osteoarthritis may have an inherited form of the disease or may have experienced continuous irritation from an unrepaired torn meniscus or other injury. Rheumatoid arthritis often affects people at an earlier age than osteoarthritis.

Signs and Diagnosis

Someone who has arthritis of the knee may experience pain, swelling, and a decrease in knee motion. A common symptom is morning stiffness that lessens as the person moves around. Sometimes the joint locks or clicks when the knee is bent and straightened, but these signs may occur in other knee disorders as well. The doctor may confirm the diagnosis by performing a physical examination and examining x-rays, which typically show a loss of joint space. Blood tests may be helpful for diagnosing rheumatoid arthritis, but other tests may be needed too. Analyzing fluid from the knee joint may be helpful in diagnosing some kinds of arthritis. The doctor may use arthroscopy to directly see damage to cartilage, tendons, and ligaments and to confirm a diagnosis, but arthroscopy is usually done only if a repair procedure is to be performed.

Treatment

Most often osteoarthritis of the knee is treated with pain-reducing medicines, such as aspirin or acetaminophen (Tylenol); nonsteroidal anti-inflammatory drugs (NSAIDs), such as ibuprofen (Motrin, Nuprin, Advil); and exercises to restore joint movement and strengthen the knee. Glucosamine, a dietary supplement, has been shown in multiple studies to reduce pain and improve joint quality. However, it may take one to two months to work. Losing excess weight can also help people with osteoarthritis.

Rheumatoid arthritis of the knee may require physical therapy and more powerful medications. In people with arthritis of the knee, a seriously damaged joint may need to be replaced with an artificial one. (A new procedure designed to stimulate the growth of cartilage by using a patient's own cartilage cells is being used experimentally to repair cartilage injuries at the end of the femur at the knee. It is not, however, a treatment for arthritis.)

Cartilage Injuries and Disorders

Chondromalacia (KON-dro-mah-LAY-she-ah), also called chondromalaciapatellae, refers to softening of the articular cartilage of the knee cap. This disorder occurs most often in young adults and can be caused by injury, overuse, parts out of alignment, or muscle weakness. Instead of gliding smoothly across the lower end of the thigh bone, the knee cap rubs against it, thereby roughening the cartilage underneath the knee cap. The damage may range from a slightly abnormal surface of the cartilage to a surface that has been worn away to the bone. Chondromalacia related to injury occurs when a blow to the knee cap tears off either a small piece of cartilage or a large fragment containing a piece of bone (osteochondral fracture).

Symptoms and Diagnosis

The most frequent symptom is a dull pain around or under the knee cap that worsens when walking down stairs or hills. A person may also feel pain when climbing stairs or when the knee bears weight as it straightens. The disorder is common in runners and is also seen in skiers, cyclists, and soccer players. A patient's description of symptoms and a follow-up x-ray usually help the doctor make a diagnosis. Although arthroscopy can confirm the diagnosis, it's not performed unless the condition requires extensive treatment.

Treatment

Many doctors recommend that patients with chondromalacia perform low-impact exercises that strengthen muscles, particularly the inner part of the quadriceps, without injuring joints. Swimming, riding a stationary bicycle, and using a cross-country ski machine are acceptable as long as the knee doesn't bend more than 90 degrees. Electrical stimulation may also be used to strengthen the muscles. If these treatments don't improve the condition, the doctor may perform arthroscopic surgery to smooth the surface of the cartilage and "wash out" the cartilage fragments that cause the joint to catch during bending and straightening. In more severe cases, surgery may be necessary to correct the angle of the knee cap and relieve friction with the cartilage or to reposition parts that are out of alignment.

Injuries to the Meniscus

The meniscus is easily injured by the force of rotating the knee while bearing weight. A partial or total tear may occur when a person quickly twists or rotates the upper leg while the foot stays still (for example, when dribbling a basketball around an opponent or turning to hit a tennis ball). If the tear is tiny, the meniscus stays connected to the front and back of the knee; if the tear is large, the meniscus may be left hanging by a thread of cartilage. The seriousness of a tear depends on its location and extent.

Symptoms

Generally, when people injure a meniscus, they feel some pain, particularly when the knee is straightened. If the pain is mild, the person may continue moving. Severe pain may occur if a fragment of the meniscus catches between the femur and the tibia. Swelling may occur soon after injury if blood vessels are disrupted, or swelling may occur several hours later if the joint fills with fluid produced by the joint lining (synovium) as a result of inflammation. If the synovium is injured, it may become inflamed and produce fluid to protect itself. This makes the knee swell. Sometimes, an injury that occurred in the past but was not treated becomes painful months or years later, particularly if the knee is injured a second time. After any injury, the knee may click, lock, or feel weak. Although symptoms of meniscal injury may disappear on their own, they frequently persist or return and require treatment.

Diagnosis

In addition to listening to the patient's description of the onset of pain and swelling, the doctor may perform a physical examination and take x-rays of the knee. The examination may include a test in which the doctor bends the leg, then rotates the leg outward and inward while extending it. Pain or an audible click suggests a meniscal tear. An MRI may be recommended to confirm the diagnosis. Occasionally, the doctor may use arthroscopy to help diagnose and treat a meniscal tear.

Treatment

If the tear is minor and the pain and other symptoms go away, the doctor may recommend a muscle-strengthening program. Exercises for meniscal problems are best started with guidance from a doctor and physical therapist or exercise therapist. The therapist will make sure that the patient does the exercises properly and without risking new or repeat injury. The following exercises after injury to the meniscus are designed to build up the quadriceps and hamstring muscles and increase flexibility and strength.

- Warming up the joint by riding a stationary bicycle, then straightening and raising the leg (but not straightening it too much).

- Extending the leg while sitting (a weight may be worn on the ankle for this exercise).

- Raising the leg while lying on the stomach.

- Exercising in a pool (walking as fast as possible in chest-deep water, performing small flutter kicks while holding onto the side of the pool, and raising each leg to 90 degrees in chest-deep water while pressing the back against the side of the pool).

If the tear is more extensive, the doctor may perform arthroscopic or open surgery to see the extent of injury and to repair the tear. The doctor can sew the meniscus back in place if the patient is relatively young, if the injury is in an area with a good blood supply, and if the ligaments are intact. Most young athletes are able to return to active sports after meniscus repair.

If the patient is elderly or the tear is in an area with a poor blood supply, the doctor may cut off a small portion of the meniscus to even the surface. In some cases, the doctor removes the entire meniscus. However, osteoarthritis is more likely to develop in the knee if the meniscus is removed. Medical researchers are investigating a procedure called an allograft, in which the surgeon replaces the meniscus with one from a cadaver. A grafted meniscus is fragile and will shrink and tear easily. Researchers have also attempted to replace a meniscus with an artificial one, but this procedure is even less successful than an allograft.

Recovery after surgical repair takes several weeks, and postoperative activity is slightly more restricted than when the meniscus is removed. Nevertheless, putting weight on the joint actually fosters recovery. Regardless of the form of surgery, rehabilitation usually includes walking, bending the legs, and doing exercises that stretch and build up leg muscles. The best results of treatment for meniscal injury are obtained in people who do not show articular cartilage changes and who have an intact ACL.

Ligament Injuries

What Are the Causes of Anterior and Posterior Cruciate Ligament Injuries?

Injury to the cruciate ligaments is sometimes referred to as a "sprain." The ACL is most often stretched or torn (or both) by a sudden twisting motion (for example, when the feet are planted one way and the knees are turned another).

The PCL is most often injured by a direct impact, such as in an automobile accident or football tackle.

Symptoms and Diagnosis

Injury to a cruciate ligament may not cause pain. Rather, the person may hear a popping sound, and the leg may buckle when he or she tries to stand on it. The doctor may perform several tests to see whether the parts of the knee stay in proper position when pressure is applied in different directions. A thorough examination is essential. A MRI is very accurate in detecting a complete tear, but arthroscopy may be the only reliable means of detecting a partial one.

Treatment

For an incomplete tear, the doctor may recommend that the patient begin an exercise program to strengthen surrounding muscles. The doctor may also prescribe a brace to protect the knee during activity. For a completely torn ACL in an active athlete and motivated person, the doctor is likely to recommend surgery. The surgeon may reattach the torn ends of the ligament or reconstruct the torn ligament by using a piece (graft) of healthy ligament from the patient (autograft) or from a cadaver (allograft). Although synthetic ligaments have been tried in experiments, the results have not been as good as with human tissue. One of the most important elements in a patient's successful recovery after cruciate ligament surgery is a 4-6 month exercise and rehabilitation program that may involve using special exercise equipment at a rehabilitation or sports center. Successful surgery and rehabilitation will allow the patient to return to a normal lifestyle.

What Is the Most Common Cause of Medial and Lateral Collateral Ligament Injuries?

The MCL is more easily injured than the LCL. The cause is most often a blow to the outer side of the knee that stretches and tears the ligament on the inner side of the knee. Such blows frequently occur in contact sports like football or hockey.

Symptoms and Diagnosis

When injury to the MCL occurs, a person may feel a pop and the knee may buckle sideways. Pain and swelling are common. A thorough examination is needed to determine the kind and extent of the injury. To diagnose a collateral ligament injury, the doctor exerts pressure on the side of the knee to determine the degree of pain and the looseness of the joint. A MRI is helpful in diagnosing injuries to these ligaments.

Treatment

Most sprains of the collateral ligaments will heal if the patient follows a prescribed exercise program. In addition to exercise, the doctor may recommend ice packs to reduce pain and swelling and a small sleeve-type brace to protect and stabilize the knee. A sprain may take 2 to 4 weeks to heal. A severely sprained or torn collateral ligament may be accompanied by a torn ACL, which usually requires surgical repair.

Tendon Injuries and Disorders

What Causes Tendinitis and Ruptured Tendons?

Knee tendon injuries range from tendinitis (inflammation of a tendon) to a ruptured (torn) tendon. If a person overuses a tendon during certain activities such as dancing, cycling, or running, the tendon stretches like a worn-out rubber band and becomes inflamed. Also, trying to break a fall may cause the quadriceps muscles to contract and tear the quadriceps tendon above the patella or the patellar tendon below the patella. This type of injury is most likely to happen in older people whose tendons tend to be weaker. Tendinitis of the patellar tendon is sometimes called jumper's knee because in sports that require jumping, such as basketball, the muscle contraction and force of hitting the ground after a jump strain the tendon. After repeated stress, the tendon may become inflamed or tear.

Symptoms and Diagnosis

People with tendinitis often have tenderness at the point where the patellar tendon meets the bone. In addition, they may feel pain during running, hurried walking, or jumping. A complete rupture of the quadriceps or patellar tendon is not only painful, but also makes it difficult for a person to bend, extend, or lift the leg against gravity. If there is not much swelling, the doctor will be able to feel a defect in the tendon near the tear during a physical examination. An x-ray will show that the patella is lower than normal in a quadriceps tendon tear and higher than normal in a patellar tendon tear. The doctor may use a MRI to confirm a partial or total tear.

Treatment

Initially, the doctor may ask a patient with tendinitis to rest, elevate, and apply ice to the knee and to take medicines such as aspirin or ibuprofen to relieve pain and decrease inflammation and swelling. If the quadriceps or patellar tendon is completely ruptured, a surgeon will reattach the ends. After surgery, the patient will wear a cast for 3 to 6 weeks and use crutches. For a partial tear, the doctor might apply a cast without performing surgery.

Rehabilitating a partial or complete tear of a tendon requires an exercise program that is similar to but less vigorous than that prescribed for ligament injuries. The goals of exercise are to restore the ability to bend and straighten the knee and to strengthen the leg to prevent repeat injury. A rehabilitation program may last 6 months, although the patient can return to many activities before then.

What Causes Osgood-Schlatter Disease?

Osgood-Schlatter disease is caused by repetitive stress or tension on part of the growth area of the upper tibia (the apophysis). It is characterized by inflammation of the patellar tendon and surrounding soft tissues at the point where the tendon attaches to the tibia. The disease may also be associated with an injury in which the tendon is stretched so much that it tears away from the tibia and takes a fragment of bone with it. The disease most commonly affects active young people, particularly boys between the ages of 10 and 15, who play games or sports that include frequent running and jumping.

Symptoms and Diagnosis

People with this disease experience pain just below the knee joint that usually worsens with activity and is relieved by rest. A bony bump that is particularly painful when pressed may appear on the upper edge of the tibia (below the knee cap). Usually, the motion of the knee is not affected. Pain may last a few months and may recur until the child's growth is completed.

Osgood-Schlatter disease is most often diagnosed by the symptoms. An x-ray may be normal, or show an injury, or, more typically, show that the growth area is in fragments.

Treatment

Usually, the disease resolves without treatment. Applying ice to the knee when pain begins helps relieve inflammation and is sometimes used along with stretching and strengthening exercises. The doctor may advise the patient to limit participation in vigorous sports. Children who wish to continue moderate or less stressful sports activities may need to wear knee pads for protection and apply ice to the knee after activity. If there is a great deal of pain, sports activities may be limited until discomfort becomes tolerable.

What Causes Iliotibial Band Syndrome?

This is an overuse condition in which inflammation results when a band of a tendon rubs over the outer bone (lateral condyle) of the knee. Although iliotibial band syndrome may be caused by direct injury to the knee, it is most often caused by the stress of long-term overuse, such as sometimes occurs in sports training.

Symptoms and Diagnosis

A person with this syndrome feels an ache or burning sensation at the side of the knee during activity. Pain may be localized at the side of the knee or radiate up the side of the thigh. A person may also feel a snap when the knee is bent and then straightened. Swelling is usually absent and knee motion is normal. The diagnosis of this disorder is typically based on the symptoms, such as pain at the outer bone, and exclusion of other conditions with similar symptoms.

Treatment

Usually, iliotibial band syndrome disappears if the person reduces activity and performs stretching exercises followed by muscle-strengthening exercises. In rare cases when the syndrome doesn't disappear, surgery may be necessary to split the tendon so it isn't stretched too tightly over the bone.

Other Knee Injuries

What Is Osteochondritis Dissecans?

Osteochondritis dissecans results from a loss of the blood supply to an area of bone underneath a joint surface and usually involves the knee. The affected bone and its covering of cartilage gradually loosen and cause pain. This problem usually arises spontaneously in an active adolescent or young adult. It may be due to a slight blockage of a small artery or to an unrecognized injury or tiny fracture that damages the overlying cartilage. A person with this condition may eventually develop osteoarthritis.

Lack of a blood supply can cause bone to break down (avascular necrosis). The involvement of several joints or the appearance of osteochondritis dissecans in several family members may indicate that the disorder is inherited.

Symptoms and Diagnosis

If normal healing doesn't occur, cartilage separates from the diseased bone and a fragment breaks loose into the knee joint, causing weakness, sharp pain, and locking of the joint. An x-ray, MRI, or arthroscopy can determine the condition of the cartilage and can be used to diagnose osteochondritis dissecans.

Treatment

If cartilage fragments have not broken loose, a surgeon may fix them in place with pins or screws that are sunk into the cartilage to stimulate a new blood supply.

If fragments are loose, the surgeon may scrape down the cavity to reach fresh bone and add a bone graft and fix the fragments in position. Fragments that cannot be mended are removed, and the cavity is drilled or scraped to stimulate new cartilage growth. Research is being done to assess the use of cartilage cell and other tissue transplants to treat this disorder.

What Is Plica Syndrome?

Plica (PLI-kah) syndrome occurs when plicae (bands of synovial tissue) are irritated by overuse or injury. Synovial plicae are the remains of tissue pouches found in the early stages of fetal development.

As the fetus develops, these pouches normally combine to form one large synovial cavity. If this process is incomplete, plicae remain as four folds or bands of synovial tissue within the knee. Injury, chronic overuse, or inflammatory conditions are associated with this syndrome.

Symptoms and Diagnosis

People with this syndrome are likely to experience pain and swelling, a clicking sensation, and locking and weakness of the knee. Because the symptoms are similar to those of some other knee problems, plica syndrome is often misdiagnosed. Diagnosis usually depends on excluding other conditions that cause similar symptoms.

Treatment

The goal of treatment is to reduce inflammation of the synovium and thickening of the plicae. The doctor usually prescribes medicine such as ibuprofen to reduce inflammation. The patient is also advised to reduce activity, apply ice and an elastic bandage to the knee, and do strengthening exercises. A cortisone injection into the plica folds helps about half of those treated. If treatment fails to relieve symptoms within 3 months, the doctor may recommend arthroscopic or open surgery to remove the plicae.

What Kinds of Doctors Treat Knee Problems?

Extensive injuries and diseases of the knees are usually treated by an orthopaedic surgeon, a doctor who has been trained in the nonsurgical and surgical treatment of bones, joints, and soft tissues such as ligaments, tendons, and muscles. Patients seeking nonsurgical treatment of arthritis of the knee may also consult a rheumatologist (a doctor specializing in the diagnosis and treatment of arthritis and related disorders).

How Can People Prevent Knee Problems?

Some knee problems, such as those resulting from an accident, can't be foreseen or prevented. However, a person can prevent many knee problems by following these suggestions:

- Before exercising or participating in sports, warm up by walking or riding a stationary bicycle, then do stretches. Stretching the muscles in the front of the thigh (quadriceps) and back of the thigh (hamstrings) reduces tension on the tendons and relieves pressure on the knee during activity.

- Strengthen the leg muscles by doing specific exercises (for example, by walking up stairs or hills, or by riding a stationary bicycle). A supervised workout with weights is another way to strengthen the leg muscles that support the knee.

- Avoid sudden changes in the intensity of exercise. Increase the force or duration of activity gradually.

- Wear shoes that both fit properly and are in good condition to help maintain balance and leg alignment when walking or running. Knee problems can be caused by flat feet or overpronated feet (feet that roll inward). People can often reduce some of these problems by wearing special shoe inserts (orthotics). Maintain a healthy weight to reduce stress on the knee. Obesity increases the risk of degenerative (wearing) conditions such as osteoarthritis of the knee.

What Types of Exercise Are Most Suitable for Someone with Knee Problems?

Three types of exercise are best for people with arthritis:

- Range-of-motion exercises help maintain normal joint movement and relieve stiffness. This type of exercise helps maintain or increase flexibility.

- Strengthening exercises help keep or increase muscle strength. Strong muscles help support and protect joints affected by arthritis.

- Aerobic or endurance exercises improve function of the heart and circulation and help control weight. Weight control can be important to people who have arthritis because extra weight puts pressure on many joints. Some studies show that aerobic exercise can reduce inflammation in some joints.

Additional Information

National Institute of Arthritis and Musculoskeletal and Skin Diseases Information Clearinghouse
National Institutes of Health
1 AMS Circle
Bethesda, MD 20892-3675
Toll-Free: 877-22-NIAMS (226-4267)
Tel: 301-495-4484
TTY: 301-565-2966   *(continued)*

Fax: 301-718-6366
Website: www.niams.nih.gov
E-mail: niamsinfo@mail.nih.gov

The clearinghouse provides information about various forms of arthritis and rheumatic disease and bone, muscle, and skin diseases. It distributes patient and professional education materials and refers people to other sources of information. Additional information and updates can also be found on the NIAMS website.

American Academy of Orthopaedic Surgeons
6300 North River Road
Rosemont, IL 60018-4262
Toll-Free: 800-346-AAOS
Tel: 847-823-7186
Fax: 847-823-8125
Website: www.aaos.org

The academy publishes several brochures on the knee. Single copies of a brochure are available free of charge by sending a self-addressed, stamped (business-size) envelope to (name of brochure) at the address above.

American College of Rheumatology
1800 Century Place, Suite 250
Atlanta, GA 30329
Tel: 404-633-3777
Fax: 404-633-1870
Website: www.rheumatology.org
E-mail: acr@rheumatology.org

This national professional organization can provide referrals to rheumatologists and allied health professionals, such as physical therapists. One-page fact sheets are available on various forms of arthritis. Lists of specialists by geographic area and fact sheets are also available on this website.

American Physical Therapy Association
1111 N. Fairfax Street
Alexandria, VA 22314
Toll-Free: 800-999-APTA (2782)
Tel: 703-684-2783

(continued)

Fax: 703-683-6748
TDD: 703-683-6748
Website: www.apta.org

The association publishes a free brochure titled "Taking Care of the Knees."

Arthritis Foundation
1330 West Peachtree Street
Atlanta, GA 30309
Toll-Free: 800-283-7800
Tel: 404-872-7100 or call your local chapter (listed in the local telephone directory)
Website: www.arthritis.org

The foundation has several free brochures about coping with arthritis, taking nonsteroid and steroid medicines, and exercise. A free brochure on protecting your joints is titled "Using Your Joints Wisely." The foundation also can provide addresses and phone numbers for local chapters and physician and clinic referrals.

Chapter 16

Neck Injuries

Definition: Injury to the neck or spinal cord.

Important Information about Neck and Spinal Injuries

When someone has a spinal injury, additional movement may cause further damage to the spine. The purpose of first aid is to prevent further harm to the victim until you can obtain medical help.

- If in doubt about whether a person has received a spinal injury, assume he or she has.

- A spinal cord injury is very serious because it can mean the loss of sensation and function in the parts of the body below the site of the injury.

Causes

- awkward positioning of the body
- bullet or stab wound
- direct trauma to the face, neck, head, or back

This chapter includes "Spinal/Neck Injury," © A.D.A.M. Inc., revised 10/8/99 by: Alan Greene, MD, CMO, adam.com., reprinted with permission; "Whiplash Information Page," National Institute of Neurological Disorders and Stroke (NINDS), reviewed 01-19-2001; and "Burners," Reprinted with permission from http://www.familydoctor.org/handouts/478.html; Revised February 2000. Copyright © American Academy of Family Physicians. All Rights Reserved.

- diving accident
- electric shock
- exertion
- twisting of the trunk

Symptoms

- stiff neck
- head held in unusual position
- weakness
- difficulty walking
- shock (with pale, clammy skin; bluish lip and fingernails; and decreased consciousness)
- paralysis of extremities
- headache, neck pain, abdominal pain, or back pain
- numbness or tingling that radiates down an arm or leg
- loss of bladder or bowel control

Do not

- bend, twist, or lift the victim's head or body
- attempt to move the victim before medical help arrives unless it is absolutely necessary
- remove a helmet if a spinal injury is suspected.

Call your healthcare provider if

- there has been any injury to the neck or spinal cord. Keep the victim absolutely immobile. Unless there is urgent danger, keep the victim in the position where he or she was found.

First Aid

1. Check the victim's airway, breathing, and circulation. If necessary, begin rescue breathing and CPR. If you think the victim might have a head, neck, or spinal injury; lift the chin rather than tilt the head back when attempting to open the airway. Keep the victim's head, neck, and back in line and roll him or her as a unit.

2.   Immobilize the victim's head and torso in the position in which they were found. Do not attempt to reposition the neck.

3.   If the victim must be moved, get several people to help. Use a sturdy support (such as a plank) as a stretcher. Together, roll the victim's entire body as a unit—keeping the head, neck, and back in a straight line—onto the stretcher.

4.   Immobilize the victim's head and torso in the position found. Place rolled-up towels, clothing, or blankets around the victim's head and torso. Use ropes, belts, tape, or strips of cloth to hold the victim in place on the stretcher. Carry the stretcher as horizontally as possible.

5.   If a stretcher is not available and the injured person must be turned over, use the logrolling technique. One rescuer stationed at the victim's head keeps the head and shoulders in a fixed position while the second rescuer extends the victim's arm (the one on the side the victim will be rolled toward) above his head. Then the first rescuer takes this arm and uses it as additional support for the head. Both rescuers gently roll the victim without moving his neck.

6.   If you are the only rescuer and the victim must be moved, use the clothes drag technique with victim lying face up or face down (however he or she was found).

7.   If the victim vomits or is choking on blood, carefully roll him or her on one side. Vomiting can signal internal injuries.

8.   Keep the victim warm to help prevent shock.

9.   Give first aid for obvious injuries, but keep the victim in the position found.

Prevention

- Regular exercise, good posture, and lifting heavy objects correctly (letting your leg muscles do most of the work) all help prevent back problems.

- Wear seat belts.

- Avoid alcohol with driving.

- Avoid diving into lakes, rivers, and surf.

- Avoid motorcycles and all-terrain vehicles.
- Avoid football.
- Back pain, if it occurs, should be discussed with the doctor.

What Is Whiplash?

Whiplash—a soft tissue injury to the neck—is also called neck sprain or neck strain. It is characterized by a collection of symptoms that occur following damage to the neck, usually because of sudden extension and flexion. The disorder commonly occurs as the result of an automobile accident and may include injury to intervertebral joints, discs, and ligaments, cervical muscles, and nerve roots. Symptoms such as neck pain may be present directly after the injury or may be delayed for several days. In addition to neck pain, other symptoms may include neck stiffness, injuries to the muscles and ligaments (myofascial injuries), headache, dizziness, abnormal sensations such as burning or prickling (paresthesias), or shoulder or back pain. In addition, some people experience cognitive, somatic, or psychological conditions such as memory loss, concentration impairment, nervousness/irritability, sleep disturbances, fatigue, or depression.

Is There Any Treatment?

Treatment for individuals with whiplash may include pain medications, nonsteroidal anti-inflammatory drugs, antidepressants, muscle relaxants, and a cervical collar (usually worn for 2 to 3 weeks). Range of motion exercises, physical therapy, and cervical traction may also be prescribed. Supplemental heat application may relieve muscle tension.

What Is the Prognosis?

Generally, prognosis for individuals with whiplash is good. The neck and head pain clears within a few days or weeks. Most patients recover within 3 months after the injury, however, some may continue to have residual neck pain and headaches.

Burners

A "burner" is an injury to one or more nerves between your neck and shoulder. It is also called a "stinger." It usually happens in sports like football. It's not a serious neck injury.

What Causes a Burner?

If you play football, you can get a burner when you tackle or block another player. One of 3 things happens:

- Your shoulder is pushed down at the same time that your head is forced to the opposite side. This stretches nerves between your neck and shoulder.

- Your head is quickly moved to one side. This pinches nerves on that side.

- The area above your collarbone is hit directly. This bruises nerves.

How Do I Know if I Have a Burner?

You'll have a burning or stinging feeling between your neck and shoulder, and probably in your arm. Your shoulder and arm may feel numb, tingly, or weak.

Your doctor will ask questions and examine you. Burners happen in only one arm at a time. If both of your arms or one arm and a leg are hurt, you may have a serious neck injury, not a burner. Your doctor will then protect your neck and get x-rays.

How Are Burners Treated?

Burners get better on their own. You may need physical therapy to stretch and strengthen your muscles.

Some burners last a few minutes. Others take several days or weeks to heal. If your burner lasts more than a few weeks, you may have a test called an electromyogram (EMG). This test can show that you have a burner and give an idea about how long it will last.

When Can I Return to My Sport?

Before you go back to playing, you must have no pain, numbness, or tingling. You must be able to move your neck in all directions. Your strength must be back to normal. You must be able to play your sport without problems from the injury.

Can I Get Another Burner?

Yes, but daily stretching exercises can help prevent burners. Tilt your head up, down, left, and right. Turn your head left and right to look over your shoulders. Hold each stretch for 20 seconds. If you play football, wear extra neck protection.

An Important Point!

Don't just assume that you have a burner. You might have a serious neck injury. If you have burning, stinging, numbness, or tingling in your arms or legs, stop what you're doing. Slowly lie down on the ground and wait for a trainer or a doctor to examine you. (Rev. February 2000)

This information provides a general overview on this topic and may not apply to everyone. To find out if this applies to you and to get more information on this subject, talk to your family doctor. Visit familydoctor.org for information on this and many other health-related topics.

Additional Information

American Chronic Pain Association (ACPA)
P.O. Box 850
Rocklin, CA 95677-0850
Tel: 916-632-0922
Fax: 916-632-3208
Website: www.theacpa.org
E-mail: ACPA@pacbell.net

National Chronic Pain Outreach Association (NCPOA)
7979 Old Georgetown Road, Suite 100
Bethesda, MD 20814-2429
Tel: 301-652-4948
Fax: 301-907-0745
E-mail: ncpoa@cfw.com

National Headache Foundation
428 W. St. James Pl., 2nd Floor
Chicago IL 60614-2750
Toll-Free: 888-NHF-5552 (643-5552)
Tel: 773-388-6399
Fax: 773-525-735
Website: www.headaches.org
E-mail: info@headaches.org

Chapter 17

Shoulder Injuries

This chapter first answers general questions about the shoulder and shoulder problems. It then answers questions about specific shoulder problems (dislocation, separation, tendinitis, bursitis, impingement syndrome, torn rotator cuff, frozen shoulder, and fracture) as well as shoulder pain caused by arthritis of the shoulder.

How Common Are Shoulder Problems?

According to the American Academy of Orthopaedic Surgeons, about 4 million people in the United States seek medical care each year for shoulder sprain, strain, dislocation, or other problems. Each year, shoulder problems account for about 1.5 million visits to orthopaedic surgeons—doctors who treat disorders of the bones, muscles, and related structures.

What Are the Structures of the Shoulder and How Does the Shoulder Function?

The shoulder joint is composed of three bones: the clavicle (collarbone), the scapula (shoulder blade), and the humerus (upper arm bone). Two joints facilitate shoulder movement. The acromioclavicular (AC) joint is located between the acromion (part of the scapula that

"Questions and Answers about Shoulder Problems," National Institute of Arthritis and Musculoskeletal and Skin Diseases (NIAMS), NIH Publication No. 01-4865, May 2001.

forms the highest point of the shoulder) and the clavicle. The gleno-humeral joint, commonly called the shoulder joint, is a ball-and-socket type joint that helps move the shoulder forward and backward and allows the arm to rotate in a circular fashion or hinge out and up away from the body. (The "ball" is the top, rounded portion of the upper arm bone or humerus; the "socket," or glenoid, is a dish-shaped part of the outer edge of the scapula into which the ball fits.) The capsule is a soft tissue envelope that encircles the glenohumeral joint. It is lined by a thin, smooth synovial membrane.

The bones of the shoulder are held in place by muscles, tendons, and ligaments. Tendons are tough cords of tissue that attach the shoulder muscles to bone and assist the muscles in moving the shoulder. Ligaments attach shoulder bones to each other, providing stability. For example, the front of the joint capsule is anchored by three gleno-humeral ligaments.

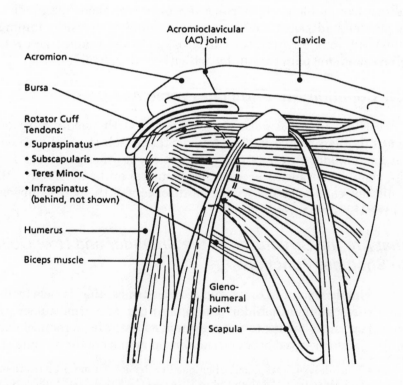

Figure 17.1. Structure of the Shoulder

The rotator cuff is a structure composed of tendons that, with associated muscles, holds the ball at the top of the humerus in the glenoid socket and provides mobility and strength to the shoulder joint.

Two filmy sac-like structures called bursae permit smooth gliding between bone, muscle, and tendon. They cushion and protect the rotator cuff from the bony arch of the acromion.

What Are the Origin and Causes of Shoulder Problems?

The shoulder is the most movable joint in the body. However, it is an unstable joint because of the range of motion allowed. It is easily subject to injury because the ball of the upper arm is larger than the shoulder socket that holds it. To remain stable, the shoulder must be anchored by its muscles, tendons, and ligaments. Some shoulder problems arise from the disruption of these soft tissues as a result of injury or from overuse or underuse of the shoulder. Other problems arise from a degenerative process in which tissues break down and no longer function well.

Shoulder pain may be localized or may be referred to areas around the shoulder or down the arm. Disease within the body (such as gallbladder, liver, or heart disease, or disease of the cervical spine of the neck) also may generate pain that travels along nerves to the shoulder.

How Are Shoulder Problems Diagnosed?

Following are some of the ways doctors diagnose shoulder problems:

- **Medical history** (the patient tells the doctor about an injury or other condition that might be causing the pain).

- **Physical examination** to feel for injury and discover the limits of movement, location of pain, and extent of joint instability.

- **Tests** to confirm the diagnosis of certain conditions. Some of these tests include:

  - x-ray

  - arthrogram—Diagnostic record that can be seen on an x-ray after injection of a contrast fluid into the shoulder joint to outline structures such as the rotator cuff. In disease or injury, this contrast fluid may either leak into an area where it does not belong, indicating a tear or opening, or be blocked from entering an area where there normally is an opening.

- MRI (magnetic resonance imaging)—A non-invasive procedure in which a machine produces a series of cross-sectional images of the shoulder.

- Other diagnostic tests, such as injection of an anesthetic into and around the shoulder joint, are discussed in specific sections of this chapter.

Dislocation

What Is a Shoulder Dislocation?

The shoulder joint is the most frequently dislocated major joint of the body. In a typical case of a dislocated shoulder, a strong force that pulls the shoulder outward (abduction) or extreme rotation of the joint pops the ball of the humerus out of the shoulder socket. Dislocation commonly occurs when there is a backward pull on the arm that either catches the muscles unprepared to resist or overwhelms the muscles. When a shoulder dislocates frequently, the condition is referred to as shoulder instability. A partial dislocation where the upper arm bone is partially in and partially out of the socket is called a subluxation.

What Are the Signs of a Dislocation and How Is It Diagnosed?

The shoulder can dislocate either forward, backward, or downward. Not only does the arm appear out of position when the shoulder dislocates, but the dislocation also produces pain. Muscle spasms may increase the intensity of pain. Swelling, numbness, weakness, and bruising are likely to develop. Problems seen with a dislocated shoulder are tearing of the ligaments or tendons reinforcing the joint capsule and, less commonly, nerve damage. Doctors usually diagnose a dislocation by a physical examination, and x-rays may be taken to confirm the diagnosis and to rule out a related fracture.

How Is a Dislocated Shoulder Treated?

Doctors treat a dislocation by putting the ball of the humerus back into the joint socket—a procedure called a reduction. The arm is then immobilized in a sling or a device called a shoulder immobilizer for several weeks. Usually the doctor recommends resting the shoulder and applying ice three or four times a day. After pain and swelling have been controlled, the patient enters a rehabilitation program that includes exercises to restore the range of motion of the shoulder and strengthen the muscles to prevent future dislocations. These exercises may progress from simple motion to the use of weights.

After treatment and recovery, a previously dislocated shoulder may remain more susceptible to reinjury, especially in young, active individuals. Ligaments may have been stretched or torn, and the shoulder may tend to dislocate again. A shoulder that dislocates severely or often, injuring surrounding tissues or nerves, usually requires surgical repair to tighten stretched ligaments or reattach torn ones.

Sometimes the doctor performs surgery through a tiny incision into which a small scope (arthroscope) is inserted to observe the inside of the joint. After this procedure, called arthroscopic surgery, the shoulder is generally immobilized for about 6 weeks and full recovery takes several months. Arthroscopic techniques involving the shoulder are relatively new and many surgeons prefer to repair a recurrent dislocating shoulder by the time-tested open surgery under direct vision. There are usually fewer repeat dislocations and improved movement following open surgery, but it may take a little longer to regain motion.

Separation

What Is a Shoulder Separation?

A shoulder separation occurs where the collarbone (clavicle) meets the shoulder blade (scapula). When ligaments that hold the joint together are partially or completely torn, the outer end of the clavicle may slip out of place, preventing it from properly meeting the scapula. Most often the injury is caused by a blow to the shoulder or by falling on an outstretched hand.

What Are the Signs of a Shoulder Separation and How Is It Diagnosed?

Shoulder pain or tenderness and, occasionally, a bump in the middle of the top of the shoulder (over the AC joint) are signs that a separation may have occurred. Sometimes the severity of a separation can be detected by taking x-rays while the patient holds a light weight that pulls on the muscles, making a separation more pronounced.

How Is a Shoulder Separation Treated?

A shoulder separation is usually treated conservatively by rest and wearing a sling. Soon after injury, an ice bag may be applied to relieve pain and swelling. After a period of rest, a therapist helps the patient perform exercises that put the shoulder through its range of motion. Most shoulder separations heal within 2 or 3 months without further intervention. However, if ligaments are severely torn, surgical repair may be required to hold the clavicle in place. A doctor may wait to see if conservative treatment works before deciding whether surgery is required.

Tendinitis, Bursitis, and Impingement Syndrome

What Are Tendinitis, Bursitis, and Impingement Syndrome of the Shoulder?

These conditions are closely related and may occur alone or in combination. If the rotator cuff and bursa are irritated, inflamed, and swollen, they may become squeezed between the head of the humerus and the acromion. Repeated motion involving the arms, or the aging process involving shoulder motion over many years, may also irritate and wear down the tendons, muscles, and surrounding structures. Tendinitis is inflammation (redness, soreness, and swelling) of a tendon. In tendinitis of the shoulder, the rotator cuff and/or biceps tendon become inflamed, usually as a result of being pinched by surrounding structures. The injury may vary from mild inflammation to involvement of most of the rotator cuff. When the rotator cuff tendon becomes inflamed and thickened, it may get trapped under the acromion. Squeezing of the rotator cuff is called impingement syndrome.

Tendinitis and impingement syndrome are often accompanied by inflammation of the bursa sacs that protect the shoulder. An inflamed bursa is called bursitis. Inflammation caused by a disease such as rheumatoid arthritis may cause rotator cuff tendinitis and bursitis. Sports involving overuse of the shoulder and occupations requiring frequent overhead reaching are other potential causes of irritation to the rotator cuff or bursa and may lead to inflammation and impingement.

What Are the Signs of Tendinitis and Bursitis?

Signs of these conditions include the slow onset of discomfort and pain in the upper shoulder or upper third of the arm and/or difficulty sleeping on the shoulder. Tendinitis and bursitis also cause pain when the arm is lifted away from the body or overhead. If tendinitis involves the biceps tendon (the tendon located in front of the shoulder that helps bend the elbow and turn the forearm), pain will occur in the front or side of the shoulder and may travel down to the elbow and forearm. Pain may also occur when the arm is forcefully pushed upward overhead.

How Are These Conditions Diagnosed?

Diagnosis of tendinitis and bursitis begins with a medical history and physical examination. X-rays do not show tendons or the bursae but may be helpful in ruling out bony abnormalities or arthritis. The doctor may remove and test fluid from the inflamed area to rule out infection. Impingement syndrome may be confirmed when injection of a small amount of anesthetic (lidocaine hydrochloride) into the space under the acromion relieves pain.

How Are Tendinitis, Bursitis, and Impingement Syndrome Treated?

The first step in treating these conditions is to reduce pain and inflammation with rest, ice, and anti-inflammatory medicines such as aspirin, naproxen (Naprosyn), ibuprofen (Advil, Motrin, or Nuprin), or cox-2 inhibitors (Celebrex, Vioxx, or Mobic). In some cases the doctor or therapist will use ultrasound (gentle sound-wave vibrations) to warm deep tissues and improve blood flow. Gentle stretching and strengthening exercises are added gradually. These may be preceded or followed by use of an ice pack. If there is no improvement, the doctor may inject a corticosteroid medicine into the space under the acromion. While steroid injections are a common treatment, they must be used with caution because they may lead to tendon rupture. If there is still no improvement after 6 to 12 months, the doctor may perform either arthroscopic or open surgery to repair damage and relieve pressure on the tendons and bursae.

Torn Rotator Cuff

What Is a Torn Rotator Cuff?

One or more rotator cuff tendons may become inflamed from overuse, aging, a fall on an outstretched hand, or a collision. Sports requiring repeated overhead arm motion or occupations requiring heavy lifting also place a strain on rotator cuff tendons and muscles. Normally, tendons are strong, but a longstanding wearing down process may lead to a tear.

What Are the Signs of a Torn Rotator Cuff?

Typically, a person with a rotator cuff injury feels pain over the deltoid muscle at the top and outer side of the shoulder, especially when the arm is raised or extended out from the side of the body. Motions like those involved in getting dressed can be painful. The shoulder may feel weak, especially when trying to lift the arm into a horizontal position. A person may also feel or hear a click or pop when the shoulder is moved.

How Is a Torn Rotator Cuff Diagnosed?

Pain or weakness on outward or inward rotation of the arm may indicate a tear in a rotator cuff tendon. The patient also feels pain when lowering the arm to the side after the shoulder is moved backward and the arm is raised. A doctor may detect weakness but may not be able to determine from a physical examination where the tear is located. X-rays, if taken, may appear normal. A MRI can help detect a full tendon tear, but does not detect partial tears. If the pain disappears after the doctor injects a small amount of anesthetic into the area, impingement is likely to be present. If there is no response to treatment, the doctor may use an arthrogram, rather than a MRI, to inspect the injured area and confirm the diagnosis.

How Is a Torn Rotator Cuff Treated?

Doctors usually recommend that patients with a rotator cuff injury rest the shoulder, apply heat or cold to the sore area, and take medicine to relieve pain and inflammation. Other treatments might be added, such as electrical stimulation of muscles and nerves, ultrasound, or a cortisone injection near the inflamed area of the rotator cuff. The patient may need to wear a sling for a few days. If surgery is not an immediate consideration, exercises are added to the treatment program to build flexibility and strength and restore the shoulder's function. If there is no improvement with these conservative treatments and functional impairment persists, the doctor may perform arthroscopic or open surgical repair of the torn rotator cuff.

Frozen Shoulder (Adhesive Capsulitis)

What Is a Frozen Shoulder?

As the name implies, movement of the shoulder is severely restricted in people with a "frozen shoulder." This condition, which doctors call adhesive capsulitis, is frequently caused by injury that leads to lack of use due to pain. Rheumatic disease progression and recent shoulder surgery can also cause frozen shoulder. Intermittent periods of use may cause inflammation. Adhesions (abnormal bands of tissue) grow between the joint surfaces, restricting motion. There is also a lack of synovial fluid, which normally lubricates the gap between the arm bone and socket to help the shoulder joint move. It is this restricted space between the capsule and ball of the humerus that distinguishes adhesive capsulitis from a less complicated painful, stiff shoulder. People with diabetes, stroke, lung disease, rheumatoid arthritis, and heart disease, or who have been in an accident, are at a higher risk for frozen shoulder. The condition rarely appears in people under 40 years old.

What Are the Signs of a Frozen Shoulder and How Is It Diagnosed?

With a frozen shoulder, the joint becomes so tight and stiff that it is nearly impossible to carry out simple movements, such as raising the arm. People complain that the stiffness and discomfort worsen at night. A doctor may suspect the patient has a frozen shoulder if a physical examination reveals limited shoulder movement. An arthrogram may confirm the diagnosis.

How Is a Frozen Shoulder Treated?

Treatment of this disorder focuses on restoring joint movement and reducing shoulder pain. Usually, treatment begins with nonsteroidal anti-inflammatory drugs and the application of heat, followed by gentle stretching exercises. These stretching exercises, which may be performed in the home with the help of a therapist, are the treatment of choice. In some cases, transcutaneous electrical nerve stimulation (TENS) with a small battery-operated unit may be used to reduce pain by blocking nerve impulses. If these measures are unsuccessful, the doctor may recommend manipulation of the shoulder under general anesthesia. Surgery to cut the adhesions is only necessary in some cases.

Fracture

What Happens When the Shoulder Is Fractured?

A fracture involves a partial or total crack through a bone. The break in a bone usually occurs as a result of an impact injury, such as a fall or blow to the shoulder. A fracture usually involves the clavicle or the neck (area below the ball) of the humerus.

What Are the Signs of a Shoulder Fracture and How Is It Diagnosed?

A shoulder fracture that occurs after a major injury is usually accompanied by severe pain. Within a short time, there may be redness and bruising around the area. Sometimes a fracture is obvious because the bones appear out of position. Both diagnosis and severity can be confirmed by x-rays.

How Is a Shoulder Fracture Treated?

When a fracture occurs, the doctor tries to bring the bones into a position that will promote healing and restore arm movement. If the clavicle is fractured, the patient must at first wear a strap and sling around the chest to keep the clavicle in place. After removing the strap and sling, the doctor will prescribe exercises to strengthen the shoulder and restore movement. Surgery is occasionally needed for certain clavicle fractures. Fracture of the neck of the humerus is usually treated with a sling or shoulder immobilizer. If the bones are out of position, surgery may be necessary to reset them. Exercises are also part of restoring shoulder strength and motion.

Arthritis of the Shoulder

What Is Arthritis of the Shoulder?

Arthritis is a degenerative disease caused by either wear and tear of the cartilage (osteoarthritis) or an inflammation (rheumatoid arthritis) of one or more joints. Arthritis not only affects joints; it may also affect supporting structures such as muscles, tendons, and ligaments.

What Are the Signs of Shoulder Arthritis and How Is It Diagnosed?

The usual signs of arthritis of the shoulder are pain, particularly over the AC joint, and a decrease in shoulder motion. A doctor may suspect the patient has arthritis when there is both pain and swelling in the joint. The diagnosis may be confirmed by a physical examination and x-rays. Blood tests may be helpful for diagnosing rheumatoid arthritis, but other tests may be needed as well. Analysis of synovial fluid from the shoulder joint may be helpful in diagnosing some kinds of arthritis. Although arthroscopy permits direct visualization of damage to cartilage, tendons, and ligaments, and may confirm a diagnosis, it is usually done only if a repair procedure is to be performed.

How Is Arthritis of the Shoulder Treated?

Most often osteoarthritis of the shoulder is treated with non-steroidal anti-inflammatory drugs, such as aspirin, ibuprofen, or cox-2 inhibitors. (Rheumatoid arthritis of the shoulder may require physical therapy and additional medicine, such as corticosteroids.) When non-operative treatment of arthritis of the shoulder fails to relieve pain or improve function, or when there is severe wear and tear of the joint causing parts to loosen and move out of place, shoulder joint replacement (arthroplasty) may provide better results. In this operation, a surgeon replaces the shoulder joint with an artificial ball for the top of the humerus and a cap (glenoid) for the scapula. Passive shoulder exercises (where someone else moves the arm to rotate the shoulder joint) are started soon after surgery. Patients begin exercising on their own about 3 to 6 weeks after surgery. Eventually, stretching and strengthening exercises become a major part of the rehabilitation program. The success of the operation often depends on the condition of rotator cuff muscles prior to surgery and the degree to which the patient follows the exercise program.

If you receive a shoulder injury, here's what you can do:

RICE = Rest, Ice, Compression, and Elevation

- **Rest**—Reduce or stop using the injured area for 48 hours.

- **Ice**—Put an ice pack on the injured area for 20 minutes at a time, 4 to 8 times per day. Use a cold pack, ice bag, or a plastic bag filled with crushed ice that has been wrapped in a towel.

- **Compression**—Compression may help reduce the swelling. Compress the area with bandages, such as an elastic wrap, to help stabilize the shoulder.

- **Elevation**—Keep the injured area elevated above the level of the heart. Use a pillow to help elevate the injury.

If pain and stiffness persist, see a doctor.

Additional Information

National Institute of Arthritis and Musculoskeletal and Skin Diseases Information Clearinghouse
National Institutes of Health
1 AMS Circle
Bethesda, MD 20892-3675
Toll-Free: 877-22-NIAMS (226-4267)
Tel: 301-495-4484
TTY: 301-565-2966
Fax: 301-718-6366
Website: www.niams.nih.gov

The clearinghouse provides information about various forms of arthritis and rheumatic disease and bone, muscle, and skin diseases. It distributes patient and professional education materials and refers people to other sources of information. Additional information and updates can also be found on the NIAMS website.

American Academy of Orthopaedic Surgeons
6300 North River Road
Rosemont, IL 60018-4262
Toll-Free: 800-346-AAOS
Tel: 847-823-7186
Fax: 847-823-8125
Website: www.aaos.org

The academy publishes brochures on total joint replacement, arthritis, arthroscopy, and other subjects. Single copies of a brochure are available free of charge by sending a self-addressed, stamped (business-size) envelope to (name of brochure) at the address above.

American College of Rheumatology
1800 Century Place, Suite 250
Atlanta, GA 30345
Tel: 404-633-3777
Fax: 404-633-1870
Website: www.rheumatology.org
E-mail: acr@rheumatology.org

This national professional organization can provide referrals to rheumatologists and allied health specialists, such as physical therapists. One-page fact sheets are also available on various forms of arthritis.

Lists of specialists by geographic area and fact sheets are also available on their website.

American Physical Therapy Association
1111 North Fairfax Street
Alexandria, VA 22314-1488
Toll-Free: 800-999-2782, ext. 3395
Tel: 703-684-2783
Fax: 703-683-6748
TDD: 703-683-6748
Website: www.apta.org

This national professional organization represents physical therapists, allied personnel, and students. Its objectives are to improve research, public understanding, and education in the physical therapies. A free brochure titled "Taking Care of Your Shoulder: A Physical Therapist's Perspective" is available on the association's website or by sending a business-size, stamped, self-addressed envelope to the address above.

Arthritis Foundation
1330 West Peachtree Street
Atlanta, GA 30309
Toll-Free: 800-283-7800
Tel: 404-872-7100 or call your local chapter (listed in the telephone directory)
Website: www.arthritis.org

This is the major voluntary organization devoted to arthritis. The foundation publishes pamphlets on arthritis, such as "Arthritis Answers," that may be obtained by calling the toll-free telephone number. The foundation also can provide physician and clinic referrals. Local chapters also provide information and organize exercise programs for people who have arthritis.

Acknowledgments

The NIAMS gratefully acknowledges the assistance of James Panagis, M.D., M.P.H., of the NIAMS; Frank A. Pettrone, M.D., of Arlington, Virginia; and Thomas J. Neviaser, M.D., of Fairfax, Virginia, in the preparation and review of this information.

Chapter 18

Sprains and Strains

This chapter contains general information about sprains and strains, which are both very common injuries. Individual sections describe what sprains and strains are, where they usually occur, what their signs and symptoms are, how they are treated, and how they can be prevented. At the end is a list of key words to help you understand the terms used in the chapter. If you have further questions, you may wish to discuss them with your doctor.

What Is the Difference between a Sprain and a Strain?

A sprain is an injury to a ligament—a stretching or a tearing. One or more ligaments can be injured during a sprain. The severity of the injury will depend on the extent of injury to a single ligament (whether the tear is partial or complete) and the number of ligaments involved.

A strain is an injury to either a muscle or a tendon. Depending on the severity of the injury, a strain may be a simple overstretch of the muscle or tendon, or it can result in a partial or complete tear.

What Causes a Sprain?

A sprain can result from a fall, a sudden twist, or a blow to the body that forces a joint out of its normal position. This results in an

"Questions and Answers about Sprains and Strains," National Institute of Arthritis and Musculoskeletal and Skin Diseases (NIAMS), December 1999.

overstretch or tear of the ligament supporting that joint. Typically, sprains occur when people fall and land on an outstretched arm, slide into base, land on the side of their foot, or twist a knee with the foot planted firmly on the ground.

Where Do Sprains Usually Occur?

Although sprains can occur in both the upper and lower parts of the body, the most common site is the ankle. Ankle sprains are the most common injury in the United States and often occur during sports or recreational activities. Approximately 1 million ankle injuries occur each year, and 85 percent of them are sprains.

The talus bone and the ends of two of the lower leg bones (tibia and fibula) form the ankle joint. This joint is supported by several lateral (outside) ligaments and medial (inside) ligaments. Most ankle sprains happen when the foot turns inward as a person runs, turns,

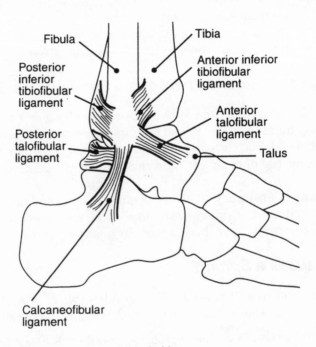

Figure 18.1. *Lateral View of the Ankle*

falls, or lands on the ankle after a jump. This type of sprain is called an inversion injury. One or more of the lateral ligaments are injured, usually the anterior talofibular ligament. The calcaneofibular ligament is the second most frequently torn ligament.

The knee is another common site for a sprain. A blow to the knee or a fall is often the cause; sudden twisting can also result in a sprain.

Sprains frequently occur at the wrist, typically when people fall and land on an outstretched hand.

What Are the Signs and Symptoms of a Sprain?

The usual signs and symptoms include pain, swelling, bruising, and loss of the ability to move and use the joint (called functional ability). However, these signs and symptoms can vary in intensity, depending on the severity of the sprain. Sometimes people feel a pop or tear when the injury happens.

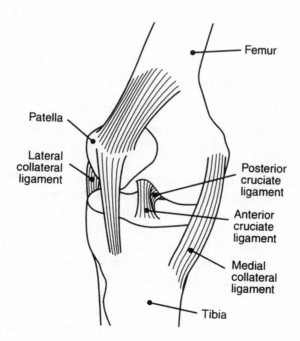

Figure 18.2. *Lateral View of the Knee*

Doctors use many criteria to diagnose the severity of a sprain. In general, **a grade I or mild sprain** causes overstretching or slight tearing of the ligaments with no joint instability. A person with a mild sprain usually experiences minimal pain, swelling, and little or no loss of functional ability. Bruising is absent or slight, and the person is usually able to put weight on the affected joint. People with mild sprains usually do not need an x-ray, but one is sometimes performed if the diagnosis is unclear.

When to See a Doctor for a Sprain

- You have severe pain and cannot put any weight on the injured joint.
- The area over the injured joint or next to it is very tender when you touch it.
- The injured area looks crooked or has lumps and bumps (other than swelling) that you do not see on the uninjured joint.
- You cannot move the injured joint.
- You cannot walk more than four steps without significant pain.
- Your limb buckles or gives way when you try to use the joint.
- You have numbness in any part of the injured area.
- You see redness or red streaks spreading out from the injury.
- You injure an area that has been injured several times before.
- You have pain, swelling, or redness over a bony part of your foot.
- You are in doubt about the seriousness of the injury or how to care for it.

A grade II or moderate sprain causes partial tearing of the ligament and is characterized by bruising, moderate pain, and swelling. A person with a moderate sprain usually has some difficulty putting weight on the affected joint and experiences some loss of function. An x-ray may be needed to help the doctor determine if a fracture is causing the pain and swelling. Magnetic resonance imaging is occasionally used to help differentiate between a significant partial injury and a complete tear in a ligament.

People who sustain a grade III or severe sprain completely tear or rupture a ligament. Pain, swelling, and bruising are usually severe, and the patient is unable to put weight on the joint. An x-ray is usually taken to rule out a broken bone.

When diagnosing any sprain, the doctor will ask the patient to explain how the injury happened. The doctor will examine the affected joint and check its stability and its ability to move and bear weight.

What Causes a Strain?

A strain is caused by twisting or pulling a muscle or tendon. Strains can be acute or chronic. An acute strain is caused by trauma or an injury such as a blow to the body; it can also be caused by improperly lifting heavy objects or overstressing the muscles. Chronic strains are usually the result of overuse—prolonged, repetitive movement of the muscles and tendons.

Where Do Strains Usually Occur?

Two common sites for a strain are the back and the hamstring muscle (located in the back of the thigh). Contact sports such as soccer, football, hockey, boxing, and wrestling put people at risk for strains. Gymnastics, tennis, rowing, golf, and other sports that require extensive gripping can increase the risk of hand and forearm strains. Elbow strains sometimes occur in people who participate in racquet sports, throwing, and contact sports.

What Are the Signs and Symptoms of a Strain?

Typically, people with a strain experience pain, muscle spasm, and muscle weakness. They can also have localized swelling, cramping, or inflammation, and with a minor or moderate strain, usually some loss of muscle function. Patients typically have pain in the injured area and general weakness of the muscle when they attempt to move it. Severe strains that partially or completely tear the muscle or tendon are often very painful and disabling.

How Are Sprains and Strains Treated?

Reduce Swelling and Pain

Treatment for sprains and strains is similar and can be thought of as having two stages. The goal during the first stage is to reduce swelling and pain. At this stage, doctors usually advise patients to follow a formula of rest, ice, compression, and elevation (RICE) for the first 24 to 48 hours after the injury. The doctor may also recommend an over-the-counter or prescription nonsteroidal anti-inflammatory drug, such as aspirin or ibuprofen, to help decrease pain and inflammation.

For people with a moderate or severe sprain, particularly of the ankle, a hard cast may be applied. Severe sprains and strains may require surgery to repair the torn ligaments, muscle, or tendons. Surgery is usually performed by an orthopaedic surgeon.

It is important that moderate and severe sprains and strains be evaluated by a doctor to allow prompt, appropriate treatment to begin. A person who has any concerns about the seriousness of a sprain or strain should always contact a doctor for advice.

RICE Therapy

Rest: Reduce regular exercise or activities of daily living as needed. Your doctor may advise you to put no weight on an injured area for 48 hours. If you cannot put weight on an ankle or knee, crutches may help. If you use a cane or one crutch for an ankle injury, use it on the uninjured side to help you lean away and relieve weight on the injured ankle.

Ice: Apply an ice pack to the injured area for 20 minutes at a time, 4 to 8 times a day. A cold pack, ice bag, or plastic bag filled with crushed ice and wrapped in a towel can be used. To avoid cold injury and frostbite, do not apply the ice for more than 20 minutes.

Compression: Compression of an injured ankle, knee, or wrist may help reduce swelling. Examples of compression bandages are elastic wraps, special boots, air casts, and splints. Ask your doctor for advice on which one to use.

Elevation: If possible, keep the injured ankle, knee, elbow, or wrist elevated on a pillow, above the level of the heart, to help decrease swelling.

Begin Rehabilitation

The second stage of treating a sprain or strain is rehabilitation. The overall goal is to improve the condition of the injured part and restore its function. The health care provider will prescribe an exercise program designed to prevent stiffness, improve range of motion, and restore the joint's normal flexibility and strength. Some patients may need physical therapy during this stage.

When the acute pain and swelling have diminished, the health care provider or physical therapist will instruct the patient to do a series of exercises several times a day. These are very important because they help reduce swelling, prevent stiffness, and restore normal, pain-free range of motion. The health care provider can recommend many different types of exercises, depending on the injury. For example, people with an ankle sprain may be told to rest their heel on the floor and write the alphabet in the air with their big toe. A patient with an injured knee or foot will work on weight-bearing and balancing exercises. The duration of the program depends on the extent of the injury, but the regimen commonly lasts for several weeks.

Another goal of rehabilitation is to increase strength and regain flexibility. Depending on the patient's rate of recovery, this process begins about the second week after the injury. The health care provider or physical therapist will instruct the patient to do a series of exercises designed to meet these goals. During this phase of rehabilitation, patients progress to more demanding exercises as pain decreases and function improves.

The final goal is the return to full daily activities, including sports when appropriate. Patients must work closely with their health care provider or physical therapist to determine their readiness to return to full activity. Sometimes people are tempted to resume full activity or play sports despite pain or muscle soreness. Returning to full activity before regaining normal range of motion, flexibility, and strength increases the chance of reinjury and may lead to a chronic problem.

The amount of rehabilitation and the time needed for full recovery after a sprain or strain depend on the severity of the injury and individual rates of healing. For example, a moderate ankle sprain may require 3 to 6 weeks of rehabilitation before a person can return to full activity. With a severe sprain, it can take 8 to 12 months before the ligament is fully healed. Extra care should be taken to avoid reinjury.

Can Sprains and Strains Be Prevented?

There are many things people can do to help lower their risk of sprains and strains:

- Maintain a healthy, well-balanced diet to keep muscles strong.
- Maintain a healthy weight.

169

- Practice safety measures to help prevent falls (for example, keep stairways, walkways, yards, and driveways free of clutter, and salt or sand icy patches in the winter).

- Wear shoes that fit properly.

- Replace athletic shoes as soon as the tread wears out or the heel wears down on one side. Do stretching exercises daily.

- Be in proper physical condition to play a sport.

- Warm up and stretch before participating in any sports or exercise.

- Wear protective equipment when playing.

- Avoid exercising or playing sports when tired or in pain.

- Run on even surfaces.

Additional Information

National Institute of Arthritis and Musculoskeletal and Skin Diseases Information Clearinghouse

NIAMS/National Institutes of Health
1 AMS Circle
Bethesda, MD 20892-3675
Toll-Free: 877-22-NIAMS
Tel: 301-495-4484
TTY: 301-565-2966
Fax: 301-718-6366
Website: www.nih.gov/niams
E-mail: niamsinfo@mail.nih.gov

American Academy of Orthopaedic Surgeons

6300 North River Road
Rosemont, IL 60018-4262
Toll-Free: 800-346-2267
Tel: 847-823-7186
Fax: 847-823-8125
Fax on Demand: 800-999-2939
Website: www.aaos.org

This professional association of orthopaedic surgeons publishes a variety of patient education brochures on common orthopaedic problems.

Key Words

Acute: An illness or injury that lasts for a short time and may be intense.

Chronic: An illness or injury that lasts for a long time.

Femur: The upper leg or thigh bone, which extends into the hip socket at its upper end and down to the knee at its lower end.

Fibula: The thin, outer bone of the leg that forms part of the ankle joint at its lower end.

Inflammation: A characteristic reaction of tissues to disease or injury; it is marked by four signs: swelling, redness, heat, and pain.

Joint: A junction where two bones meet.

Ligament: A band of tough, fibrous tissue that connects two or more bones at a joint and prevents excessive movement of the joint.

Muscle: Tissue composed of bundles of specialized cells that contract and produce movement when stimulated by nerve impulses.

Range of motion: The arc of movement of a joint from one extreme position to the other; range-of-motion exercises help increase or maintain flexibility and movement in muscles, tendons, ligaments, and joints.

Tendons: Tough, fibrous cords of tissue that connect muscle to bone.

Tibia: The thick, long bone of the lower leg (also called the shin) that forms part of the knee joint at its upper end and the ankle joint at its lower end.

Acknowledgments

The NIAMS gratefully acknowledges the assistance of James S. Panagis, M.D., M.P.H., of NIAMS; Jo A. Hannafin, M.D., Ph.D., of the Hospital for Special Surgery, New York, NY; and Harold B. Kitaoka, M.D., of the Mayo Clinic, Rochester, MN, in the preparation and review of this document.

Part Three

Trauma Injuries

Chapter 19

Trauma, Burn, Shock, and Injury Facts and Figures

Trauma

Trauma is defined as an injury caused by a physical force; examples include the consequences of motor vehicle accidents, falls, drowning, gunshots, fires and burns, and stabbing or other physical assault. Trauma kills more people between the ages of 1 and 44 than any other disease or illness. According to the National Center for Health Statistics, trauma (including unintentional injuries and homicides) causes:

- 43 percent of all deaths from ages 1-4
- 48 percent of all deaths from ages 5-14
- 62 percent of all deaths from ages 15-24

According to the American Trauma Society, 100,000 Americans of all ages die from trauma each year.

- Surgical procedures are considered a form of controlled injury, so many of the medical complications faced by surgery patients are very similar to those faced by trauma victims.

Shock

- Shock is defined as "circulatory collapse," when the arterial blood pressure is too low to maintain an adequate supply of

National Institute of General Medical Sciences (NIGMS), updated March 13, 2001.

blood to the body's tissues. Shock is characterized by cold and sweaty skin, weak and rapid pulse, irregular breathing, dry mouth, dilated pupils, and reduced flow of urine.

- Shock can be caused by internal or external bleeding (hypovolemic shock), dehydration, burns, or severe vomiting and/or diarrhea—all of which involve the loss of large amounts of bodily fluids.

- Other causes of shock include: the presence of microorganisms in the bloodstream (called bacteremic or septic shock), a severe allergic reaction (called anaphylactic shock), drug overdose (such as with narcotics or barbiturates), alterations in the ability of the heart to pump blood effectively (cardiogenic shock), and extreme emotional upset due to personal tragedy or disaster (neurogenic shock).

Burn

Burn is defined as tissue damage caused by a variety of agents, such as heat, chemicals, electricity, sunlight, or nuclear radiation. Most common are burns caused by scalds, building fires, and flammable liquids and gases.

- First-degree burns affect only the outer layer (called the epidermis) of the skin.

- Second-degree burns damage the epidermis and the layer beneath it (called the dermis).

- Third-degree burns involve damage or complete destruction of the skin to its full depth and damage to underlying tissues. People who experience such burns often require skin grafting.

- The swelling and blistering characteristic of burns are caused by the loss of fluid from damaged blood vessels.

- In severe cases, such fluid loss can cause shock, requiring immediate transfusion of the patient with blood or a physiological salt solution to restore adequate fluid levels to maintain blood pressure.

- Burns often lead to infection, due to damage to the skin's protective barrier. In many cases, topical antibiotics (creams or ointments applied to the skin) can prevent or treat such infection. The three topical antibiotics that are most widely used are silver sulfadiazene cream, mafenide acetate cream, and silver nitrate.

- According to the American Burn Association, each year in the United States, 1.25 million burn injuries require medical attention.

  - Approximately 50,000 of these require hospitalization, and roughly half of those burn patients are admitted to a specialized burn unit.

  - Each year, approximately 4,500 of these people die.

- Up to 10,000 people in the United States die every year of burn-related infections; pneumonia is the most common infectious complication among hospitalized burn patients.

  - Twenty years ago, burns covering half the body were routinely fatal; today, patients with burns covering 90 percent of the body can survive (but often with permanent impairments).

  - Practices that have contributed to this improvement include advances in resuscitation, wound cleaning and follow-up care, nutritional support, and infection control.

  - Grafting with natural or artificial materials can also speed the healing process.

- Complications following injury, shock, or burns may occur long after the initial incident, often when the patient is in an intensive care unit (ICU). Many ICU patients face similar medical problems regardless of the reason for their admission into the unit.

- The leading causes of death in ICUs are multiple organ system dysfunction, in which several of the body's organs fail at once, and adult respiratory distress syndrome, in which the lungs in particular fail. In both conditions, the organs of the body are ravaged by the patient's own immune system, leading to severe, debilitating, and uncontrolled inflammation.

- Improving methods of wound healing and tissue repair offers tremendous opportunities to enhance the quality of life for trauma and burn patients, and may also help to reduce health care costs.

• Scientists are investigating ways to treat wounds caused by trauma, burns, or surgical interventions with biological agents (e.g. growth factors) or new drugs.

• The National Institute of General Medical Sciences (NIGMS), one of the National Institutes of Health (NIH), sponsors research—mostly basic but some clinical—in the areas of burn, shock, and trauma. Other NIH components support or conduct research in aspects of trauma, burn, and injury related to their missions, as well.

Additional Information

National Institute of General Medical Sciences, NIH
45 Center Drive MSC 6200
Bethesda, MD 20892-6200
Tel: 301-496-7301
Website: www.nigms.nih.gov
E-mail: pub_info@nigms.nih.gov

Please review Chapter 62, "Directory of Resources," for additional resource listings.

Chapter 20

Abuse

Chapter Contents

Section 20.1

Combating Family Violence

"Combating Family Violence," *Office of Justice Programs Annual Report FY 2000,* Chapter 4, Office of Justice Programs.

The nature and extent of violence within the family is tragic and alarming. Family violence—intimate partner violence, child maltreatment, and elder abuse—is still a significant problem that often results in an increase in the use of criminal and civil justice processes. However, progress is being made in addressing this problem.

Building Knowledge about Violence against Women

Violence against women by intimate partners fell by 21 percent from 1993 through 1998, according to the Intimate Partner Violence report released by the Bureau of Justice Statistics (BJS) in May 2000. The data are from BJS's National Crime Victimization Survey, in which a nationally representative sample of men and women age 12 years old and older are interviewed twice a year. The report provides information on violence by intimates (current or former spouses, girlfriends, or boyfriends) and covers trends in intimate violence, characteristics of victims (race, sex, age, income, ethnicity, and whether the victims live in urban, suburban, or rural areas), type of crime (physical assault, verbal threats), and trends for reporting to police. Intimate victimizations measured include rape, sexual assault, robbery, aggravated assault, and simple assault. Data on murder by intimates are also given.

According to the report, an estimated 876,340 violent victimizations against women by intimate partners occurred during 1998 down from 1.1 million in 1993. In both 1993 and 1998 men were the victims of about 160,000 violent crimes by an intimate partner. On average each year from 1993-1998, 22 percent of all female victims of violence in the United States were attacked by an intimate partner, compared to 3 percent of all male violence victims.

Other highlights from the *Intimate Partner Violence* report include:

- Intimate partners committed fewer murders in 1996, 1997, or 1998 than in any other year since 1976;

- Between 1976 and 1998 the number of male victims of intimate partner murder fell an average 4 percent per year, and the number of female victims fell an average 1 percent;

- During 1998 women were the victims of intimate partner violence about five times more often than males, and;

- There were 767 female victims of intimate partner violence per 100,000 women in 1998, compared to 146 male victims.

According to data contained in the Federal Bureau of Investigation's Supplementary Homicide Reports:

- about 11 percent of all murders in 1998 (1,830 homicides) were the result of intimate partner violence, compared to about 3,000 such homicides in 1976;

- in 72 percent of the intimate partner homicides, the victim was female (1,320 incidents) compared to 50 percent in 1976;

- the number of white female intimate partner homicide victims rose 3 percent between 1976 and 1998;

- the number of black females killed by intimates fell 45 percent, black males fell 74 percent, and white males fell 44 percent;

- between 1997 and 1998, the number of white females murdered by an intimate partner increased 15 percent;

- between 1993 and 1998, women from 16 to 24 years old experienced the highest per capita rates of intimate victimization— 19.6 per 1,000 women;

- about half of the intimate partner violence against women was reported to police during the 6-year period; black women were more likely than other women to report such violence;

- among victims of violence by a domestic partner, the percentage of women who reported the violence to police was higher in 1998 (59 percent) than in 1993 (48 percent);

- half of the female intimate violence victims told the survey they were physically injured, and 37 percent of these victims sought professional medical treatment;

- about 45 percent of the female intimate violence victims lived in households with children younger than 12 years old; and

- among all U.S. households, 27 percent were homes of children younger than 12 years. However, it is not known to what extent young children in households with intimate violence witnessed that violence.

Although the incidence of family violence has shown a decline, family violence continues to occur across the country. In July 2000, OJP's National Institute of Justice and the Department of Health and Human Service's Centers for Disease Control and Prevention (CDCP) released the report, *Extent, Nature, and Consequences of Intimate Partner Violence: Findings from the National Violence Against Women Survey* (NVAWS). This study, which followed the release of the BJS *Intimate Partner Violence* report containing NCVS data, used a different method to collect the data. The NCVS asked respondents specifically about their experiences with crime, whereas the NVAWS was administered in the context of a personal safety survey. As a result, the surveys showed both similarities and differences in their findings. For example, both surveys indicate that women are much more likely to be victimized than men and are more likely to suffer injuries as a result of victimization. However, the surveys differ in the number of victimizations reported by survey respondents and the proportions of those reporting their victimization to the police. Both surveys are part of the Justice Department's efforts to develop multiple measures to improve understanding of violence between intimates and formulate more effective policy, including prevention and intervention tools.

According to the NVAWS report, nearly 25 percent of surveyed women and about 7 percent of surveyed men said they have been raped and/or physically assaulted by a current or former spouse or partner at some time in their lives. The NVAWS compared victimization rates among women and men, specific racial and ethnic groups, and same-sex and opposite-sex couples.

The NVAWS found the following:

- violence perpetrated against women by intimates is often accompanied by emotionally abusive and controlling behavior;

- women whose partners were jealous, controlling, or verbally abusive were significantly more likely to report being victimized;

- verbal abuse was found to be the behavior most likely to predict intimate partner victimization;

- rates of reported intimate partner violence varied significantly among women of different racial backgrounds;

- African-American and American Indian/Alaska Native women and men tended to report higher rates of intimate partner violence than women and men from other backgrounds;

- Asian/Pacific Islander women and men tended to report lower rates;

- women experience more chronic and injurious physical assaults in intimate partner relationships than do men;

- women who were physically assaulted by an intimate partner averaged 6.9 physical assaults by the same partner and men averaged 4.4 assaults; and

- more than 40 percent of women who were assaulted experienced an injury during their most recent assault, compared to 20 percent of the men.

Section 20.2

Dating Violence

National Center for Injury Prevention and Control (NCIPC),
reviewed January 27, 2000.

Dating violence may be defined as the perpetration or threat of an act of violence by at least one member of an unmarried couple on the other member within the context of dating or courtship.[1] This violence encompasses any form of sexual assault, physical violence, and verbal or emotional abuse.

Scope of the Problem

Violent behavior that takes place in a context of dating or courtship is not a rare event. Estimates vary because studies and surveys use different methods and definitions of the problem.

- A review of dating violence research found that prevalence rates of nonsexual, courtship violence range from 9% to 65%, depending on whether threats and emotional or verbal aggression were included in the definition.[1]

- Data from a study of 8th and 9th grade male and female students indicated that 25% had been victims of nonsexual dating violence and 8% had been victims of sexual dating violence.[2]

- Summarizing many studies, the average prevalence rate for nonsexual dating violence is 22% among male and female high school students and 32% among college students. Females are somewhat more likely than males to report being victims of violence.[1]

- In a national study of college students, 27.5% of the women surveyed said that they had suffered rape or attempted rape at least once since age 14.[3] Only 5% of those experiences were reported to the police.[3] The term "hidden rape" has emerged because this survey and many other studies found that sexual assaults are seldom reported to the police.[3,4,5,6,7]

- Over half of a representative sample of more than 1,000 female students at a large urban university had experienced some form of unwanted sex. Twelve percent of these acts were perpetrated by casual dates and 43% by steady dating partners.[8]

- Studies of college students [9,10] and high school students [11] suggest that both males and females inflict and receive dating violence in equal proportion, but the motivation for violence by women is more often for defensive purposes.[10,12] Other studies have found that women and girls were victims of dating violence twice as often as men and boys,[12,13] and that females suffer significantly more injuries than males.[12,13]

- A National Crime Victimization survey found that women were 6 times more likely than men to experience violence at the hands of an intimate partner.[14] Intimate partners include current or former spouses, boyfriends, girlfriends, dating partners, regardless of whether they are cohabiting or not.

- Nearly half of the 500,000 rapes and sexual assaults reported to the police by women of all ages were committed by friends or acquaintances.[14] From 80% to 95% of the rapes that occur on college campuses are committed by someone known to the victim.[8,15]

Risk Factors

Characteristics of Victims

- Young women aged 12-18 who are victims of violence are more likely than older women to report that their offenders were acquaintances, friends, or intimate partners.[14]

- The likelihood of becoming a victim of dating violence is associated with having female peers who have been sexually victimized,[16] lower church attendance,[17] greater number of past dating partners,[11] acceptance of dating violence,[11] and personally having experienced a previous sexual assault.[18]

Characteristics of Perpetrators

- Studies have found the following to be associated with sexual assault perpetration: the male having sexually aggressive peers; [18,19,20,21,22] heavy alcohol or drug use;[23,24] and the man's acceptance of dating violence,[11] the male's assumption of key roles in dating such as initiating the date, being the driver, and paying dating expenses; miscommunication about sex; previous sexual intimacy with the victim; interpersonal violence, traditional sex roles, adversarial attitudes about relationships, and rape myths.[23,24]

- Men who have a family history of observing or experiencing abuse are more likely to inflict abuse, violence, and sexual aggression.[16]

- As the consumption of alcohol by either the victim or perpetrator increases, the rate of serious injuries associated with dating violence also increases.[25]

References

1. Sugarman, D. B. and Hotaling, G. T. *Dating violence: prevalence, context and risk markers.* In: Pirog-Good, M. A. and Stets, J. E. (Eds.) Violence in dating relationships. New York: Praeger; 1989:3-32.

2. Foshee, V.A.; Linder, G.F.; Bauman, K.E.; Langwick, S.A.; Arriaga, X.B.; Heath, J.L.; McMahon, P.M.; Bangdiwala, S. The Safe Dates Project: Theoretical Basis, Evaluation Design,

and Selected Baseline Findings. Youth Violence Prevention: Description and baseline data from 13 evaluation projects (K. Powell; D. Hawkins, Eds.). *American Journal of Preventive Medicine, Supplement,* 1996; 12 (5):39-47.

3. Koss, M. P.; Gidycz, C. A.; and Wisniewski, N. The scope of rape: incidence and prevalence of sexual aggression and victimization in a national sample of higher education students. *J. Consult Clin. Psychology* 1987; 55:162-170.

4. Koss, M. P. The hidden rape victim: personality, attitudinal and situational characteristics. *Psychology of Women Quarterly* 1985;9:193-212.

5. Koss, M. P. Defending Date Rape. *Journal of Interpersonal Violence* 1992;7(1) 121-126.

6. Kilpatrick, D. G.; Best, C. L.; Veronen, L. J.; Amick, A. E.; Villeponteaux, L. A.; and Ruff, G. A. Mental health correlates of criminal victimization: A random community survey. *Journal of Consulting and Clinical Psychology* 1985; 53:866-873.

7. Russell, D. E. H. *Sexual exploitation: rape, child sexual abuse and workplace harrassment.* Beverly Hills, CA: Sage Publications; 1984.

8. Abbey, A.; Ross, L. T.; Mcduffie, D.; Mcauslan, P. Alcohol and dating risk factors for sexual assault among college women. *Psychology of Women Quarterly* 1996; 20(1)147-169.

9. Arias, I.; Samios, M.; and O'Leary, K. Daniel. Prevalence and correlates of physical aggression during courtship. *Journal of Interpersonal Violence* 1987;2(No. 1, March):82-90.

10. White, J. W. and Koss, M. P. *Courtship violence: incidence in a national sample of higher education students.* Violence and Victims 1991;6(4):247-256.

11. Gray, H.M.; Foshee, V. Adolescent Dating Violence: Differences between one-sided and mutually violent profiles. *Journal of Interpersonal Violence* 1997;12(1)126-141.

12. Makepeace, J. M. Gender differences in courtship violence victimization. *Family Relations* 1986;35:383-388.

13. Makepeace, J. M. Life events, stress and courtship violence. *Family Relations* 1983;32:101-109.

14. Bachman, R; Saltzman, L.E. *Violence Against Women: Estimates from the redesigned survey*, Bureau of Justice Statistics, Special Report, U.S. Department of Justice, August 1995.

15. Abbey, A. Acquaintance rape and alcohol consumption on college campuses: How are they linked? *College Health*. 1991; 39(January):165-169.

16. Gwartney-Gibbs, P. A.; Stockard, J.; and Bohmer, S. Learning courtship aggression: The influence of parents, peers and personal experiences. *Family Relations* 1987; 36:276-282.

17. Makepeace, J. M. Social factor and victim-offender differences in courtship violence. *Family Relations* 1987; 36:87-91.

18. Ageton, S. Sexual Assault Among Adolescents. Lexington, MA: Heath; 1983.

19. Adler, C. *An exploration of self-reported sexually aggressive behavior*. Crime and Delinquency1985;31: 301-331.

20. DeKeseredy, W. S. *Woman abuse in dating relationships*. Toronto, CA: Canadian Scholars' Press, Inc.; 1988.

21. Gwartney-Gibbs, P.; and Stockard, J. *Courtship aggression and mixed-sex peer groups*. In: Pirog-Good, Maureen A. and Stets, Jan E. (Eds.) Violence in Dating Relationships. New York, NY: Praeger Publishers; 1989: 185-204.

22. Kanin, E. J. *Date rapists: differential sexual socialization and relative deprivation*. Archives of Sexual Behavior 1985; 14:219-231.

23. Kanin, E.J. Date rape: unofficial criminals and victims. *Victimology: An International Journal* 1984;9(1): 95-108.

24. Muehlenhard, C. L.; Linton, M. A. Date rape and sexual aggression in dating situations: Incidence and risk factors. *J. Counseling Psychology* 1987;34:186-196.

25. Makepeace, J. M., *The severity of courtship violence and the effectiveness of individual precautions*. Family Abuse and Its Consequences. New Directions in Research (Gerald T. Hotaling, David Finkelhor, John T. Kirkpatrick, Murray A. Straus, Eds.) 1988: 297-311.

Section 20.3

Child Abuse

"Highlights from *Child Maltreatment 1999*," National Clearinghouse on Child Abuse and Neglect Information, updated April 2001; "The ABC's of Safe and Healthy Child Care," Division of Healthcare Quality Promotion (DHQP), January 1997; "The Co-Occurrence of Intimate Partner Violence Against Mothers and Abuse of Children" National Center for Injury Prevention and Control, 1999; and "FAQs about Child Fatalities," National Clearinghouse on Child Abuse and Neglect Information, updated April 2001.

This section presents highlights from the Federal publication *Child Maltreatment 1999*. The highlights are based on responses from the States to the 1999 National Child Abuse and Neglect Reporting System (NCANDS). Data were collected in aggregate through the Summary Data Component Survey or at the case level through the Detailed Case Data Component of NCANDS.

Referrals and Reports

As referrals of possible child maltreatment come to the attention of child protective services (CPS), they either are winnowed from consideration or transmitted further for investigation or assessment ("screened in" or "screened out") For those reports screened in, a further determination is made about whether to investigate. The role of the CPS agency includes deciding whether to take further protective actions on behalf of a child.

- Of the estimated 2,974,000 referrals received, approximately three-fifths (60.4%) were transferred for investigation or assessment and two-fifths (39.6%) were screened out.

- More than half of child abuse and neglect reports (54.7) were received from professionals. The remaining 45.3 percent of reports were submitted by nonprofessionals, including family and community members.

- Most States have established time standards for initiating the investigation of reports. The average response time to initiate investigating reports was 63.8 hours.*

- Slightly fewer than one-third of investigations (29.2%) resulted in a disposition of either substantiated or indicated child maltreatment. More than half (54.7%) resulted in a finding that child maltreatment was not substantiated.*

- The average annual workload of CPS investigation and assessment workers was 72 investigations.*

Child Maltreatment Victims

Victims of maltreatment are defined as children who are found to have experienced substantiated or indicated maltreatment or are found to be at risk of experiencing maltreatment.

- There were an estimated 826,000 victims of maltreatment nationwide. The 1999 rate of victimization, 11.8 per 1,000 children, decreased from the 1998 rate of 12.6.*

- Almost three-fifths of all victims (58.4%) suffered neglect, while one-fifth (21.3%) suffered physical abuse; 11.3 percent were sexually abused. More than one-third (35.9%) of all victims were reported to be victims of other or additional types of maltreatment.

- The highest victimization rates were for the 0-3 age group (13.9 maltreatments per 1,000 children of this age in the population), and rates declined as age increased.

- Rates of many types of maltreatment were similar for male and female children, but the sexual abuse rate for female children (1.6 female children for every 1,000 female children in the population) was higher than the sexual abuse rate for male children (0.4 male children per 1,000).

- Victimization rates by race/ethnicity ranged from a low of 4.4 Asian/Pacific Islander victims per 1,000 children of the same race in the population to 25.2 African-American victims per 1,000 children of the same race in the population.

- Children who had been victimized prior to 1999 were almost three times more likely to experience recurrence during the 6 months following their first victimization in 1999 than children without a prior history of victimization.

Perpetrators

A perpetrator of child abuse and/or neglect is a person who has maltreated a child while in a caretaking relationship to that child.

- Three-fifths (61.8%) of perpetrators were female. Female perpetrators were typically younger than their male counterparts—41.5 percent of female perpetrators were younger than 30 compared with 31.2 percent of male perpetrators who were younger than 30.

- Almost nine-tenths (87.3%) of all victims were maltreated by at least one parent. The most common pattern of maltreatment was a child victimized by a female parent acting alone (44.7%).

- Female parents were identified as the perpetrators of neglect and physical abuse for the highest percentage of child victims. In contrast, male parents were identified as the perpetrators of sexual abuse for the highest percentage of victims.

Fatalities

Child fatality estimates are based on data recorded by CPS agencies and/or other agencies.

- An estimated 1,100 children died of abuse and neglect, a rate of approximately 1.62 deaths per 100,000 children in the general population.*

- Slightly more than 2 percent (2.1%) of all fatalities occurred while the victim was in foster care.*

- Children younger than a year old accounted for 42.6 percent of the fatalities, and 86.1 percent were younger than 6 years of age.

- Maltreatment deaths were more often associated with neglect (38.2%) than with any other type of abuse.

- Slightly more than one-tenth (12.5%) of the families of child fatalities had received family preservation services in the 5 years prior to the deaths, while only 2.7 percent of the child fatality victims had been returned to the care of their families prior to their deaths.*

Services Provided

CPS agencies provide services to prevent future instances of child abuse and neglect and to remedy harm that has occurred as a result of child maltreatment. Preventive services are provided to parents whose children are at risk of abuse or neglect. Remedial or post-investigative services are offered to families that have experienced a child maltreatment episode.

- Nationwide, an estimated 1,563,000 children (22.3 out of every 1,000 children in the population) received preventive services.*

- The average time from the start of investigation to provision of service was 47.4 days.*

- Nationally, 55.8 percent of child victims (an estimated 461,000) received post-investigative services, and an additional 14.2 percent of children with unsubstantiated reports (an estimated 217,000) also received services.*

- Nationally, an estimated 171,000 child victims were placed in foster care. An estimated additional 49,000 children who were not victims (i.e., children with unsubstantiated reports) were placed in foster care.*

- About one-fifth (21.2%) of victims had received family preservation services within the previous 5 years, while more than 5 percent (5.1% of victims) had been reunited with their families in the previous five years.*

- Court actions were initiated for an estimated 26.1 percent of maltreatment victims. Four-fifths of these victims (79.3%) were provided with court-appointed representatives.*

*Findings required by the Child Abuse Prevention and Treatment Act, as amended in 1996, to be included in all annual State data reports to the Secretary of Health and Human Services. Because this is only the third year that many of these data have been required, not all States were able to provide data on every item.

Source: U.S. Department of Health and Human Services. *Child Maltreatment 1999: Reports from the States to the National Child Abuse and Neglect Data System.* (Washington, DC: U.S. Government Printing Office, 2001).

Intentional Injuries

Child abuse is harm to, or neglect of, a child by another person, whether adult or child. Child abuse happens in all cultural, ethnic, and income groups. Child abuse can be physical, emotional/verbal, sexual, or through neglect. Abuse may cause serious injury to the child and may even result in death. Signs of possible abuse include:

Physical Abuse

- Unexplained or repeated injuries such as welts, bruises, or burns. Injuries that are in the shape of an object (belt buckle, electric cord, etc.)

- Injuries not likely to happen given the age or ability of the child. For example, broken bones in a child too young to walk or climb.

- Disagreement between the child's and the parent's explanation of the injury.

- Unreasonable explanation of the injury.

- Obvious neglect of the child (dirty, undernourished, inappropriate clothes for the weather, lack of medical or dental care).

- Fearful behavior.

Emotional/Verbal Abuse

- Aggressive or withdrawn behavior.
- Shying away from physical contact with parents or adults.
- Afraid to go home.

Sexual Abuse

- Child tells you he/she was sexually mistreated.
- Child has physical signs such as:
  - difficulty in walking or sitting.
  - stained or bloody underwear.
  - genital or rectal pain, itching, swelling, redness, or discharge bruises or other injuries in the genital or rectal area.

- Child has behavioral and emotional signs such as:
  - difficulty eating or sleeping.
  - soiling or wetting pants or bed after being potty trained.
  - acting like a much younger child.
  - excessive crying or sadness.
  - withdrawing from activities and others.
  - talking about or acting out sexual acts beyond normal sex play for age.

Abuse can happen in any family, regardless of any special characteristics. However, in dealing with parents, be aware of characteristics of families in which abuse may be more likely:

- Families who are isolated and have no friends, relatives, church or other support systems.
- Parents who tell you they were abused as children.
- Families who are often in crisis (have money problems, move often).
- Parents who abuse drugs or alcohol.
- Parents who are very critical of their child.
- Parents who are very rigid in disciplining their child.
- Parents who show too much or too little concern for their child.
- Parents who feel they have a difficult child.
- Parents who are under a lot of stress.

If you suspect child abuse of any kind, you should:

- Take the child to a quiet, private area.
- Gently encourage the child to give you enough information to evaluate whether abuse may have occurred.
- Remain calm so as not to upset the child.
- If the child reveals the abuse, reassure him/her that you believe him/her, that he/she is right to tell you, and that he/she is not bad.
- Tell the child you are going to talk to persons who can help him/her.

- Return the child to the group (if appropriate).

- Record all information.

- Immediately report the suspected abuse to the proper local authorities. In most states, reporting suspected abuse is required by law.

If you employ other providers or accept volunteers to help you care for the children in your facility, you should check their background for a past history of child abuse or other criminal activity. Contact your local police department. Many states require that childcare providers have background and criminal history checks.

Dealing with child abuse is emotionally difficult for a provider. As a child care provider, you should get training in recognizing and reporting child abuse before you are confronted with a suspected case. If you suspect a case of child abuse, you may need to seek support from your local health department, child support services department, or other sources within your area.

Child Fatalities

Children are one of the most vulnerable groups in our society. Child fatalities due to maltreatment represent the worst case scenario in attempts to protect children. Despite the efforts of the child protection system, child fatalities remain a serious problem. Although the untimely deaths of children due to illness and accidents have been closely monitored, the same cannot be said of children who have died as the result of physical assault or severe neglect. Intervention strategies targeted at resolving this problem face complex challenges.

Child Fatalities Due to Maltreatment Are Increasing

Although child deaths caused by abuse and/or neglect are relatively infrequent, the rate of child maltreatment fatalities, confirmed by Child Protective Services (CPS) to have been the result of child maltreatment, has steadily increased over the last decade. The National Child Abuse and Neglect Data System (NCANDS) reported that in 1997 there were an estimated 1,196 child fatalities, or 1.7 children per 100,000 in the general population. (This estimate was based on reports from 41 States that reported a total of 967 fatalities.) The U.S. Advisory Board on Child Abuse and Neglect in *A Nation's Shame: Fatal Child Abuse and Neglect in the United States*, reported that a more realistic estimate of annual child deaths as a result of abuse and neglect, both known and unknown to CPS agencies, is about 2,000, or approximately five children per day. Experts such as Ryan Rainey from the National Center for Prosecution of Child Abuse believe that the number of child deaths from maltreatment per year may be as high as 5,000.

The Actual Number of Child Fatalities May Be Underreported

Determining the actual numbers of children who die annually from abuse is complex. Many researchers and practitioners believe that child fatalities are underreported because some deaths labeled as accidents, child homicides, and/or Sudden Infant Death Syndrome (SIDS) might be attributed to child maltreatment if more comprehensive investigations were conducted. It is difficult to distinguish a child who has been suffocated from a child who has died as a result of SIDS, or a child who was dropped, pushed, or thrown from a child who dies from a legitimate fall. Some researchers and practitioners have gone so far as to estimate that there may be twice the number of deaths as a result of abuse and/or neglect as are reported by NCANDS if cases unknown to CPS agencies are included.

There Is a Lack of Standard Terminology for Child Fatalities

To further complicate the issue, different terminology is used to discuss child fatalities, sometimes interchangeably. NCANDS defines "child fatality" as a child dying from abuse or neglect, because either (a) the injury from the abuse or neglect was the cause of death, or (b) the abuse and/or neglect was a contributing factor to the cause of death. Researchers such as Finkelhor and Christoffel use the term "child abuse homicide" to define a childhood death resulting from maltreatment (either assault or neglect) by a responsible caretaker. Law enforcement and criminal justice agencies also use the term "child abuse homicide," but their definition, while including the caretaker as perpetrator, also includes the "criminal act of homicide by non-caretakers" (death at the hands of another, felony child endangerment, and criminal neglect). More specifically, the term "infanticide" is increasingly used to define the murdering of children younger than 6 or 12 months by their parents.

Young Children Are the Most Vulnerable

Research supports that very young children (age 5 and younger) are the most frequent victims of child fatalities. NCANDS data for 1997 from a subset of States demonstrated that children 3 or younger accounted for 77 percent of fatalities. This population is the most vulnerable for many reasons including their small size and inability to defend themselves. The fatal abuse usually occurs in one of two ways: repeated abuse and/or neglect over a period of time (battered child syndrome) or in a single, impulsive incident of assault (drowning, suffocating, or shaking the baby, for example).

Primary Caretakers Are the Most Frequent Perpetrators

No matter how the fatal abuse occurs, one fact of great concern is that most of the perpetrators are, by definition, primary caretakers such as parents and other relatives.

Though there is no single profile for the perpetrator of fatal child abuse, there are consistent characteristics that reappear in studies. Frequently the perpetrator is a young adult in his/her mid-20s without a high school diploma, living at or below the poverty level, depressed, and who may have difficulty coping with stressful situations. In many instances, the perpetrator has experienced violence first-hand.

The Response to Fatal Child Abuse or Neglect Is Complex

The response to the problem is often hampered by inconsistencies:

- The inaccurate reporting of the number of children who die each year as a result of abuse and neglect

- The lack of national standards for child autopsies or death investigations

- The different roles that CPS agencies play in the investigation process

- The use in many States of an elected coroner who is not required to have any medical or child abuse and neglect training rather than a medical examiner.

Child Fatality Review Teams

To address some of these inconsistencies, multidisciplinary/multiagency Child Fatality Review Teams have emerged in many States to provide a coordinated approach to the investigation of child deaths. These teams are comprised of prosecutors, coroners or medical examiners, law enforcement personnel, CPS workers, public health care providers, and others.

The teams review cases of child deaths and facilitate appropriate follow-up. The follow-up may include assuring that services are provided for surviving family members, providing information to assist in the prosecution of perpetrators, and developing recommendations to improve child protection and community support systems. In addition, teams can assist in determining avenues for prevention efforts and improving training for front-line workers. Well-designed, properly organized Child Fatality Review Teams appear to offer the greatest hope for defining the underlying nature and scope of fatalities due to child abuse and neglect and for offering solutions.

Prevention Services Are Key

When addressing the issue of child maltreatment, and especially child fatalities, prevention is a recurring theme. In 1995, the U.S. Advisory Board on Child Abuse and Neglect recommended a universal approach to the prevention of child fatalities that would reach out to all families through the implementation of several key strategies. These efforts would begin by providing services such as home visitation by trained professionals or paraprofessionals, hospital-linked outreach to parents of infants and toddlers, community-based programs designed for the specific needs of neighborhoods, and effective public education campaigns.

References

Christoffel, K.K. (1992). Child abuse fatalities. In S. Ludwig, & A.E. Kornberg. (Eds.), *Child abuse. A medical reference* (2nd ed.). New York: Churchill Livingstone, Inc.

Department of Justice. Office of Juvenile Justice and Delinquency Programs. (1994, February 16–17). *Child fatality review teams: A multi-agency approach.* (Participant Guide). National Training Teleconference.

Finkelhor, D. (1997). In G. Kaufman Kantor, & J. Jasinski (Eds.), *Out of the darkness: Contemporary perspectives on family violence.* Thousand Oaks, CA: Sage Publications.

Kaplan S.R. (1996). *Child fatalities and child fatality review teams.* Washington, DC: ABA Center on Children and the Law.

Lewit, E.M. (1994). Reported child abuse and neglect. *In The future of children (Sexual Abuse of Children)*,(4)2.

U.S. Advisory Board on Child Abuse and Neglect. (1995). *A nation's shame: Fatal child abuse and neglect in the United States*. Washington, DC: U.S. Department of Health and Human Services.

U.S. Department of Health and Human Services, Children's Bureau. (1999). *Child maltreatment 1997: Reports from the states to the national child abuse and neglect data system*. Washington, DC: U.S. Government Printing Office.

National Center on Child Abuse and Neglect. (1992). *National child abuse and neglect data system: 1990 summary data component, Working Paper 1*. Washington, DC: U.S. Department of Health and Human Services.

Walsh, B. (1994). Section II: Criminal Investigation of Physical Abuse and Neglect. In J. Briere, L. Berliner, J.A. Bulkley, C. Jenny, & T. Reid (Eds.), *The APSAC handbook on child maltreatment*. Chicago, IL: American Professional Society on the Abuse of Children (APSAC).

Wang, C.T., & Daro, D. (1998). *Current trends in child abuse reporting and fatalities: The results of the 1997 Annual Fifty State Survey*. Chicago, IL: National Committee to Prevent Child Abuse.

The Co-Occurrence of Intimate Partner Violence against Mothers and Abuse of Children

Violence against mothers by their intimate partners is a serious risk factor for child abuse.[1] Conversely, mothers of abused children are at higher risk of being abused than mothers of non-abused children.[2] Co-occurrence of violence against mothers and their children by intimate partners of women is critical for community advocates, child protection workers, educators and maternal and child health care providers and others to address the safety of mothers and their children.[3,4]

Scope of the Problem

The concurrence "rate" of child abuse and intimate partner violence against mothers is defined as the proportion of families in the population or sample in which a woman and her child are both victims of violence by an intimate. In the mother's case, the intimate is her partner: the child may be abused by the mother's intimate partner or the battered mother. Concurrence rates vary widely in the literature; however, the quality of these studies, their data sources and their definitions of abuse also vary considerably. Approximately 20 studies exist with original data on concurrence rates.

The four most rigorous studies describe concurrence rates of approximately 50%. These four studies utilized samples representative of the U.S. population, multivariate analyses or control samples.[2, 5, 6, 7] Selected results are presented.

McKibben and colleagues,[2] the only study to use a control population, found that 40%-60% of mothers of 32 abused children were also victimized compared to 13% of mothers of 32 matched children with no record of abuse in an urban public hospital. A fifth study supports the results of the smaller, controlled study. Stark and Flitcraft (n=116; concurrence rate=32-45%) used a retrospective hospital record review and a similar data classification method.[8]

Ross' analysis[7] of 3,363 American parents interviewed for the 1985 National Family Violence Survey [6] indicates that each additional act of violence toward a spouse increases the probability of the violent spouse also being abusive to the child, particularly for fathers. Women who were the most chronically violent to their spouse had a 38% probability of also physically abusing a male child, the gender most often physically abused. However, the most chronically violent husbands had a nearly 100% probability of also physically abusing their male children.

The Ross[7] results suggests that measurement of concurrence rates will vary significantly by gender of the abusive partner as well as the child, and by intensity of the abuse. Future studies should include these risk factors in the analyses.

References

1. Stark E, Flitcraft A. Spouse Abuse (p. 142) in *Violence in America: a Public Health Approach* Eds. Rosenberg and Fenley: Oxford University Press, 1991.

2. McKibben L, DeVos E, Newberger E. Victimization of Mothers of Abused Children: A Controlled Study. *Pediatrics* 1989;84:531-535.

3. Wright RJ, Wright RO, Isaac NE. Response to battered mothers in the pediatric emergency department: a call for an interdisciplinary approach to family violence. *Pediatrics* 1997;99:186-192.

4. Peled E. The battered women's movement response to children of battered women: a critical analysis. *Violence Against Women* 1997;3:424-446.

5. Straus M, Gelles RJ, Steinmetz SK. 1980. *Behind Closed Doors: Violence in the American Family.* New York: Doubleday/Anchor.

6. Straus M, Gelles. 1990. *Physical violence in American families: Risk Factors and adaptations to violence in 8,145 families.* New Brunswick, NJ: Transaction Publishers.

7. Ross S. Risk of Physical Abuse to Children of Spouse Abusing Parents. *Child Abuse and Neglect* 1996;20:589-598.

8. Stark E, Flitcraft AH. Women and children at risk: a feminist perspective on child abuse. *International Journal of Health Service* 1988;18:97-118.

9. Nudelman J, Durborow N, Gramb M, Letellier P. Best Practices: Innovative Domestic Violence Programs in Health Care Settings. The Family Violence Prevention Fund, 1997.(Ph: (415) 252-8900; Website: www.fvpf.org/health/)

10. Hangen, E. (1994) *DSS (Dept. of Social Services) Interagency Domestic Violence Team Pilot Project: Program data evaluation.* Boston: Massachusetts Department of Social Services.

Section 20.4

Elder Abuse

This section includes an excerpt from "Elder Abuse Prevention," Fact Sheet, Administration on Aging, 2001; "What Is Elder Abuse?" National Center on Elder Abuse (NCEA); and Table 4-14 of "The National Elder Abuse Incidence Study; Final Report," Administration on Aging, September 1998.

Elder Abuse Is a Serious Problem

Each year hundreds of thousands of older persons are abused, neglected, and exploited by family members and others. Many victims are people who are older, frail, vulnerable, and who cannot help themselves and depend on others to meet their most basic needs.

Legislatures in all 50 states have passed some form of elder abuse prevention laws. Laws and definitions of terms vary considerably from one state to another, but all states have set up reporting systems. Generally, adult protective services (APS) agencies receive and investigate reports of suspected elder abuse.

National Elder Abuse Incidence Study

Reports to APS agencies of domestic elder abuse increased 150 percent between 1986 and 1996. This increase dramatically exceeded the 10 percent increase in the older population over the same period.

A national incidence study conducted in 1996 found the following:

- 551,011 persons, aged 60 and over, experienced abuse, neglect, and/or self-neglect in a one-year period;

- Almost four times as many new incidents of abuse, neglect, and/ or self-neglect were not reported as those that were reported to and substantiated by adult protective services agencies;

- Persons, aged 80 years and older, suffered abuse and neglect two to three times their proportion of the older population; and

- Among known perpetrators of abuse and neglect, the perpetrator was a family member in 90 percent of cases. Two-thirds of the perpetrators were adult children or spouses.

What Are the Major Types of Elder Abuse?

Federal definitions of elder abuse, neglect, and exploitation appeared for the first time in the 1987 Amendments to the Older Americans Act. These definitions were provided in the law only as guidelines for identifying the problems and not for enforcement purposes. Currently, elder abuse is defined by state laws, and state definitions vary considerably from one jurisdiction to another in terms of what constitutes the abuse, neglect, or exploitation of the elderly. In addition, researchers have used many different definitions to study the problem. Broadly defined, however, there are three basic categories of elder abuse:

1. domestic elder abuse;
2. institutional elder abuse; and
3. self-neglect or self-abuse.

In most cases, state statutes addressing elder abuse provide the definitions of these different categories of elder abuse, with varying degrees of specificity.

Domestic elder abuse generally refers to any of several forms of maltreatment of an older person by someone who has a special relationship with the elder (e.g., a spouse, a sibling, a child, a friend, or a caregiver in the older person's own home or in the home of a caregiver.)

Institutional abuse, on the other hand, generally refers to any of the above-mentioned forms of abuse that occur in residential facilities for older persons (e.g., nursing homes, foster homes, group homes, board and care facilities). Perpetrators of institutional abuse usually are persons who have a legal or contractual obligation to provide elder victims with care and protection (e.g., paid caregivers, staff, professionals).

Definitions and legal terms vary from state to state in regards to the types of domestic elder abuse that NCEA recognizes as well as their signs and symptoms.

Physical Abuse

Physical abuse is defined as the use of physical force that may result in bodily injury, physical pain, or impairment. Physical abuse may include but is not limited to such acts of violence as striking (with or without an object), hitting, beating, pushing, shoving, shaking, slapping, kicking, pinching, and burning. In addition, the inappropriate use of drugs and physical restraints, force-feeding, and physical punishment of any kind also are examples of physical abuse.

Signs and symptoms of physical abuse include but are not limited to:

- bruises, black eyes, welts, lacerations, and rope marks;
- bone fractures, broken bones, and skull fractures;
- open wounds, cuts, punctures, untreated injuries in various stages of healing;
- sprains, dislocations, and internal injuries/bleeding;
- broken eyeglasses/frames, physical signs of being subjected to punishment, and signs of being restrained;
- laboratory findings of medication overdose or under utilization of prescribed drugs;
- an elder's report of being hit, slapped, kicked, or mistreated;
- an elder's sudden change in behavior;
- and the caregiver's refusal to allow visitors to see an elder alone.

Sexual Abuse

Sexual abuse is defined as non-consensual sexual contact of any kind with an elderly person. Sexual contact with any person incapable of giving consent is also considered sexual abuse. It includes but is not limited to unwanted touching, all types of sexual assault or battery, such as rape, sodomy, coerced nudity, and sexually explicit photographing.

Signs and symptoms of sexual abuse include but are not limited to:

- bruises around the breasts or genital area;
- unexplained venereal disease or genital infections;
- unexplained vaginal or anal bleeding;

- torn, stained, or bloody underclothing;
- and an elder's report of being sexually assaulted or raped.

Emotional or Psychological Abuse

Emotional or psychological abuse is defined as the infliction of anguish, pain, or distress through verbal or nonverbal acts. Emotional/psychological abuse includes but is not limited to verbal assaults, insults, threats, intimidation, humiliation, and harassment. In addition, treating an older person like an infant; isolating an elderly person from his/her family, friends, or regular activities; giving an older person the "silent treatment;" and enforced social isolation are examples of emotional/psychological abuse.

Signs and symptoms of emotional/psychological abuse include but are not limited to:

- being emotionally upset or agitated;
- being extremely withdrawn and non-communicative or non-responsive;
- unusual behavior usually attributed to dementia (e.g., sucking, biting, rocking);
- and an elder's report of being verbally or emotionally mistreated.

Neglect

Neglect is defined as the refusal or failure to fulfill any part of a person's obligations or duties to an elder. Neglect may also include failure of a person who has fiduciary responsibilities to provide care for an elder (e.g., pay for necessary home care services) or the failure on the part of an in-home service provider to provide necessary care. Neglect typically means the refusal or failure to provide an elderly person with such life necessities as food, water, clothing, shelter, personal hygiene, medicine, comfort, personal safety, and other essentials included in an implied or agreed-upon responsibility to an elder.

Signs and symptoms of neglect include but are not limited to:

- dehydration, malnutrition, untreated bed sores, and poor personal hygiene;
- unattended or untreated health problems;
- hazardous or unsafe living condition/arrangements (e.g., improper wiring, no heat, or no running water);

- unsanitary and unclean living conditions (e.g. dirt, fleas, lice on person, soiled bedding, fecal/urine smell, inadequate clothing); and

- an elder's report of being mistreated.

Abandonment

Abandonment is defined as the desertion of an elderly person by an individual who has assumed responsibility for providing care for an elder, or by a person with physical custody of an elder.

Signs and symptoms of abandonment include but are not limited to:

- the desertion of an elder at a hospital, a nursing facility, or other similar institution;

- the desertion of an elder at a shopping center or other public location; and

- an elder's own report of being abandoned.

Financial or Material Exploitation

Financial or material exploitation is defined as the illegal or improper use of an elder's funds, property, or assets. Examples include but are not limited to cashing an elderly person's checks without authorization/permission; forging an older person's signature; misusing or stealing an older person's money or possessions; coercing or deceiving an older person into signing any document (e.g., contracts or will); and the improper use of conservatorship, guardianship, or power of attorney.

Signs and symptoms of financial or material exploitation include but are not limited to:

- sudden changes in bank account or banking practice, including an unexplained withdrawal of large sums of money by a person accompanying the elder;

- the inclusion of additional names on an elder's bank signature card;

- unauthorized withdrawal of the elder's funds using the elder's ATM card;

- abrupt changes in a will or other financial documents;

- unexplained disappearance of funds or valuable possessions;

- substandard care being provided or bills unpaid despite the availability of adequate financial resources;

- discovery of an elder's signature being forged for financial transactions or for the titles of his/her possessions;

- sudden appearance of previously uninvolved relatives claiming their rights to an elder's affairs and possessions;

- unexplained sudden transfer of assets to a family member or someone outside the family;

- the provision of services that are not necessary; and

- an elder's report of financial exploitation.

Self-Neglect

Self-neglect is characterized as the behavior of an elderly person that threatens his/her own health or safety. Self-neglect generally manifests itself in an older person as a refusal or failure to provide himself/herself with adequate food, water, clothing, shelter, personal hygiene, medication (when indicated), and safety precautions. The definition of self-neglect excludes a situation in which a mentally competent older person, who understands the consequences of his/her decisions, makes a conscious and voluntary decision to engage in acts that threaten his/her health or safety as a matter of personal choice.

Signs and symptoms of self-neglect include but are not limited to:

- dehydration, malnutrition, untreated or improperly attended medical conditions, and poor personal hygiene;

- hazardous or unsafe living conditions/arrangements (e.g., improper wiring, no indoor plumbing, no heat, no running water);

- unsanitary or unclean living quarters (e.g., animal/insect infestation, no functioning toilet, fecal/urine smell);

- inappropriate and/or inadequate clothing, lack of the necessary medical aids (e.g., eyeglasses, hearing aids, dentures); and

- grossly inadequate housing or homelessness.

Why Does Elder Abuse Occur and Who are the Perpetrators?

Elder abuse, like other types of domestic violence, is extremely complex. Generally a combination of psychological, social, and economic factors, along with the mental and physical conditions of the victim and the perpetrator, contribute to the occurrence of elder maltreatment. Although the factors listed below cannot explain all types of elder maltreatment because it is likely that different types (as well as each single incident) involve different casual factors, they are some of the causes researchers say are important.

Caregiver Stress

Caring for frail older people is a very difficult and stress-provoking task. This is particularly true when older people are mentally or physically impaired, when the caregiver is ill-prepared for the task, or when the needed resources are lacking. Under these circumstances, the increased stress and frustration of a caregiver may lead to abuse or willful neglect.

Impairment of Dependent Elder

Some researchers have found that elders in poor health are more likely to be abused than those in good health. They have also found that abuse tends to occur when the stress level of the caregiver is heightened as a result of a worsening of the elder's impairment.

Cycle of Violence

Some families are more prone to violence than others because violence is a learned behavior and is transmitted from one generation to another. In these families, abusive behavior is the normal response to tension or conflict because they have not learned any other ways to respond.

Personal Problems of Abusers

Researchers have found that abusers of the elderly (typically adult children) tend to have more personal problems than do non-abusers. Adult children who abuse their parents frequently suffer from such problems as mental and emotional disorders, alcoholism, drug addiction, and financial difficulty. Because of these problems, these adult children are often dependent on the elders for their support. Abuse in these cases may be an inappropriate response by the children to the sense of their own inadequacies.

Who Are the Abusers?

More than two-thirds of elder abuse perpetrators are family members of the victims, typically serving in a caregiving role.

Table 20.1. Relationship of Perpetrators to Victims of Domestic Elder Abuse for Selected Types of Maltreatment[1]

Income Category	Neglect	Emotional/ Psychological	Physical abuse	Financial/ Material	Abandon- ment
Child	43.2%	53.9%	48.6%	60.4%	79.5%
Sibling	8.7%*	1.8%*	4.7%*	1.3%*	0.0%
Grandchild	8.8%*	8.9%*	5.6%*	9.2%*	6.6%*
Parent	0.5%*	0.0%*	0.8%*	0.0%*	0.0%*
Spouse	30.3%*	12.6%	23.4%	4.9%*	6.4%*
Other Relative	3.7%*	11.7%*	5.4%*	9.7%*	0.0%*
Friend or Neighbor	1.6%*	10.3%	10.2%	8.7%	*0.0%*
In-home service provider	4.2%*	0.9%*	0.2%*	1.7%*	7.4%*
Out-of-home service provider	0.0%*	0.0%*	1.2%*	4.1%*	0.0%*
Percentage of total perpetrators	47.8%	36.1%	26.9%	30.4%	4.2%*

[1]Based on an estimated 59,218 substantiated incidents of elder abuse. Some entries have missing values.

*The confidence band for these numbers is wide, relative to the size of the estimate. The true number may be close to zero or much larger than the estimate.

Is Elder Abuse a Crime?

Depending on the statute of a given state, elder abuse may or may not be a crime. However, most physical, sexual, and financial/material abuses are considered crimes in all states. In addition, depending on the type of the perpetrator's conduct and its consequences for the victims, certain emotional abuse and neglect cases are subject to criminal prosecution. However, self-neglect is not a crime in all jurisdictions, and, in fact, elder abuse laws of some states do not address self-neglect.

For Help Regarding Elder Abuse

When domestic elder abuse occurs, it can be addressed—if it comes to the attention of authorities. Although each state has a different system to address elder abuse, the following are some of the agencies that have been established by federal, state, and local governments to help.

Which State and Local Agencies are Helping Victims and Their Families Involved in Elder Abuse?

In most states, the APS (Adult Protective Services) agency, typically located within the human service agency, is the principal public agency responsible for both investigating reported cases of elder abuse and for providing victims and their families with treatment and protective services. In most jurisdictions, the county departments of social services maintain an APS unit that serves the need of local communities.

However, many other public and private agencies and organizations are actively involved in efforts to protect vulnerable older persons from abuse, neglect, and exploitation. Some of these agencies include:

- the state unit on aging;

- the law enforcement agency (e.g., the police department, the district attorney's office, the court system, the sheriff's department);

- the medical examiner/coroner's office;

- hospitals and medical clinics;

- the state long-term care ombudsman's office;

- the public health agency; the area agency on aging;

- the mental health agency; and the facility licensing/certification agency.

Depending on the state law governing elder abuse, the exact roles and functions of these agencies vary widely from one jurisdiction to another.

Although most APS agencies also handle adult abuse cases (where clients are between 18 and 59 years of age), nearly 70 percent of their caseloads involve elder abuse. The APS community is relatively small compared with the groups working for other human service programs, but it is composed of a few thousand professionals, nationwide.

Section 20.5

Alcohol, Violence, and Aggression

Alcohol Alert No. 38-1997, National Institute on Alcohol Abuse and Alcoholism (NIAAA).

Scientists and nonscientists alike have long recognized a two-way association between alcohol consumption and violent or aggressive behavior.[1] Not only may alcohol consumption promote aggressiveness, but victimization may lead to excessive alcohol consumption. Violence may be defined as behavior that intentionally inflicts, or attempts to inflict, physical harm. Violence falls within the broader category of aggression, which also includes behaviors that are threatening, hostile, or damaging in a nonphysical way.[2] This section explores the association between alcohol consumption, violence, and aggression and the role of the brain in regulating these behaviors. Understanding the nature of these associations is essential to breaking the cycle of alcohol misuse and violence.

Extent of the Alcohol-Violence Association

Based on published studies, Roizen[3] summarized the percentages of violent offenders who were drinking at the time of the offense as follows: up to 86 percent of homicide offenders, 37 percent of assault offenders, 60 percent of sexual offenders, up to 57 percent of men and 27 percent of women involved in marital violence, and 13 percent of child abusers. These figures are the upper limits of a wide range of estimates. In a community-based study, Pernanen[4] found that 42 percent of violent crimes reported to the police involved alcohol, although 51 percent of the victims interviewed believed that their assailants had been drinking.

Alcohol-Violence Relationships

Several models have been proposed to explain the complex relationships between violence or aggression and alcohol consumption. To avoid exposing human or animal subjects to potentially serious injury, research results discussed below are largely based on experiments on nonphysical aggression. Other studies involving humans are based on epidemiological surveys or data obtained from archival or official sources.

Alcohol Misuse Preceding Violence

Direct Effects of Alcohol. Alcohol may encourage aggression or violence by disrupting normal brain function. According to the disinhibition hypothesis, for example, alcohol weakens brain mechanisms that normally restrain impulsive behaviors, including inappropriate aggression.[5] By impairing information processing, alcohol can also lead a person to misjudge social cues, thereby overreacting to a perceived threat.[6] Simultaneously, a narrowing of attention may lead to an inaccurate assessment of the future risks of acting on an immediate violent impulse.[7]

Many researchers have explored the relationship of alcohol to aggression using variations of an experimental approach developed more than 35 years ago.[8,9] In a typical example, a subject administers electric shocks or other painful stimuli to an unseen "opponent," ostensibly as part of a competitive task involving learning and reaction time. Unknown to the subject, the reactions of the nonexistent opponent are simulated by a computer. Subjects perform both while sober and after consuming alcohol. In many studies, subjects exhibited increased aggressiveness (e.g., by administering stronger shocks) in proportion to increasing alcohol consumption.[10]

These findings suggest that alcohol may facilitate aggressive behavior. However, subjects rarely increased their aggression unless they felt threatened or provoked. Moreover, neither intoxicated nor sober participants administered painful stimuli when nonaggressive means of communication (e.g., a signal lamp) were also available.[5,9]

These results are consistent with the real-world observation that intoxication alone does not cause violence.[4] The following subsections explore some mechanisms whereby alcohol's direct effects may interact with other factors to influence the expression of aggression.

Social and Cultural Expectancies. Alcohol consumption may promote aggression because people expect it to.[5] For example, research using real and mock alcoholic beverages shows that people who believe they have consumed alcohol begin to act more aggressively, regardless of which beverage they actually consumed.[10] Alcohol-related expectancies that promote male aggressiveness, combined with the widespread perception of intoxicated women as sexually receptive and less able to defend themselves, could account for the association between drinking and date rape.[11]

In addition, a person who intends to engage in a violent act may drink to bolster his or her courage or in hopes of evading punishment or censure.[12,13] The motive of drinking to avoid censure is encouraged by the popular view of intoxication as a "time-out," during which one is not subject to the same rules of conduct as when sober.[14,15]

Violence Preceding Alcohol Misuse

Childhood Victimization. A history of childhood sexual abuse[16] or neglect[17] is more likely among women with alcohol problems than among women without alcohol problems. Widom and colleagues[17] found no relationship between childhood victimization and subsequent alcohol misuse in men. Even children who only witness family violence may learn to imitate the roles of aggressors or victims, setting the stage for alcohol abuse and violence to persist over generations.[18] Finally, obstetric complications that damage the nervous system at birth, combined with subsequent parental neglect such as might occur in an alcoholic family, may predispose one to violence, crime, and other behavioral problems by age 18.[19,20]

Violent Lifestyles. Violence may precede alcohol misuse in offenders as well as victims. For example, violent people may be more likely than nonviolent people to select or encounter social situations and subcultures that encourage heavy drinking.[21] In summary, violence may contribute to alcohol consumption, which in turn may perpetuate violence.

Common Causes for Alcohol Misuse and Violence

In many cases, abuse of alcohol and a propensity to violence may stem from a common cause.[22] This cause may be a temperamental trait, such as a risk-seeking personality, or a social environment (e.g., delinquent peers or lack of parental supervision) that encourages or contributes to deviant behavior.[21]

Another example of a common cause relates to the frequent co-occurrence of antisocial personality disorder (ASPD) and early-onset (i.e., type II) alcoholism.[23] ASPD is a psychiatric disorder characterized by a disregard for the rights of others, often manifested as a violent or criminal lifestyle. Type II alcoholism is characterized by high inheritability from father to son; early onset of alcoholism (often during adolescence); and antisocial, sometimes violent, behavioral traits.[24] Type II alcoholics and persons with ASPD overlap in their tendency to violence and excessive alcohol consumption and may share a genetic basis.[23]

Spurious Associations

Spurious associations between alcohol consumption and violence may arise by chance or coincidence, with no direct or common cause. For example, drinking is a common social activity for many adult Americans, especially those most likely to commit violent acts. Therefore, drinking and violence may occur together by chance.[5] In addition, violent criminals who drink heavily are more likely than less intoxicated offenders to be caught and consequently are overrepresented in samples of convicts or arrestees.[7] Spurious associations may sometimes be difficult to distinguish from common-cause associations.

Physiology of Violence

Although individual behavior is shaped in part by the environment, it is also influenced by biological factors (e.g., hormones) and ultimately planned and directed by the brain. Individual differences in brain chemistry may explain the observation that excessive alcohol consumption may consistently promote aggression in some persons, but not in others.[25] The following subsections highlight some areas of intensive study.

Serotonin

Serotonin, a chemical messenger in the brain, is thought to function as a behavioral inhibitor. Thus, decreased serotonin activity is associated with increased impulsivity and aggressiveness[26] as well as with early-onset alcoholism among men.[27]

Researchers have developed an animal model that simulates many of the characteristics of alcoholism in humans. Rhesus macaque monkeys sometimes consume alcohol in sufficient quantities to become intoxicated. Macaques with low serotonin activity consume alcohol at elevated rates;[25] these monkeys also demonstrate impaired impulse control, resulting in excessive and inappropriate aggression.[25,27] This behavior and brain chemistry closely resemble that of type II alcoholics. Interestingly, among both macaques and humans, parental neglect leads to early-onset aggression and excessive alcohol consumption in the offspring, again correlated with decreased serotonin activity.[27]

Although data are inconclusive, the alcohol-violence link may be mediated by chemical messengers in addition to serotonin, such as dopamine and norepinephrine.[28] There is also considerable overlap among nerve cell pathways in the brain that regulate aspects of aggression,[29] sexual behavior, and alcohol consumption.[30] These observations suggest a biological basis for the frequent co-occurrence of alcohol intoxication and sexual violence.

Testosterone

The steroid hormone testosterone is responsible for the development of male primary and secondary sexual characteristics. High testosterone concentrations in criminals have been associated with violence, suspiciousness, and hostility.[31,32] In animal experiments, alcohol administration increased aggressive behavior in socially dominant squirrel monkeys, who already exhibited high levels of aggression and testosterone.[33] Alcohol did not, however, increase aggression in subordinate monkeys, which exhibited low levels of aggression and testosterone.[6]

These findings may shed some light on the life cycle of violence in humans. In humans, violence occurs largely among adolescent and young adult males, who tend to have high levels of testosterone compared with the general population. Young men who exhibit antisocial behaviors often "burn out" with age, becoming less aggressive when they reach their forties.[34] By that age, testosterone concentrations are decreasing, while serotonin concentrations are increasing, both factors that tend to restrain violent behavior.[35]

Conclusion

No one model can account for all individuals or types of violence. Alcohol apparently may increase the risk of violent behavior only for certain individuals or subpopulations and only under some situations and social/cultural influences.[4,36]

Although much remains to be learned, research suggests that some violent behavior may be amenable to treatment and some may be preventable. One study found decreased levels of marital violence in couples who completed behavioral marital therapy for alcoholism and remained sober during follow-up.[37] Results of another study[7] suggest that a 10-percent increase in the beer tax could reduce murder by 0.3 percent, rape by 1.32 percent, and robbery by 0.9 percent. Although these results are modest, they indicate a direction for future research. In addition, preliminary experiments have identified medications that have the potential to reduce violent behavior. Such medications include certain anticonvulsants (e.g., carbamazepine);[38] mood stabilizers (e.g., lithium);[39] and antidepressants, especially those that increase serotonin activity (e.g., fluoxetine).[40,41] However, these studies either did not differentiate alcoholic from nonalcoholic subjects or excluded alcoholics from participation.

References

1. Reiss, A.J., Jr., & Roth, J.A., eds. *Understanding and Preventing Violence*. Vol. 3. Washington, DC: National Academy Press, 1994.

2. Moss, H.B., & Tarter, R.E. Substance abuse, aggression, and violence. *Am J Addict* 2(2):149-160, 1993.

3. Roizen, J. Epidemiological issues in alcohol-related violence. In: Galanter, M., ed. *Recent Developments in Alcoholism*. Vol. 13. New York: Plenum Press, 1997. pp. 7-40.

4. Pernanen, K. *Alcohol in Human Violence*. New York: Guilford Press, 1991.

5. Gustafson, R. Alcohol and aggression. *J Offender Rehabil* 21(3/4):41-80, 1994.

6. Miczek, K.A., et al. Alcohol, GABAA-benzodiazepine receptor complex, and aggression. In: Galanter, M., ed. *Recent*

Developments in Alcoholism. Vol. 13. New York: Plenum Press, 1997. pp. 139-171.

7. Cook, P.J., & Moore, M.J. Economic perspectives on reducing alcohol-related violence. In: Martin, S.E., ed. *Alcohol and Interpersonal Violence.* NIAAA Research Monograph No. 24. NIH Pub. No. 93-3496. Rockville, MD: NIAAA, 1993. pp. 193-212.

8. Buss, A.H. *The Psychology of Aggression.* New York: Wiley, 1961.

9. Gustafson, R. What do experimental paradigms tell us about alcohol-related aggressive responding? *J Stud Alcohol* 11(suppl):20-29, 1993.

10. Bushman, B.J. Effects of alcohol on human aggression: Validity of proposed explanations. In: Galanter, M., ed. *Recent Developments in Alcoholism.* Vol. 13. New York: Plenum Press, 1997. pp. 227-243.

11. Lang, A.R. Alcohol-related violence: Psychological perspectives. In: Martin, S.E., ed. *Alcohol and Interpersonal Violence.* NIAAA Research Monograph No. 24. NIH Pub. No. 93-3496. Rockville, MD: NIAAA, 1993. pp. 121-148.

12. Collins, J.J. Alcohol and interpersonal violence: Less than meets the eye. In: Wolfgang, M.E., eds. *Pathways to Criminal Violence.* Newbury Park, CA: Sage Publications, 1989. pp. 49-67.

13. Fagan, J. Intoxication and aggression. In: Tonry, M., & Wilson, J.Q., eds. *Crime and Justice.* Vol. 13. Chicago: Univ. of Chicago Press, 1990. pp. 241-320.

14. MacAndrew, C., & Edgerton, R.B. *Drunken Comportment.* Chicago: Aldine Publishing, 1969.

15. Zack, M., & Vogel-Sprott, M. Drunk or sober? Learned conformity to a behavioral standard. *J Stud Alcohol* 58(5):495-501, 1997.

16. Miller, B.A. Investigating links between childhood victimization and alcohol problems. In: Martin, S.E., ed. *Alcohol and Interpersonal Violence.* NIAAA Research Monograph No. 24. NIH Pub. No. 93-3496. Rockville, MD: NIAAA, 1993. pp. 315-323.

17. Widom, C.S., et al. Alcohol abuse in abused and neglected children followed-up: Are they at increased risk? *J Stud Alcohol* 56(2):207-217, 1995.

18. Brookoff, D., et al. Characteristics of participants in domestic violence: Assessment at the scene of domestic assault. *JAMA* 277(17):1369-1373, 1997.

19. Raine, A., et al. Birth complications combined with early maternal rejection at age 1 year predispose to violent crime at age 18 years. *Arch Gen Psychiatry* 51(12):984-988, 1994.

20. Raine, A., et al. High rates of violence, crime, academic problems, and behavioral problems in males with both early neuromotor deficits and unstable family environments. *Arch Gen Psychiatry* 53(6):544-549, 1996.

21. White, H.R. Longitudinal perspective on alcohol use and aggression during adolescence. In: Galanter, M., ed. *Recent Developments in Alcoholism*. Vol. 13. New York: Plenum Press, 1997. pp. 81-103.

22. Jessor, R., & Jessor, S.L. *Problem Behavior and Psychosocial Development*. New York: Academic Press, 1977.

23. Virkkunen, M., et al. *Serotonin in alcoholic violent offenders*. Ciba Foundation Symposium 194:168-182, 1995.

24. Cloninger, C.R., et al. Inheritance of alcohol abuse: Cross-fostering analysis of adopted men. *Arch Gen Ps ychiatry* 38:861-868, 1981.

25. Higley, J.D., et al. A nonhuman primate model of type II excessive alcohol consumption? Part 1. Low cerebrospinal fluid 5-hydroxyindoleacetic acid concentrations and diminished social competence correlate with excessive alcohol consumption. *Alcohol Clin Exp Res* 20(4):629-642, 1996.

26. Virkkunen, M., & Linnoila, M. Serotonin and glucose metabolism in impulsively violent alcoholic offenders. In: Stoff, D.M., & Cairns, R.B., eds. *Aggression and Violence*. Mahwah, NJ: Lawrence Erlbaum, 1996. pp. 87-100.

27. Higley, J.D., & Linnoila, M. A nonhuman primate model of excessive alcohol intake: Personality and neurobiological parallels of type I- and type II-like alcoholism. In: Galanter, M., ed.

Recent Developments in Alcoholism. Vol. 13. New York: Plenum Press, 1997. pp. 192-219.

28. Coccaro, E.F., & Kavoussi, R.J. Neurotransmitter correlates of impulsive aggression. In: Stoff, D.M., & Cairns, R.B., eds. *Aggression and Violence.* Mahwah, NJ: Lawrence Erlbaum, 1996. pp. 67-86.

29. Alexander, G., et al. Parallel organization of functionally segregated circuits linking basal ganglia and cortex. *Annu Rev Neurosci* 9:357-381, 1986.

30. Modell, J.G., et al. Basal ganglia/limbic striatal and thalamocortical involvement in craving and loss of control in alcoholism. *J Neuropsychiatry Clin Neurosci* 2(2):123-144, 1990.

31. Dabbs, J.M., Jr., et al. Salivary testosterone and cortisol among late adolescent male offenders. *J Abnorm Child Psychol* 19(4):469-478, 1991.

32. Virkkunen, M., et al. CSF biochemistries, glucose metabolism, and diurnal activity rhythms in alcoholic, violent offenders, fire setters, and healthy volunteers. *Arch Gen Psychiatry* 51:20-27, 1994.

33. Miczek, K.A., et al. Alcohol, drugs of abuse, aggression, and violence. In: Reiss, A.J., & Roth, J.A., eds. *Understanding and Preventing Violence.* Vol. 3. Washington, DC: National Academy Press, 1994. pp. 377-570.

34. Robins, L.N. Deviant Children Grown Up. Baltimore: Williams & Wilkins, 1996.

35. Brown, G.L., & Linnoila, M.I. CSF serotonin metabolite (5-HIAA) studies in depression, impulsivity, and violence. *J Clin Psychiatry* 51(4)(suppl):31-43, 1990.

36. Lipsey, M.W., et al. Is there a causal relationship between alcohol use and violence? A synthesis of evidence. In: Galanter, M., ed. *Recent Developments in Alcoholism.* Vol. 13. New York: Plenum Press, 1997. pp. 245-282.

37. O'Farrell, T.J., & Murphy, C.M. Marital violence before and after alcoholism treatment. *J Consult Clin Psychol* 63:256-262, 1995.

38. Gardner, D.L., & Cowdry, R.W. Positive effects of carbamazepine on behavioral dyscontrol in borderline personality disorder. *Am J Psychiatry* 143(4):519-522, 1986.

39. Sheard, M.H., et al. The effect of lithium on impulsive behavior in man. *Am J Psychiatry* 133:1409-1413, 1976.

40. Coccaro, E.F., et al. Fluoxetine treatment of compulsive aggression in DSM-III-R personality disorder patients. *J Clin Psychopharm* 10:373-375, 1990.

41. Salzman, C., et al. Effect of fluoxetine on anger in symptomatic volunteers with borderline personality disorder. *J Clin Psychopharm* 15(1):23-19, 1995.

Chapter 21

Severe Burn
Injuries and Treatment

Burn Incidence

Estimate: Over 1 million burn injuries per year.

Trend: The incidence of burn injury in the United States has declined significantly from the 2 million annual injuries estimated in the first report of the National Health Interview Survey (NHIS), drawn from 1957-61 data. As of the early 1990s, the rate of reportable burn injuries in the U.S. had declined from about 10/10,000 to 4.2/10,000.

Sources: An estimate of total burn incidence is extracted and made available every 8-10 years by the National Health Interview Survey (NHIS) from data collected in its ongoing health survey of a sample of American households. The last NHIS estimate of 1.129 million burns is drawn from 1991-93 data.

Fire and Burn Deaths

Estimate: 4,500 fire and burn deaths per year. This total includes an estimated 3,750 deaths from fires and 750 from motor vehicle and

This chapter includes "Burn Incidence and Treatment in the U.S.: 2000 Fact Sheet," © 2000 American Burn Association, reprinted with permission; "Emergency Treatment of Burns," © 1988-2001 Shriners Hospitals for Children, reprinted with permission; "Injury Facts, Burn Injury," SAFE KIDS, 2000; and "Living Skin Grafts Enhance Burn Treatment," by Alison Davis, National Institute of General Medical Sciences (NIGMS), October 26, 2001.

aircraft crashes, contact with electricity, chemicals or hot liquids and substances, and other sources of burn injury. Since the respective role of flame and smoke in fire deaths is often not determined by autopsy, "burn" death totals cannot be distinguished from those which result from smoke poisoning.

Trend: Fire and burn deaths in the United States declined about 50% from 1971 to 1998. Since the U.S. population grew 25% during that period, the decline in the death rate was over 60%.

Sources: Annual survey of fire departments by the National Fire Protection Association (to 1997); annual Vital and Health Statistics reports of the National Center for Health Statistics (to 1994).

Hospital Admissions and Emergency Department Visits

Estimates: 45,000 hospitalizations per year, about half to 125 specialized burn treatment centers and half to the nation's 5,000 other hospitals. 700,000 annual emergency department visits @ 1.2 per injury. (Burn center hospitals average 200 burn admissions a year, other hospitals less than five.)

Trend: Total acute hospitalizations resulting from burn injury have declined 50% since 1971. The decline partly reflects fewer repeat hospitalizations during acute treatment and more accurate coding. Burn center admissions meanwhile have doubled, increasing their share from 13% to 50% of all burn patients. Since emergency departments have only been surveyed since 1992, the outpatient burn trend is not yet clear.

Sources: Hospital admissions: National Hospital Discharge Survey (1995-98 data); Agency for Health Care Policy and Research (1990-93 HCUP-II data); DRG Handbook (1996 data). Burn Center Admissions: American Burn Association (1991 admissions data). Emergency Department visits: National Hospital Ambulatory Medical Care Survey (1992-95 data). Injuries represented in Emergency Department Visits: National Medical Expenditure Survey (1987 data).

Severity of Burn Injuries

Estimate: The average size of a burn injury admitted to a burn center is about 14% of total body surface area (% TBSA). (1991-93)

Burns of 10% TBSA or less account for 54% of burn center admissions, while burns of 60% TBSA or more account for 4% of admissions. About 6% of burn center admissions do not survive, most of whom have suffered severe inhalation injury in fires.

Trend: Since 1965, the proportion of burn center admissions with burns of 10% TBSA or less has more than doubled, from 26% to 54%, while large burns (60% TBSA or greater) have declined from 10% to less than 4% of total admissions. This trend reflects both an absolute decline in large burn injuries and increasing recognition of the importance of specialized facilities and experience in treating significant burn injuries of all sizes.

Sources: A survey of 28 burn centers contributing data to the American Burn Association burn patient registry (1991-93); data from the National Burn Information Exchange (1965-85). Thanks to the Burn Foundation, Philadelphia, PA, for report preparation. Revised August 7, 2000.

Emergency Treatment of Burns

Thermal Burns

Thermal burns are caused by contact with open flames, hot liquids, hot surfaces, and other sources of high heat.

1. Stop the burning. Remove the victim from the heat source.
2. Cool the burn with cold water.
3. Check breathing. Stop bleeding.
4. Cover the burn with a sterile pad or clean sheet.
5. Maintain body temperature and take victim to the nearest medical facility.

Note: Do not apply oils, sprays, or ointments to a serious burn.

- Sunburn may also be cooled with water. If the sunburn is severe or is very extensive, seek medical attention.

Chemical Burns

1. Flush skin with water for at least 20 minutes.

2. Remove contaminated clothing, but avoid spreading the chemical to unaffected areas.

3. If the victim's eyes are involved, flush the eyes continuously with water until medical help is obtained. Remove contact lenses.

4. Follow steps 3 to 5 for thermal burns (check breathing, stop bleeding, cover burn, maintain body temperature, and transport to medical facility).

Note: In cases involving some powdered or dry chemicals, it may not be appropriate to flush with water. If a dry chemical is involved, carefully brush the chemical off the skin and check the package or package insert for emergency information.

Electrical Burns

1. Pull the plug at the wall or shut off the current. Do not touch the victim while they are in contact with electricity.

2. Follow steps 3 to 5 for thermal burns.

3. All electrical injuries should receive medical attention.

- In homes where young children are present, consider using "tamperproof" or child-proof receptacles or receptacle covers.

- Limit your use of extension cords.

General Considerations

- Remove rings, belts, shoes, and tight clothing before swelling occurs.

- If clothing is stuck to the burn, ***do not remove it***. Carefully cut around the stuck fabric to remove loose fabric.

- Burns on the face, hands, and feet should always be considered serious and should receive prompt medical attention.

Treatment for Burns

Minor Burns

- Hold burned area under cool running water for 15 minutes.

- Do not apply ointments or butter.

- Cover the area with dry gauze.

- Do not pop blisters.

Consult a doctor if burns occur on the face, hands, genitalia, feet, or for any burn on an infant.

Severe Burns

- Have one person call 911 or the local emergency number while another person runs cool water over the burned area. Do not use ice.

- Do not put ointment or grease on the burn and do not try to remove pieces of cloth from the burned area.

- Do not break blisters.

- Do not give the victim anything to eat or drink.

- Do raise the burned limbs to minimize swelling.

- Do keep the victim from being chilled or overheated.

Children and Burn Injuries

Thousands of children suffer burn-related injuries each year. Children ages 4 and under are at the greatest risk, with an injury rate more than four times that of children ages 5 to 14.

Burns have long been recognized as among the most painful and devastating injuries a person can sustain and survive. Burns often require long periods of rehabilitation, multiple skin grafts, and painful physical therapy, and they can leave victims with lifelong physical and psychological trauma.

Scald burn injury (caused by hot liquids or steam) is the most common type of burn-related injury among young children, while flame burns (caused by direct contact with fire) are more prevalent among older children. All children are also at risk for contact, electrical, and chemical burns. Because young children have thinner skin than that of older children and adults, their skin burns at lower temperatures and more deeply. A child exposed to hot tap water at 140 degrees Fahrenheit for three seconds will sustain a third-degree burn, an injury requiring hospitalization and skin grafts.

Children, especially ages 4 and under, may not perceive danger, have less control of their environment, may lack the ability to escape a life-threatening burn situation, and may not be able to tolerate the physical stress of a post-burn injury.

Deaths and Injuries

- In 1998, 608 children ages 14 and under died due to fire- and burn-related injury. It is estimated that flames and burns are responsible for one-fourth of all fire-related deaths.

- In 1999, an estimated 99,500 children ages 14 and under were treated in hospital emergency rooms for burn-related injuries. Of these injuries, 62,580 were thermal burns, 23,620 were scald burns, 9,430 were chemical burns, and 2,250 were electrical burns.

- An average of nine children ages 14 and under die from scald burn-related injuries each year. Children ages 4 and under account for nearly all of these deaths.

- Among children ages 4 and under hospitalized for burn-related injuries, it is estimated that 65 percent are treated for scald burns and 20 percent for contact burns.

- In 1999, nearly 3,800 children ages 14 and under were treated in hospital emergency rooms for fireworks-related injuries.

How and Where Burn Deaths and Injuries Occur

- Child-play fires are the leading cause of residential fire-related death and injury among children ages 5 and under.

- Among children ages 14 and under, hair curlers and curling irons, room heaters, ovens and ranges, irons, gasoline, and fireworks are the most common causes of product-related thermal burn injuries.

- The majority of scald burns to children, especially among those ages 6 months to 2 years, are from hot foods and liquids spilled in the kitchen or other places where food is prepared and served.

- Hot tap water accounts for nearly one-fourth of all scald burns among children and is associated with more deaths and hospitalizations than other hot liquid burns. Tap-water burns most often occur in the bathroom and tend to be more severe and cover a larger portion of the body than other scald burns.

- Burns account for approximately 55 percent of all fireworks-related injuries and primarily occur to the hands, head, and eyes. Fireworks-related injuries peak during the month surrounding July 4, when 75 percent of them occur.

- Nearly two-thirds of electrical burn injuries among children ages 12 and under are associated with household electrical cords and extension cords. Wall outlets are associated with an additional 14 percent of these injuries.

- The vast majority (95 percent) of microwave burns among children are scald burns. Microwave burns are typically caused by spilling hot liquids or food, and injuries are primarily associated with the trunk or the face.

Who Is at Risk

- Children ages 4 and under and children with disabilities are at the greatest risk of burn-related death and injury. These children are especially at risk from scald and contact burns.

- Male children are at higher risk of burn-related death and injury than female children.

- Children in homes without smoke alarms are at greater risk of fires and fire-related death and injury.

- Males, especially those ages 10 to 14, are at the highest risk of fireworks-related injuries. However, children ages 4 and under are at the highest risk for sparkler-related injuries.

Burn Prevention Effectiveness

- Smoke alarms are extremely effective at preventing fire-related death and injury. The chances of dying in a residential fire are cut in half when a smoke alarm is present. Smoke alarms and sprinkler systems combined could reduce fire-related deaths by 82 percent and injuries by 46 percent.

- More than 75 percent of all scald burn-related injuries among children ages 2 and under could be prevented through behavioral and environmental modifications. Hot tap water scalds can be prevented by lowering the setting on water heater thermostats to 120 degrees Fahrenheit or below, and by installing anti-scald devices in water faucets and showerheads.

Burn Protection Laws

Many states and the District of Columbia have laws that require smoke alarms to be used in both new and existing dwellings. Some states have no comprehensive smoke alarm laws. Other states have a variety of laws covering specific situations such as new dwellings or multi-occupancy dwellings only.

In 1994, the U.S. Consumer Product Safety Commission issued a mandatory safety standard requiring disposable and novelty cigarette lighters to be child-resistant. Since this standard has been in effect, the number of child-play lighter fires has declined 42 percent, and the number of deaths and injuries associated with these fires has declined 31 percent and 26 percent, respectively.

Many communities have established local ordinances or building codes which require the installation of anti-scald plumbing devices in all new construction. Such legislation has been effective in reducing the number of scald burn deaths and injuries associated with hot tap water.

Health Care Costs and Savings

The total annual cost of scald burn-related deaths and injuries among children ages 14 and under is approximately $2.1 billion. Children ages 4 and under account for $1.3 billion, or more than 60 percent, of these costs. Total charges for pediatric admissions to burn centers average $22,700 per case.

Prevention Tips

- Never leave a child alone, especially in the bathroom or kitchen. If you must leave the room, take the child with you.

- Install smoke alarms in your home on every level and in every sleeping area. Test them once a month, replace the batteries at least once a year (unless the batteries are designed for longer life), and replace the alarms every 10 years. Ten-year lithium alarms are also available and do not require an annual battery change.

- Set your water heater thermostat to 120 degrees Fahrenheit or below. Consider installing water faucets and showerheads containing anti-scald technology.

- Keep matches, gasoline, lighters, and all other flammable materials locked away and out of children's reach.

- Use back burners and turn pot handles to the back of the stove when cooking. Keep appliance cords out of children's reach, especially if the appliances contain hot foods or liquids. Cover unused electrical outlets with safety devices.

- Keep hot foods and liquids away from table and counter edges. Never carry or hold children and hot foods and/or liquids at the same time.

- Never allow children to handle fireworks.

Living Skin Grafts Enhance Burn Treatment

In the United States, 1.25 million people seek medical attention for burns every year, according to the American Burn Association. Third-degree burns, which extend to the deepest of the skin's layers, require immediate care to prevent infection and dangerous fluid loss that can lead to shock. A quarter-century ago, NIH-funded burn surgeons determined that badly burned skin should be removed as quickly as possible (rather than letting it slough off over time), followed by immediate and permanent replacement of the lost skin. This seemingly simple idea ultimately became standard practice for treating major burn injuries and led to the development of what is now an artificial skin system called Integra ®. After removing the damaged skin, surgeons blanket a burn wound with a covering like Integra ®, then apply a skin graft on top of this biomaterial to coax the growth of new skin to close the wound. While ideally surgeons obtain skin grafts from the burned patient, in the case of severe burns covering 80 to 90 percent of the body surface, there is not enough remaining skin to use for this purpose.

Dr. Steven T. Boyce at the University of Cincinnati and the Cincinnati Shriner's Burns Hospital has succeeded in growing skin cells from a burned patient and adding them to a polymer sheet to create living skin grafts in the laboratory. In an effort to permanently close burn wounds, Boyce and his coworkers placed the laboratory-grown skin grafts on top of Integra ® and bathed everything with a nutritious mix of growth factors and antibiotics to help prod the growth of new blood vessels and control infection. The researchers tested this technique on three children who had been badly burned in fires. The results were promising, showing that the new method offers an advantage over other currently available technologies, such as using non-living epidermal substitutes that cannot as accurately restore the structure and function of native skin. In each test case, the patient's new skin was a lighter color than before, but it had returned to its original softness, smoothness, and strength—with minimal scarring.

The new method may improve the treatment of severely burned patients who have lost more than half of their skin to third-degree burns, because the availability of skin for grafting the burn wounds of these patients is often limiting to recovery. This approach to wound treatment may also decrease treatment costs and hospitalization times associated with the treatment of severe burns, though more studies are needed to formally test these predictions. Finally, the method succeeded in regaining much of the cosmetic appearance of the burn-damaged skin of these young patients—a crucial element in helping burn victims return to a normal life.

Reference

Boyce ST, Kagan RJ, Meyer NA, Yakuboff KP, and Warden GD: Cultured skin substitutes combined with Integra Artificial Skin to replace native skin autograft and allograft for the closure of excised full-thickness burns. *J. Burn Care Rehab.* 1999;20:453-61.

Additional Information

Shriners Hospitals for Children
International Shrine Headquarters
2900 Rocky Point Dr.
Tampa, FL 33607-1460
Toll-Free: 800-237-5055
Tel: 813-281-0300
Website: www.shrinershq.org

American Burn Association
625 N. Michigan Ave.
Suite 1530
Chicago, IL 60611
Toll-Free: 800-548-2876
Tel: 312-642-9260
Fax: 312-642-9130
Website: www.ameriburn.org
E-mail: info@ameriburn.org

Chapter 22

Facial and Dental Trauma

Patients may not expect dental professionals to show interest, compassion, empathy, and curiosity or ask questions beyond those related to dental procedures. But they should because the discussion that ensues after the questions have been asked gives dental professionals the opportunity to educate patients. The consequences of an adult not wearing a seat belt, an infant not being properly placed and restrained in an infant seat, a bicycle accident, a sports injury, or domestic abuse leave hundreds of thousands of patients with craniofacial orodental trauma.

Craniofacial orodental trauma affects people of all ages, sexes, and cultures. This type of trauma often is unintentional and is caused by auto accidents, sports injuries, falls, or other accidents at work or in the home. In addition, violence, including domestic and child abuse, produces thousands of craniofacial orodental injuries each year. Dental professionals are part of the prevention of these unintentional and intentional injuries and are part of the treatment of craniofacial orodental injuries.

Unintentional Trauma: Accidents

By the time children reach age 16 years, 35 percent will have sustain dental trauma at least once. Boys are twice as likely as girls to

"Compassion, Communication and Craniofacial," Insights on Human Health, National Institute of Dental and Craniofacial Research (NIDR), April 2000.

231

report dental trauma and are much more likely to experience such trauma more than once. Boys sustain their injuries most frequently at age 4 years and between ages 8 and 11 years; girls, at ages 4 and 9 years.[4]

Certain subpopulations of children are in more danger than are others. Toddlers and young adolescents have the highest injury rates. Studies by the National Institute of Child Health and Human Development have found that children of single adult households have a 40 percent increased risk of accidental injury compared with other children. Interestingly, children in childcare facilities were not at increased risk of injury, compared with children cared for by a parent or guardian. Children younger than 2 years of age whose mothers had fewer than 12 years of education and who were cared for at more than one childcare facility, however, had a fivefold increased risk of injury.[5]

In young children, craniofacial, oral, and dental trauma is mainly caused through falls. A German survey of more than 1,300 children younger than 19 years of age with facial trauma found that 68 percent had soft-tissue injuries and 24 percent had dental trauma.[6]

A hospital in Missouri found that the frequency of dental trauma in children peaked in the 1- to 2-year-old age group, and that the most predominant injury was laceration of the lip. The leading cause of trauma in this study was falls, which accounted for more than one-half of oral injuries.[7] Besides falls, young children, as well as adults, can be injured in bicycle and automobile accidents, two etiologies that can produce much more serious injuries. The advent of bicycle helmets has aided prevention; in Washington state, for example, helmets reduced the risk of injuries to the upper and middle face by more than 60 percent.[8] Still, each year more than 150,000 children are treated for bicycle-related craniofacial orodental injuries in emergency departments across the country.[9]

Currently, 15 states have some form of bicycle helmet legislation that covers children, but the Centers for Disease Control and Prevention, or CDC, estimates that 75 percent of bicycle-related fatalities among children could be prevented if all children on bicycles wore helmets. The CDC also projects that the universal use of bicycle helmets by children 4 through 15 years of age would prevent up to 45,000 craniofacial injuries and 55,000 maxillary and mandibular injuries annually.[9]

Mountain biking—either on wide dirt paths or single-track trails—has become a popular sport over the last decade. Unfortunately, it also is a dangerous one. Mountain bikers registered at the Department of

Oral and Maxillofacial Surgery at the University of Innsbruck, Austria, had more severe injury profiles than did road bicyclists. Fifty-five percent of the mountain bikers had facial fractures, compared with 35 percent of road cyclists. Zygomatic fractures were more common in road cyclists, whereas mountain bikers were more likely to sustain Le Fort I, II, and III fractures.[10]

By the time children reach adolescence, they are more likely to sustain craniofacial orodental trauma through auto accidents, sports injuries, or violence, which also are common causes of such trauma in adults. Motor vehicle crashes are the leading cause of death for people 5 to 27 years of age and tend to be the primary cause of most midface fractures and lacerations, due to the face striking a dashboard, windshield, steering wheel, or the back of the front seat.[11] Seat belt use can drastically reduce the incidence and severity of these injuries.[12] Although 16 states—plus the District of Columbia and Puerto Rico—have mandatory seat belt laws, enforcement varies. The National Highway Traffic Safety Administration estimates that if all states had standard enforcement of seat belt laws, more than 49,000 injuries could be prevented, and $3.4 billion would be saved annually.[13]

The largest proportion of adolescent injuries—not just craniofacial orodental injuries but all types—is due to motor vehicle crashes. Adolescents are far less likely to use seat belts than any other age group and are more likely than adults to have accidents at night or while under the influence of alcohol.[14]

Among older children and young adults, sports such as biking, skiing, and soccer and other contact sports can result in a significant proportion of craniofacial orodental trauma. A British survey of maxillofacial sports injuries found that such injuries were much more likely in males—more than 80 percent of injured patients were male. Most injuries were lacerations, but 10 percent of patients had dentoalveolar fractures, and 8 percent had facial fractures.[15]

Intentional Trauma: Violence

While many etiologies of craniofacial orodental trauma are accidental or unintentional injuries, all too many injuries are caused by violence. Fistfights or the use of guns, knives, bottles, or other weapons commonly affect the craniofacial orodental complex. In a survey of more than 2,400 violence-related injuries, nearly 70 percent were craniofacial.

The most common weapons are fists and feet.[16] Data from the aforementioned German survey[6] showed that more than 60 percent of craniofacial injuries in teen-agers were due to an assault. Mandibular fractures were most common, with condylar fractures making up 80 percent of all fractures to the jaw.[6]

While nasal, mandibular, and zygomatic fractures are common consequences of assaults using fists and feet,[17] penetrating craniofacial trauma caused by guns, knives, and other weapons can result in multiple fractures, soft-tissue injuries and intracranial penetration, which have lifelong consequences such as brain damage and blindness. These sequelae are in addition to the obvious cosmetic complications. Of 100 patients treated at a Brooklyn, NY hospital for gunshot wounds to the face, 38 percent had significant neurological injury, and 67 percent sustained bony injury. Ultimately, one-fourth of the patients had at least one complication such as osteomyelitis.[18]

People with assault-related injuries, like those with accident-related craniofacial orodental trauma, are predominantly male; in the study of gunshot wounds to the face, 89 of 100 patients were male.[18] Other studies have found that men constitute approximately 80 percent of assault victims who suffer craniofacial orodental trauma.[18,19]

While men seem to sustain most of the injuries caused by sports and assaults, women suffering from domestic abuse make up a substantial number of craniofacial orodental trauma victims, although domestic violence is a frequently unrecognized cause of such injury. Compared with women injured through other means, these women tend to have injuries to the head, face, and neck.[20] Of 218 women seen at a California emergency department with injuries from domestic violence, 28 percent had to be admitted as a result of the severity of their injuries. More than 85 percent of the women had been abused previously, and 40 percent had required medical care previously. Ten percent were pregnant at the time of abuse.[21]

In many cases, domestic partner abuse occurs with child abuse.[22] Using data from the 1985 National Family Violence Survey, researchers found that each act of violence toward a partner cumulatively increases the probability of the violent partner also being abusive to the child, particularly for fathers. The most chronically violent husbands (toward their spouses) had a nearly 100 percent probability of also physically abusing their male children, but not their female ones.[23] Children also can suffer craniofacial orodental trauma through domestic violence, either through direct abuse or from attempts to intervene during acts of partner abuse. Of children injured in the latter fashion, craniofacial injuries are the most common type of trauma they experience.[24]

Many injuries that result from domestic abuse are minor ones. However, by dental practitioners inquiring as to the causes of all injuries, it may be possible for them to pinpoint more cases of abuse and facilitate a process in which families seek the help they need. A young mother or child may be unwilling to discuss "private problems" with a health care provider. Then again, the dental health care provider may represent the one safe person whom these people can turn to, someone knowledgeable who will listen and maybe help them. The ADA's Principles of Ethics and Code of Professional Conduct[25] includes a statement that as dentists we have an ethical duty to become familiar with the perioral signs of child abuse and to report all suspected cases to the proper authority. More than 3 million children in the United States were reported to child protective services in 1997 as suspects of being abused. Of these, 1 million cases were substantiated, a 50 percent increase over 1989.[26]

References

1. Talbot M. The placebo prescription. *New York Times Magazine* Jan. 9, 2000:34.

2. Peabody FW. The care of the patient. *JAMA* 1927;88(12):877.

3. Thomas KB. General practice consultations: is there any point in being positive? *Br Med J* (Clin Res Ed) 1987;294(6581):1200-2.

4. Borssen E, Holm AK. Traumatic dental injuries in a cohort of 16-year-olds in northern Sweden. *Endod Dent Traumatol* 1997;13(6): 276-80.

5. National Institute of Child Health and Human Development. Division of Epidemiology, Statistics and Prevention Research: Report to council June 1997. Available at: http://www.nichd.nih.gov/publications/pubs/coun_despr.htm. Accessed Jan. 17, 2000.

6. Zerfowski M, Bremerich A. Facial trauma in children and adolescents. *Clin Oral Investig* 1998;2(3):120-4.

7. Neil DW, Clark MV, Lowe JW, Harrington MS. Oral trauma in children: a hospital survey. *Oral Surg Oral Med Oral Pathol* 1989;68(6):691-6.

8. Thompson DC, Nunn ME, Thompson RS, Rivara FP. Effectiveness of bicycle safety helmets in preventing serious facial injury. *JAMA* 1996;276(24):1974-5.

9. National Center for Injury Prevention and Control. Bicycle-related head injuries. Available at: http://www.bhsi.org/webdocs/stats.htm. Accessed Jan. 7, 2000.

10. Gassner R, Tuli T, Emshoff R, Waldhart E. Mountainbiking: a dangerous sport–comparison with bicycling on oral and maxillofacial trauma. *Int J Oral Maxillofac Surg* 1999; 28(3):188-91.

11. National Highway Transportation Safety Administration. Air bag on/off switches: questions and answers. Available at: http://www.nhtsa.gov/airbags/airbgQandA.html. Accessed Jan. 11, 2000.

12. Nicholoff TJ Jr., Del Castillo CB, Velmonte MX. Reconstructive surgery for complex midface trauma using titanium miniplates: Le Fort I fracture of the maxilla, zygomatico-maxillary complex fracture and nasomaxillary complex fracture, resulting from a motor vehicle accident. *J Philipp Dent Assoc* 1998;50(3):5-13.

13. National Highway Transportation Safety Administration. Summary: the case for standard seat belt use laws. Available at: www.nhtsa.gov/people/injury/airbags/seatbelt/Summary.htm. Accessed Jan. 11, 2000.

14. National Center for Injury Prevention and Control. Fact sheet on adolescent injury. Available at: www.cdc.gov/ncipc/factsheets/adoles.htm. Accessed Jan. 7, 2000.

15. Hill CM, Burford K, Martin A, Thomas DW. A one-year review of maxillofacial sports injuries treated at an accident and emergency department. *Br J Oral Maxillofac Surg* 1998; 36(1):44-7.

16. Brink O, Vesterby A, Jensen J. Pattern of injuries due to interpersonal violence. *Injury* 1998;29(9):705-9.

17. Shepherd JP, Shapland M, Pearce NX, Scully C. Pattern, severity and aetiology of injuries in victims of assault. *J R Soc Med* 1990;83(2):75-8.

18. Dolin J, Scalea T, Mannor L, Sclafani S, Trooskin S. The management of gunshot wounds to the face. *J Trauma* 1992;33(4): 508-14.

19. Bostrom L. Injury panorama and medical consequences for 1158 persons assaulted in the central part of Stockholm, Sweden. *Arch Orthop Trauma Surg* 1997;116(6-7): 315-20.

20. Muelleman RL, Lenaghan PA, Pakieser RA. Battered women: injury locations and types. *Ann Emerg Med* 1996;28(5):486-92.

21. Berrios DC, Grady D. Domestic violence. Risk factors and outcomes. *West J Med* 1991; 155(2):133-5.

22. Hutchison IL, Magennis P, Shepherd JP, Brown AE. The BAOMS United Kingdom survey of facial injuries: part 1, aetiology and the association with alcohol consumption. *Br J Oral Maxillofac Surg* 1998;36(1):3-13.

23. National Center for Injury Prevention and Control. The co-occurrence of intimate partner violence against mothers and abuse of children. Available at: www.cdc.gov/ncipc/dvp/dvcan.htm. Accessed Jan. 11, 2000.

24. Christian CW, Scribano P, Seidl T, Pinto-Martin JA. Pediatric injury resulting from family violence. *Pediatrics* 1997; 99(2):E8.

25. *Principles of ethics and code of professional conduct.* Chicago: American Dental Association; 1998.

26. Proceedings: Dentists C.A.R.E. (Child Abuse Recognition and Education) Conference, Chicago, July 31-Aug. 1, 1998. Chicago: American Dental Association; 1999:1-76.

Additional Information

National Highway Traffic Safety Administration
U.S. Department of Transportation
400 Seventh St., SW
Washington, D.C. 20590
General number: 202-366-0123
Auto safety hotline: 800-424-9393
Child safety seat information: 202-366-2696
Seat belt information: 202-366-9294
Air bag information: 202-366-0910
Website: www.nhtsa.dot.gov

National Center for Injury Prevention and Control
4770 Buford Highway NE
Mailstop K65
Atlanta, Ga. 30341-3724
Tel: 770-488-1506
Fax: 770-488-1667
Automated information line: 770-488-4677
Division of Unintentional Injury Prevention: 770-488-4652
Division of Violence Prevention: 770-488-4352
Website: www.cdc.gov/ncipc/ncipchm.htm
E-mail: OHCINFO@cdc.gov

National Institute of Child Health and Human Development
Building 31, Room 2A32, MSC 2425
31 Center Drive
Bethesda, Md. 20892-2425
Toll-Free: 800-370-2943
Website: www.nichd.nih.gov
E-mail: NICHDClearinghouse@mail.nih.gov

National Clearinghouse on Child Abuse and Neglect Information
P.O. Box 1182
Washington, D.C. 20013
Tel: 703-385-7565
Website: www.calib.com/nccanch

Chapter 23

Firearm Injury, Scope of the Problem

The Problem

- In 1994 there were 38,505 firearm-related deaths. These included:
    - over 17,800 firearm-related homicides
    - over 18,700 firearm-related suicides
    - over 1,300 unintentional deaths related to firearms.[1]

- It is estimated that there are approximately 3 nonfatal firearm injuries for every death associated with a firearm.[2]

- In 1990, firearm injuries cost over $20.4 billion in both direct costs for hospital and other medical care, and in indirect costs for long-term disability and premature death.[3] At least 80% of the economic costs of treating firearm injuries are paid for by taxpayer dollars.[3]

Firearm-Related Homicides

- More than 70% of homicides are committed with a firearm.[1]

- In each year since 1988, more than 80% of homicide victims 15 to 19 years of age were killed with a firearm. In 1994, nearly

"Firearm Injuries and Fatalities," National Center for Injury Prevention and Control, reviewed April 18, 2001.

90% of homicide victims 15 to 19 years of age were killed with a firearm.[1]

- Firearm assaults on family members and other intimate acquaintances are 12 times more likely to result in death than are assaults using other weapons.[4]

- In 1994, 4,211 women over 19 years of age were victims of homicide in the United States. Over half of these women (54%) were killed with a firearm.[1]

Youth and Firearms

- In 1994, firearm injuries were the second leading cause of death for young people, 10 to 24 years of age and the third leading cause of death for persons aged 25 to 34.[1]

- Nearly 29% of those who died from firearm injuries in 1994 were 15 to 24 years old.[1]

- In 1995, 7.6% or 1 in 12 students in a national survey reported carrying a firearm for fighting or self-defense at least once in the previous 30 days. In 1990, this was true of 4.1% or 1 in 24 students.[5,6]

- Between 1985 and 1994, the risk of dying from a firearm injury has more than doubled for teenagers 15 to 19 years of age.[1]

Firearm-Related Suicides

- People living in households in which guns are kept have a risk of suicide that is 5 times greater than people living in households without guns.[7]

- Between 1980 and 1994, the overall suicide rate for persons aged 15-19 increased by 29%; the increase in firearm-related suicides accounted for 96% of the increase in the overall suicide rate.[1]

Unintentional Firearm Injuries

- In 1994, there were 787 unintended firearm deaths among persons aged 10 to 29, accounting for 58% of all unintentional firearm deaths in the nation that year. Unintentional firearm deaths are those that occur when the person firing the gun does not intend to harm another.[1]

CDC's Program to Prevent Firearm-Related Injuries

- As the lead agency in injury control, CDC plays a key role in co-ordinating activities and programs in the Public Health Service to prevent firearm-related injuries.

- A nationwide system to track firearm-related injuries, *The National Electronic Injury Surveillance System (NEISS)*, was established in collaboration with the Consumer Product Safety Commission in 1992. This system collects data on firearm-related injuries from a population-based sample of 91 hospital emergency departments throughout the country.

- CDC is also supporting the development of surveillance systems in seven states to monitor firearm injuries and related risk behaviors (e.g., safe storage, carrying weapons). The information generated from these surveillance systems will help states to assess the magnitude of the firearm injury problem and evaluate programs and policies designed to prevent firearm injuries.

Other Firearm-Injury Activities

- The preparation of a surveillance summary on firearm injury and mortality in the United States.

- Risk and protective factor research on firearm violence, including formative research on weapon-carrying among youth.

- Extramural research on injury topics including studies of risk factors for gun use and injuries among young males living in inner cities.

References

1. National Summary of Injury Mortality Data, 1987-1994. Atlanta, GA: Centers for Disease Control and Prevention, National Center for Injury Prevention and Control, November, 1996.

2. Annest JL, Mercy JA, Gibson DR, Ryan GW. National estimates of nonfatal firearm-related injuries: beyond the tip of the iceberg. *JAMA* 1995;283:1749-1754.

3. Max W, Rice, DP. Shooting in the dark: estimating the cost of firearm injuries. *Health Affairs* 1993;12(4):171-185.

4. Saltzman LE, Mercy JA, O'Carroll PW, Rosenberg ML, Rhodes PH. Weapon involvement and injury outcomes in family and intimate assaults. *JAMA* 1992;267:3042-3047.

5. Kann L, Warrem CW, Harris WA, Collins JL, Williams BI, Ross JG, Kolbe LJ. Youth Risk Behavior Surveillance, 1995. Atlanta, GA: Centers for Disease Control and Prevention. CDC Surveillance Summaries, September 27, 1996.

6. *Weapon-Carrying Among High School Students—United States*, 1990. Atlanta, GA: Centers for Disease Control and Prevention, *MMWR* 1991;40:681-684.

7. Kellermann AL, Rivara FP, Somes G, Reay DT, Francisco J, Banton G, Prodzinski J, Fligner C, Hackman BB. Suicide in the home in relation to gun ownership. *New England Journal of Medicine* 1992;327:467-472.

Additional Information

National Center for Injury Prevention and Control
Mailstop K65
4770 Buford Highway NE
Atlanta, GA 30341-3724
Tel: 770-488-1506
Fax: 770-488-1667
Website: www.cdc.gov/ncipc
E-mail: DVPINFO@cdc.gov

Chapter 24

Spinal Cord Injury

Spinal cord injury (SCI) occurs when a traumatic event results in damage to cells within the spinal cord or severs the nerve tracts that relay signals up and down the spinal cord. The most common types of SCI include contusion (bruising of the spinal cord) and compression (caused by pressure on the spinal cord). Other types of injuries include lacerations (severing or tearing of some nerve fibers, such as damage caused by a gun shot wound), and central cord syndrome (specific damage to the corticospinal tracts of the cervical region of the spinal cord). Severe SCI often causes paralysis (loss of control over voluntary movement and muscles of the body) and loss of sensation and reflex function below the point of injury, including autonomic activity such as breathing and other activities such as bowel and bladder control. Other symptoms such as pain or sensitivity to stimuli, muscle spasms, and sexual dysfunction may develop over time. SCI patients are also prone to develop secondary medical problems, such as bladder infections, lung infections, and bedsores.

"Spinal Cord Injury Information Page," National Institute of Neurological Disorders and Stroke (NINDS), reviewed August 2, 2000; "Facts and Figures at a Glance," Fact Sheet published by the National Spinal Cord Injury Statistical Center, © 2001 Board of Trustees, University of Alabama, reprinted with permission; and "What You Should Know about Spinal Cord Injuries," SafeUSA, Centers for Disease Control and Prevention (CDC), 2001.

Treatment

While recent advances in emergency care and rehabilitation allow many SCI patients to survive, methods for reducing the extent of injury and for restoring function are still limited. Immediate treatment for acute SCI includes techniques to relieve cord compression, prompt (within 8 hours of the injury) drug therapy with corticosteroids such as methylprednisolone to minimize cell damage, and stabilization of the vertebrae of the spine to prevent further injury.

Prognosis

The types of disability associated with SCI vary greatly depending on the severity of the injury, the segment of the spinal cord at which the injury occurs, and which nerve fibers are damaged. Most people with SCI regain some functions between a week and 6 months after injury, but the likelihood of spontaneous recovery diminishes after 6 months. Rehabilitation strategies can minimize long-term disability.

Spinal Cord Injury Facts and Figures as of May 2001

It is estimated that the annual incidence of spinal cord injury (SCI), not including those who die at the scene of the accident, is approximately 40 cases per million population in the U. S., or approximately 11,000 new cases each year. Since there have not been any overall incidence studies of SCI in the U.S. since the 1970s it is not known if incidence has changed in recent years.

Prevalence

The number of people in the United States who are alive today and who have SCI has been estimated to be between 721 and 906 per million population. This corresponds to between 183,000 and 230,000 persons. Note: Incidence and prevalence statistics are estimates obtained from several studies. These statistics are not derived from the National SCI Database.

The National Spinal Cord Injury Database has been in existence since 1973 and captures data from an estimated 13% of new SCI cases in the U.S. Since its inception, 24 federally funded Model SCI Care Systems have contributed data to the National SCI Database. As of September, 1999 the database contained information on more than 19,648 persons who sustained traumatic spinal cord injuries. All the remaining statistics on this sheet are derived from this database or from collaborative studies conducted by the Model Systems.

Detailed discussions of all topics in this chapter may be found in a special issue of the journal, *Archives of Physical Medicine and Rehabilitation*, published in November, 1999.

Age at Injury

SCI primarily affects young adults. Fifty-five percent of SCIs occur among persons in the 16 to 30 year age group, and the average age at injury is 32.1 years. Since 1973 there has been an increase in the mean age at time of injury. Those who were injured before 1979 had a mean age of 28.6 while those injured after 1990 had a mean age of 35.3 years. Another trend is an increase in the proportion of those who were at least 61 years of age at injury. In the 1970s persons older than 60 years of age at injury comprised 4.7% of the database. Since 1990 this has increased to 10%. This trend is not surprising since the median age of the general population has increased from 27.9 years to 35.3 years during the same time period.

Gender

Overall, 81.6% of all persons in the national database are male. Although this four-to-one male to female ratio has varied little throughout the 25 years of the Model Systems data collection, since 1990, the percentage of males has decreased to 80.5% (from 81.8% in the 1970's).

Ethnic Groups

A significant trend over time has been observed in the racial distribution of persons in the Model System database. Among persons injured between 1973 and 1978, 77.5% of persons in the database were Caucasian, 13.5% were African-American, 5.7% were Hispanic, 2% were American Indian, and 0.8% were Asian. However, among those injured since 1990 only 59.1% were Caucasian, while 27.6% were African-American, 7.7% were Hispanic, 0.4% were American Indian, 2.1% were Asian (and 0.5% were unknown and 2.5% were unclassified).

Etiology

Since 1990, motor vehicle crashes account for 38.5% of the SCI cases reported. The next largest contributor is acts of violence (primarily gunshot wounds), followed by falls and recreational sporting activities. Interesting trends in the database show the proportions of injuries due to motor vehicle crashes and sporting activities have declined while the proportion of injuries from acts of violence and falls has increased steadily since 1973. Table 24.1 shows the percentage breakdown of causes.

Table 24.1. Etiology of SCI since 1990

Causes of SCI	Percents
Vehicular crashes	38.5%
Violence	24.9%
Falls	21.8%
Other causes	7.9%
Sports injuries	7.2%

Neurologic Level and Extent of Lesion

Persons with tetraplegia (51.6%) have sustained injuries to one of the eight cervical segments of the spinal cord; those with paraplegia (46.3%) have lesions in the thoracic, lumbar, or sacral regions of the spinal cord. For the remaining persons, 0.7% recover prior to discharge and 1.4% are persons for whom this information is not available.

Since 1990 the most frequent neurologic category is incomplete tetraplegia (29.5%), followed by complete paraplegia (27.3%), incomplete paraplegia (21.3%), and complete tetraplegia (18.5%). Trends over time indicate an increasing proportion of persons with incomplete paraplegia and a decreasing proportion of persons with complete tetraplegia.

Occupational Status

More than half (56.9%) of those persons with SCI admitted to a Model System reported being employed at the time of their injury. The post-injury employment picture is better among persons with paraplegia than among their tetraplegic counterparts. By post-injury year 10, 31.9% of persons with paraplegia are employed, while 24.4% of those with tetraplegia are employed during the same year.

Residence

Today 88.7% of all persons with SCI who are discharged alive from the system are sent to a private, noninstitutional residence (in most cases their homes before injury). Only 4.8% are discharged to nursing homes. The remaining are discharged to hospitals, group living situations, or other destinations.

Marital Status

Considering the youthful age of most persons with SCI, it is not surprising that most (53.4%) are single when injured. Among those who were married at the time of injury, as well as those who marry after injury, the likelihood of their marriage remaining intact is slightly lower when compared to the uninjured population. The likelihood of getting married after injury is also reduced.

Length of Stay

Overall, average days hospitalized in the acute care unit for those who enter a Model System immediately following injury has declined from 26 days in 1974 to 16 days in 1999. Similar downward trends are noted for days in the rehab unit, from 115 days to 44 days. Overall, mean days hospitalized (during acute care and rehab) were greater for persons with neurologically complete injuries.

Lifetime Costs

Average yearly health care and living expenses and the estimated lifetime costs that are directly attributable to SCI vary greatly according to severity of injury:

Table 24.2. Average Yearly Expenses (in 1999 dollars)

Severity of Injury	First Year	Each Subsequent Year
High Tetraplegia (C1-C4)	$572,178	$102,491
Low Tetraplegia (C5-C8)	$369,488	$41,983
Paraplegia	$209,074	$21,274
Incomplete Motor Functional at any Level	$168,627	$11,817

Table 24.3. Estimated Lifetime Costs by Age at Injury (discounted at 2%)

Severity of Injury	25 years old	50 years old
High Tetraplegia (C1-C4)	$2,185,667	$1,286,714
Low Tetraplegia (C5-C8)	$1,235,841	$782,628
Paraplegia	$730,277	$498,095
Incomplete Motor Functional at any Level	$487,150	$353,047

These figures do not include any indirect costs such as losses in wages, fringe benefits, and productivity which could average almost $49,312 but vary substantially based on education, severity of injury, and pre-injury employment history.

Table 24.4. Life Expectancy for Persons Who Survive the First 24 Hours

Age at Injury	No SCI	Motor Functional at any Level	Para	Low Tetra (C5-C8)	High Tetra (C1-C4)	Ventilator Dependent at any Level
20 yrs	57.2	51.6	45.2	39.4	33.8	16.2
40 yrs	38.4	33.5	27.8	23.0	18.7	7.2
60 yrs	21.2	17.5	13.0	9.6	6.8	1.2

Table 24.5. Life Expectancy for Persons Who Survive at Least 1 Year Post-Injury

Age at Injury	No SCI	Motor Functional at any Level	Para	Low Tetra (C5-C8)	High Tetra (C1-C4)	Ventilator Dependent at any Level
20 yrs	57.2	52.5	46.2	41.2	37.1	26.8
40 yrs	38.4	34.3	28.7	24.5	21.2	13.7
60 yrs	21.2	18.1	13.7	10.6	8.4	4.0

Life expectancy is the average remaining years of life for an individual. Life expectancies for persons with SCI continue to increase, but are still somewhat below life expectancies for those with no spinal cord injury. Mortality rates are significantly higher during the first year after injury than during subsequent years, particularly for severely injured persons.

Cause of Death

In years past, the leading cause of death among persons with SCI was renal failure. Today, however, significant advances in urologic management have resulted in dramatic shifts in the leading causes of death. Persons enrolled in the National SCI Database since its inception in 1973 have now been followed for 27 years after injury. During that time, the causes of death that appear to have the greatest impact on reduced life expectancy for this population are pneumonia, pulmonary emboli, and septicemia.

Preventing Spinal Cord Injuries

Each year, nearly 11,000 Americans sustain a traumatic spinal cord injury (SCI), and many of them suffer permanent disabilities. More than 190,000 persons in the U.S. live with paralysis caused by spinal cord injury. The following tips, based on information from the Centers for Disease Control and Prevention (CDC) and the Spinal Cord Injury Information Network, may reduce the risk of spinal cord injury:

- Wear a seat belt every time you drive a car or ride in one. Make sure your children are buckled into a child safety seat, booster seat, or seat belt (as appropriate for their age). Motor vehicle crashes are the number one cause of SCI.

- Keep firearms and ammunition locked in a cabinet or safe when not in use. The second leading cause of SCI is violence, most often related to firearms use.

- Prevent falls—the third leading cause of SCI—by
  - using a step stool with a grab bar to reach objects on high shelves;
  - installing handrails on stairways;
  - installing window guards to keep young children from falling out of windows;

- using safety gates at the top and bottom of stairs when young children are around.

- Play sports safely

  - Wear all required safety gear.

  - Never engage in head-first moves, such as spearing (in football, using the helmet to tackle) or sliding head-first into a base.

  - Avoid hitting the boards with your head in ice hockey.

  - Insist on spotters when performing new or difficult moves in gymnastics.

Additional Information

Please refer to Chapter 62, "Directory of Resources," for extensive resource listings.

Chapter 25

Traumatic Brain Injury

Epidemiology of Traumatic Brain Injury in the United States

Of all types of injury, those to the brain are among the most likely to result in death or permanent disability. Estimates of traumatic brain injury (TBI) incidence, severity, and cost reflect the enormous losses to individuals, their families, and society from these injuries. These data demonstrate a critical need for more effective ways to prevent brain injuries and care for those who are injured.

Incidence of traumatic brain injury (TBI). Using national data for 1995-1996, the CDC estimates that TBIs have this impact in the United States each year:

- 1 million people are treated and released from hospital emergency departments[1]
- 230,000 people are hospitalized and survive[2]
- 50,000 people die[3]

This chapter includes excerpts from "Epidemiology of Traumatic Brain Injury in the United States," National Center for Injury Prevention and Control, reviewed May 2000; "Head Injury," reprinted with permission from Neurosurgery:// ON-CALL ® at www.neurosurgery.org. © 2000, American Association of Neurological Surgeons/Congress of Neurological Surgeons; and "What You Should Know about Traumatic Brain Injury," SafeUSA, updated June 11, 2001. Please refer to Chapter 62, "Directory of Resources," for extensive resource listings.

TBI incidence rate, risk factors, and causes. Using preliminary hospitalization and mortality data collected from 12 states (Alaska, Arizona, Sacramento County [California], Colorado, Louisiana, Maryland, Missouri, New York, Oklahoma, Rhode Island, South Carolina, and Utah) during 1995-1996, CDC finds the following:[4]

- The average TBI incidence rate (combined hospitalization and mortality rate) is 95 per 100,000 population. Twenty-two percent of people who have a TBI die from their injuries.

- The risk of having a TBI is especially high among adolescents, young adults, and people older than 75 years of age.

- For persons of all ages, the risk of TBI among males is twice the risk among females.

- The leading causes of TBI are motor vehicle crashes, violence, and falls. Nearly two-thirds of firearm-related TBIs are classified as suicidal in intent.

- The leading causes of TBI vary by age: falls are the leading cause of TBI among persons aged 65 years and older, whereas transportation leads among persons aged 5 to 64 years.

- The outcome of these injuries varies greatly depending on the cause: 91% of firearm-related TBIs resulted in death, but only 11% of fall-related TBIs are fatal.

Incidence and prevalence of TBI-related disability. Based on national TBI incidence data and preliminary data from the Colorado Traumatic Brain Injury Registry that describe TBI-related disability in 1996-1997, CDC estimates the following:[5]

- Each year more than 80,000 Americans survive a hospitalization for traumatic brain injury but are discharged with TBI-related disabilities.

- 5.3 million Americans are living today with a TBI-related disability.

Note: The preliminary estimates described above are derived from provisional data that are subject to change, pending receipt of additional data. Therefore, the information contained in this outline should not be published without approval from the Centers for Disease Control and Prevention.

References

1. Guerrero J, Thurman DJ, Sniezek JE. Emergency department visits association with traumatic brain injury: United States, 1995-1996. *Brain Injury*, 2000; 14(2):181-6.

2. Thurman DJ, Guerrero J. Trends in hospitalization associated with traumatic brain injury. *JAMA*, 1999; 282(10):954-7.

3. Unpublished data from Multiple Cause of Death Public Use Data from the National Center for Health Statistics, 1996. Methods are described in Sosin DM, Sniezek JE, Waxweiler RJ. Trends in death associated with traumatic brain injury, 1979-1992. *JAMA* 1995;273(22):1778-1780.

4. Analysis by the CDC National Center for Injury Prevention and Control, using data obtained from state health departments in Alaska, Arizona, California (reporting Sacramento County only), Colorado, Louisiana, Maryland, Missouri, New York, Oklahoma, Rhode Island, South Carolina, and Utah. Methods are described in:

   • Centers for Disease Control and Prevention. Traumatic Brain Injury — Colorado, Missouri, Oklahoma, and Utah, 1990-1993. *MMWR* 1997;46(1):8-11.

   • Thurman DJ, Sniezek JE, Johnson D, Greenspan A, Smith SM. *Guidelines for Surveillance of Central Nervous System Injury*. Atlanta: Centers for Disease Control and Prevention, 1995.

5. Thurman DJ, Alverson CA, Dunn KA, Guerrero J, Sniezek JE. Traumatic brain injury in the United States: a public health perspective. *J Head Trauma Rehab*, 1999; 14(6):602-15.

Epidemiology

Head injury is a major public health problem. It occurs most commonly in teenagers and young adults who would otherwise have been productive members of society. The disabilities that many of them incur from their head injuries often make them dependent upon rehabilitation services and other special care needs for the rest of their lives. Although head injuries steal away more potentially productive years than such common illnesses as cancer, AIDS, heart disease, and diabetes, less research money is spent on head injury than on these other diseases.

Head injury is also commonly referred to as traumatic brain injury (TBI). The most common cause of TBI is motor vehicle accidents. This is also the most common mechanism in teenagers and young adults. The next most common cause is a fall, and this mechanism is most common at the extremes of age, i.e., pediatric and geriatric patients. Alcohol or other drug use contributes significantly to the occurrence of many head injuries.

Pathology

Treatment for head injury may be either surgical or non-surgical. However, these treatments are not mutually exclusive. Many of the same biochemical events that cause damage of the brain after non-operative TBI also occur in patients who undergo surgery, and an operation may not be able to stop or reverse these underlying processes.

Surgical Lesions

When discussing head-injured patients, neurosurgeons often use the term "mass lesion," which refers to an area of localized injury that may cause pressure within the brain. The most common mass lesions seen after TBI are hematomas and contusions. A hematoma is a blood clot within the brain or on its surface. A contusion may be thought of as an area of "bruised" brain. When examined under a microscope, cerebral contusions are comparable to bruises in other parts of the body. They consist of areas of injured or swollen brain mixed with blood that has leaked out of arteries, veins, or capillaries.

Hematomas and contusions can occur anywhere within the brain. Those hematomas between the skull and the dura, which is a thick membrane that surrounds the brain, are called epidural hematomas. Hematomas that are between the dura and the surface of the brain are called subdural hematomas. Intracerebral hematomas are blood clots that are located within the brain tissue itself. Contusions are seen most commonly at the base of the front parts of the brain, but they can occur anywhere.

Subarachnoid hemorrhage appears as diffuse blood spread thinly over the surface of the brain. This is seen commonly after head injury. If this is the only abnormality present on a CT scan, then observation for a short period may be the only treatment needed.

Diffuse Injuries

The hematomas and contusions described generally occur in only one or a few specific parts of a patient's brain, and they are usually easily seen on a computerized tomography (CT) scan. However, TBI can also produce microscopic changes that cannot be seen on CT scans and that are scattered throughout the brain. This category of injuries is called diffuse brain injury, which can occur with or without an associated mass lesion.

One type of diffuse brain injury is diffuse axonal injury. This refers to impaired function and gradual loss of some axons, which are the long extensions of a nerve cell that enable such cells to communicate with each other even if they are located in parts of the brain that are far apart. If enough axons are injured in this way, then the ability of nerve cells to communicate with each other and to integrate their function may be lost or greatly impaired, possibly leaving a patient with severe disabilities.

Another type of diffuse injury is ischemia, or insufficient blood supply to certain parts of the brain. It has been shown that a drop in blood supply to very low levels may occur commonly in a significant percentage of head-injured patients. This is important because a brain that has just undergone a traumatic injury is especially sensitive to even slight reductions in blood flow. For the same reason, changes in blood pressure during the first few days after head injury can have an adverse effect.

Skull Fractures

No treatment is required for most linear skull fractures, which are simple breaks or "cracks" in the skull. Of greater concern is the possibility that forces strong enough to cause a skull fracture may also have caused some damage to the underlying brain. Fractures of the base of the skull are worrisome if they cause injury to nerves, arteries, or other structures. If a fracture extends into the sinuses, there may be leakage of cerebrospinal fluid (CSF) from the nose or ears. Most such leaks will stop spontaneously. Sometimes, it may be necessary to insert a lumbar drain, which is a long, thin, flexible tube that is inserted into the CSF space in the spine of the lower back. This provides an alternate route of CSF drainage so that the dural tear that is responsible for the CSF leak in the base of the skull has time to seal.

Depressed skull fractures are those in which part of the bone presses on or into the brain. These may require surgical treatment. The damage caused by depressed skull fractures depends upon the region of the brain in which they are located and also upon the possible coexistence of any associated diffuse brain injury.

Assessment

Like all trauma patients, persons with head injury need a systematic yet rapid evaluation in the emergency room. Cardiac and pulmonary functions are the first priority. Next, a rapid examination of the entire body is performed.

Neurological Examination

An accurate neurological examination is important to categorize the severity of a patient's injuries and to plan further evaluation and possible treatment. The standard for objectively assessing the severity of head injury is the Glasgow Coma Scale (GCS) (Table 25.1). This scale assigns points to each patient based upon three categories: verbal function, eye opening, and best motor (movement) response. Patients with a GCS score of 13-15 are usually classified as having mild head injuries. Those with a GCS score of 9-12 have moderate head injuries, and those with a score of 3-8 are usually described as having severe head injuries. Any patient who is not obeying commands (for example, to follow instructions to hold up two fingers) is also often considered to have a severe head injury, even if the GCS score may be slightly higher than eight.

In addition to the GCS, the ability of the pupils to become smaller in bright light is also important after head injury. In patients with large mass lesions or with high intracranial pressure (ICP), one or both pupils may be very wide or "blown." The presence of a wide, or dilated, pupil on only one side suggests that a large mass lesion may be present on the same side as the dilated pupil.

Radiologic Assessment

CT scanning is the gold standard for the radiologic assessment of a head-injured patient. A CT scan is easy to perform and is an excellent test for detecting the presence of blood and fractures, which are the most important lesions to identify in emergency situations.

Plain x-rays of the skull are recommended by some people as a way to evaluate patients with only mild neurologic dysfunction. However, most centers in the United States have readily available CT scanning, which is a more accurate test. For this reason, the routine use of skull x-rays for head-injured patients has declined.

Magnetic resonance imaging (MRI) is not commonly performed for acute head injury because it takes longer to perform an MRI scan than a CT scan, because MRI is not as useful as CT for acute trauma, and because transporting an acutely injured patient from the emergency room to the MRI scanner is difficult. However, after a patient has stabilized, MRI may demonstrate the existence of lesions that could not be detected by CT. Such information is generally more useful for determining prognosis than for influencing treatment.

Treatment

Surgical

Many patients with moderate or severe head injuries are taken directly from the emergency room to the operating room. In many cases, surgery is performed to remove a large hematoma or contusion that is significantly compressing the brain or raising the pressure within the skull. After surgery, these patients are usually observed and monitored in the intensive care unit (ICU).

Other head-injured patients may not go to the operating room immediately, but instead are first taken from the emergency room to the ICU. However, contusions or hematomas may enlarge over the first hours or days after head injury, so that some patients are not taken to surgery until several days after an injury. Sometimes these delayed hematomas are discovered when a patient's neurologic exam worsens or when the ICP increases. On other occasions, a routine follow-up CT scan that was ordered to see if a small lesion has changed in size indicates that the hematoma or contusion has enlarged significantly. In many of these cases, removing the lesion before it enlarges and causes neurologic damage may be safest for the patient.

At surgery, the hair over the appropriate part of the head is shaved. After the scalp incision is made, the bone that is removed is usually taken out in a single piece or "flap," which is then replaced after surgery. Sometimes, however, the bone may be shattered or heavily contaminated. In these cases, the contaminated or shattered fragments may be removed and not replaced. The next structure encountered is the dura, which is carefully cut to reveal the underlying brain. After any hematoma or contusion is removed, the surgeon makes sure that the area is not bleeding. He then closes the dura, replaces the bone, and closes the scalp. (If the brain is very swollen, some surgeons may decide not to replace the bone until the swelling goes down, which may take up to several weeks.) The surgeon may elect to place an ICP monitor or other types of monitors if these were not already in place. The patient is then returned to the ICU for observation and additional care.

Medical

At the present time, there is no drug or "miracle treatment" that can be given to prevent nerve damage or promote nerve healing after TBI. The best treatment that can be performed in an ICU is to prevent any secondary injury to the brain. The "primary insult" refers to the initial trauma to the brain, whereas a "secondary insult" is any subsequent development that may contribute to neurologic injury. For example, as mentioned, an injured brain is especially sensitive and vulnerable to decreases in blood pressure that might otherwise be well tolerated. Thus, one way of avoiding secondary insults is to try to maintain the blood pressure at normal or perhaps slightly elevated levels. Likewise, increases in ICP, decreases in blood oxygenation, increases in body temperature, increases in blood glucose, and many other disturbances can potentially worsen neurologic damage. Thus, the prevention of secondary insults is a major part of the ICU management of head-injured patients.

Various monitoring devices may assist the physicians in caring for the patient. Placement of an ICP monitor into the brain itself can help detect excessive swelling of the brain. One commonly used type of ICP monitor is a ventriculostomy, which is a narrow, flexible, hollow catheter that is passed into the ventricles, or fluid spaces in the center of the brain, to monitor ICP and also to drain CSF if the ICP increases. Placement of an oxygen sensor into the jugular vein can detect how much oxygen is in the blood that is coming from the brain and in this way can give an indication of how much oxygen the brain is using. This may be related to the degree of brain damage. Many other monitoring techniques are currently under investigation to see if they can help to improve outcome after head injury or provide other critical information about caring for these patients.

Rehabilitation

Once they leave the acute care hospital, some head-injured patients may benefit from an aggressive rehabilitation program. Such patients usually had less severe initial injuries or have begun to show significant improvement from severe injuries. In some cases, their further recovery may be expedited by transfer to a rehabilitation hospital or to the rehabilitation service of a large hospital. For more severely injured patients or for those whose recovery is slow, constant vigilance is required to prevent the gradual onset of problems with joint mobility, skin integrity, respiratory status, and many other physiologic functions. Patients with moderate or mild injuries, as well as severely injured patients who have improved sufficiently, may be candidates for outpatient therapy.

Regardless of the setting, most head-injury rehabilitation centers emphasize compensatory strategies, which essentially help patients learn to reach the maximum level of function allowed by their impairments. The concept of cognitive retraining, which presumes that at least some of the brain's cognitive capacity can be restored by constant repetition of certain simple tasks, is more controversial but is also emphasized at many centers. Another major goal of head injury rehabilitation is working with patients' families to educate them about what they can realistically expect and how they can best help their injured family member.

Outcome

One of the most widely used systems to classify outcome from head injury is the Glasgow Outcome Scale (Table 25.2).

Patients with mild head injury (usually defined as Glasgow Coma Score 13-15) tend to do well. They may sometimes be troubled by headaches, dizziness, irritability, or similar symptoms, but these gradually improve in most cases.

Patients with moderate head injuries fare less well. Approximately 60% will make a good recovery, and another 25% or so will be left with a moderate degree of disability. Death or a persistent vegetative state will be the outcome in roughly 7%-10%. The remainder are left with a severe degree of disability.

Not surprisingly, the group comprised of severely head-injured patients has the worst outcomes. Only a quarter to a third of these patients have good outcomes. Moderate disability and severe disability each occur in about a sixth of patients, with moderate disability being slightly more common. Roughly a third of these patients die. The remaining few percent remain persistently vegetative.

The above statistics apply to patients with so-called closed head injuries. For penetrating head injuries, which in modern society are caused most commonly by handguns, outcomes follow a different pattern. Over half of all patients with gunshot wounds to the head who

Table 25.1. Glasgow Coma Scale

Scale Value	Best Motor Response	Best Verbal Response	Best Eye Opening Response
6	Obeys commands		
5	Localizes stimulus	Oriented	
4	Withdraws from stimulus	Conversant, but confused	Eyes open spontaneously
3	Flexes arm	States recognizable words or phrases	Eyes open to voice
2	Extends arm	Makes unintelligible sounds	Eyes open to painful stimulus
1	No response	No response	Remain closed

Table 25.2. Glasgow Outcome Scale

Outcome	Score	Description
Good Recovery (GR)	5	Minor disabilities, but able to resume normal life.
Moderate Disability (MD)	4	More significant disabilities, but still able to live independently. Can use public transportation, work in an assisted situation, etc.
Severe Disability (SD)	3	Conscious, but dependent upon others for daily care. Often institutionalized.
Persistent Vegetative State (PVS)	2	Not conscious, though eyes may be open and may "track" movement.
Death (D)	1	Self-explanatory.

are alive upon arrival at a hospital go on to die because their initial injuries are so severe. However, most of the remaining patients tend to do fairly well, largely because their injuries are relatively mild (Glasgow Coma Scale score of 13-15). Relatively few patients suffer injuries of intermediate severity (that is, with a Glasgow Coma Scale score of 6-12) from gunshot wounds, but it is this group that has the most variability in outcomes.

It must be emphasized that, despite its usefulness, the Glasgow Outcome Scale is not a good tool with which to measure subtle emotional or cognitive problems. Several months after a severe head injury, patients who have a good score on the Glasgow Outcome Scale may in fact have significant neuropsychological disabilities. Tremendous effort is being directed into finding better ways to evaluate these problems, into improving the quality of pre-hospital, acute, and rehabilitative care, and into research to learn more about the effects of head injury and their possible treatment.

Preventing Traumatic Brain Injuries

The following safety tips, provided by the Centers for Disease Control and Prevention (CDC) and the Brain Injury Association, may help reduce the chances that you or your children will have a traumatic brain injury.

- Wear a seatbelt every time you drive or ride in a car.

- Buckle your child into a child safety seat, booster seat, or seatbelt (depending on the child's age) every time the child rides in a car.

- Wear a helmet and make sure your children wear helmets when
    - riding a bike or motorcycle;
    - playing a contact sport such as football or ice hockey;
    - using in-line skates or riding a skateboard;
    - batting and running bases in baseball or softball;
    - riding a horse;
    - skiing or snowboarding.

- Keep firearms and bullets stored in a locked cabinet or safe when not in use.

- Avoid falls by
  - using a stepstool with a grab bar to reach objects on high shelves;
  - installing handrails on stairways;
  - installing window guards to keep young children from falling out of open windows;
  - using safety gates at the top and bottom of stairs when young children are around.
- Make sure the surface on your child's playground is made of shock-absorbing material (e.g., hardwood mulch, sand).

The following are common symptoms of concussion among adults:

- low-grade headaches or neck pain that won't go away
- having more trouble than usual with mental tasks (e.g., remembering, concentrating, making decisions)
- slowness in thinking, speaking, acting, or reading
- getting lost or easily confused
- feeling tired all the time, lacking energy or motivation changes in sleeping patterns (sleeping a lot more or having a hard time sleeping)
- feeling light-headed or dizzy, losing your balance
- increased sensitivity to sounds, light, or distractions
- blurred vision, eyes that tire easily
- loss of the sense of smell or taste
- ringing in the ears mood changes (e.g., feeling sad or angry for no reason)

Some symptoms that may appear in a child with a concussion include the following:
- listlessness or tiring easily
- irritability or crankiness
- changes in eating or sleeping patterns
- changes in the way the child plays

- changes in performance at school
- lack of interest in favorite toys or activities
- loss of new skills, such as toilet training
- loss of balance, unsteady walking

Tips for People with TBI

If you think you or your child may have a brain injury, see a doctor right away. The doctor will tell you what to do to help the healing process. But here are some general tips to aid in recovery:

- While healing, get lots of rest.
- Don't rush back into daily activities like work or school.
- Avoid doing anything that could cause another blow or jolt to the head.
- Ask your doctor when it's safe to drive a car, ride a bike, or use heavy equipment because your ability to react may be slower after a brain injury.
- Take only the drugs your doctor has approved, and don't drink alcohol until your doctor says it's okay.
- If you have a hard time remembering things, write them down.

If the brain injury was severe, the injured person may need therapy to learn skills that were lost, such as speaking, walking, or reading. Your doctor can help arrange rehabilitation services.

Additional Information

Please refer to Chapter 62, "Directory of Resources," for extensive resource listings.

Chapter 26

Psychological Effects of Trauma

When Disaster Strikes

Each year, disasters and traumas are an all-too-common part of life for millions throughout the world. The World Health Organization estimates that from 1900-1988, hurricanes left 1.2 million people without homes and directly affected the lives of 3.5 million people. Floods afflicted 339 million people and left 36 million homeless. Earthquakes, typhoons, and cyclones affected another 26 million people each and rendered 10 million homeless. The year 1995 was the most expensive year for disaster internationally—$150 billion dollars was lost primarily in developed countries.

Sadly, those least prepared to deal with disaster often suffer the most: the less developed an area is economically, the greater the number of deaths, injuries, and amount of damage its population sustains in a disaster—especially in more densely populated areas. Cities, states, and nations often lack the resources and insurance coverage they need to help people living in impoverished areas. However, as the 1995 earthquake in Kobe, Japan, illustrated (6,000 dead; 30,000 injured; 300,000 homeless), even industrialized countries with extensive disaster preparation are not immune.

"When Disaster Strikes," Fact Sheet, © 1997 American Psychiatric Association, reprinted with permission, and "Let's Talk Facts about Posttraumatic Stress Disorder," © 1999 American Psychiatric Association, reprinted with permission.

Disasters at Home

In 1996 alone, the American Red Cross responded to 236 major disasters in 48 states, spending a total of $216 million in assistance. The Red Cross noted that virtually every community across the nation was affected by disaster. For example, during one weekend in April 1996, 70 tornadoes hit 10 midwestern and southern states. Forest fires destroyed hundreds of homes in California, New Mexico, Arizona, and Alaska. There was widespread flooding in the eastern U.S. due to a rapid spring meltdown of snow. There also were two major aviation disasters in 1996: the ValuJet and TWA Flight 800 crashes.

Other Traumas

In addition to natural disasters, people today are exposed to a wide range of other traumas: industrial accidents, airplane crashes, and acts of violence as well as more common traumatic events such as house fires, motor vehicle accidents, and physical assaults. In total, each year 3.6 million Americans sustain severe or life-threatening injuries in motor vehicle collisions and other accidents.

Estimates tell us that almost 40 percent of Americans will be exposed to a traumatic event during their lifetimes. While the physical dangers inherent in disasters are obvious, these events are a grave threat to mental health as well.

The Psychological Effects of Disaster

Many people survive disasters without developing significant psychological symptoms. Others, however, may have a difficult time "getting over it." Survivors of trauma have reported a wide range of psychiatric problems, including depression, alcohol and drug abuse, lingering symptoms of fear and anxiety that make it hard to work or go to school, family stress, and marital conflicts. Post-Traumatic Stress Disorder (PTSD) and Acute Stress Disorder (ASD) are probably the best known psychiatric disorders following a traumatic event. People suffering with PTSD or ASD often have persistent nightmares or "flashbacks" of the trauma. They may avoid reminders of the trauma or "feel numb" and have difficulty responding normally to average life situations. They may be on edge, have trouble sleeping, have angry outbursts, or seem excessively watchful. They may become badly depressed and begin to abuse drugs and/or alcohol as a way of medicating their painful feelings. This substance abuse can become active addiction.

The effects of trauma are not limited to those affected directly by the events. Others may also suffer indirect effects from trauma—referred to as "vicarious" or "secondary" traumatization. Those at risk include spouses and loved ones of trauma victims, people who try to help victims, such as police or firemen, and health care professionals who treat trauma victims, such as therapists and emergency room personnel, as well as journalists.

Who Will Develop Problems after Trauma?

The strongest predictor of who will develop problems after trauma is if an individual has a prior history of psychiatric problems. Research into the effects of trauma have shown that, in general, the more devastating and terrifying the trauma is, the more likely it is that a person exposed to it will develop psychiatric symptoms.

Aspects of the disaster or trauma which increase the likelihood of psychiatric distress include a lack of warning about the event, injury during the trauma, death of a loved one, exposure to the grotesque (e.g., maimed bodies), darkness, experiencing the trauma alone, torture, and the possibility of recurrence. However, it should be emphasized that it is not necessary to experience torture or to see bodies and blood in order to develop psychiatric problems after trauma. Researchers are less sure, at this time, what factors protect some people from psychiatric illness following exposure to trauma.

What Treatments Can Help a Traumatized Person?

It is important that a person who has been exposed to a disaster understand that he or she will probably have some of the symptoms described above as a normal response to an abnormal situation. These symptoms usually resolve over time. However, if they persist or interfere with the person's ability to function normally, professional help should be sought. Talk about suicide, excessive guilt or anxiety, and substance abuse are warning signals that require immediate professional attention.

Psychiatrists and other mental health professionals use a variety of effective treatments for disaster-related disorders. Talking treatments—such as individual, couples, family, or group therapy—can be very helpful. Psychiatric medications can also provide relief for the symptoms of depression, anxiety, and sleep disturbances. It is very important for a psychiatrist or other mental health professional to evaluate persistent symptoms to develop a comprehensive treatment program.

How Can Friends, Family, and Co-Workers Help?

One of the most important things a friend, family member, or co-worker can do for someone who's been in a disaster or other trauma is to be a supportive, active listener.

- Listen patiently and nonjudgmentally as the person tells his or her story.

- Avoid offering direct advice other than encouraging him or her to find healthy ways—such as exercise—to cope with stress.

- Discourage such damaging ways of coping as excessive use of alcohol.

It is also important to realize that it takes weeks, months, and sometimes years before a survivor of trauma is able to put the disaster behind him or her. At times people who have resolved their symptoms following the trauma have a recurrence of traumatic symptoms during stressful times in their lives, such as retirement, divorce, or loss of a loved one.

While it is common for loved ones to become impatient and puzzled over the traumatized person's inability to get on with life, it is especially important at these times to persevere and continue to listen patiently. Many people struggle with the urge to "fix it" for their traumatized loved ones. Again, the best "fix" is non-judgmental listening.

Posttraumatic Stress Disorder (PTSD)

Posttraumatic stress disorder (PTSD)—once called shell shock—affects hundreds of thousands of people who have survived earthquakes, airplane crashes, terrorist bombings, inner-city violence, domestic abuse, rape, war, genocide, and other disasters, both natural and human made.

The Facts

Posttraumatic stress disorder (PTSD) has been called shell shock or battle fatigue syndrome. It has often been misunderstood or misdiagnosed, even though the disorder has very specific symptoms.

Ten percent of the population has been affected at some point by clinically diagnosable PTSD. Still more show some symptoms of the disorder. Although it was once thought to be mostly a disorder of war veterans who had been involved in heavy combat, researchers now know that PTSD also affects both female and male civilians, and that it strikes more females than males.

In some cases the symptoms of PTSD disappear with time, whereas in others they persist for many years. PTSD often occurs with—or leads to—other psychiatric illnesses, such as depression.

Everyone who experiences trauma does not require treatment; some recover with the help of family, friends, or clergy. But many do need professional treatment to recover from the psychological damage that can result from experiencing, witnessing, or participating in an overwhelmingly traumatic event.

Symptoms

PTSD usually appears within 3 months of the trauma, but sometimes the disorder appears later. PTSD's symptoms fall into three categories:

- Intrusion
- Avoidance
- Hyperarousal

Intrusion

In people with PTSD, memories of the trauma reoccur unexpectedly, and episodes called "flashbacks" intrude into their current lives. This happens in sudden, vivid memories that are accompanied by painful emotions that take over the victim's attention. This re-experience, or "flashback," of the trauma is a recollection. It may be so strong that individuals almost feel like they are actually experiencing the trauma again or seeing it unfold before their eyes and in nightmares.

Avoidance

Avoidance symptoms affect relationships with others: The person often avoids close emotional ties with family, colleagues, and friends. At first, the person feels numb, has diminished emotions, and can complete only routine, mechanical activities. Later, when re-experiencing the event, the individual may alternate between the flood of emotions caused by re-experiencing and the inability to feel or express emotions at all. The person with PTSD avoids situations or activities that are reminders of the original traumatic event because such exposure may cause symptoms to worsen.

The inability of people with PTSD to work out grief and anger over injury or loss during the traumatic event means the trauma can continue to affect their behavior without their being aware of it. Depression is a common product of this inability to resolve painful feelings. Some people also feel guilty because they survived a disaster while others—particularly friends or family—did not.

Hyperarousal

PTSD can cause those who have it to act as if they are constantly threatened by the trauma that caused their illness. They can become suddenly irritable or explosive, even when they are not provoked. They may have trouble concentrating or remembering current information, and, because of their terrifying nightmares, they may develop insomnia. This constant feeling that danger is near causes exaggerated startle reactions.

Finally, many people with PTSD also attempt to rid themselves of their painful re-experiences, loneliness, and panic attacks by abusing alcohol or other drugs as a "self medication" that helps them to blunt their pain and forget the trauma temporarily. A person with PTSD may show poor control over his or her impulses and may be at risk for suicide.

Treatment

Today, psychiatrists and other mental health professionals have good success in treating the very real and painful effects of PTSD. These professionals use a variety of treatment methods to help people with PTSD to work through their trauma and pain.

Behavior therapy focuses on correcting the painful and intrusive patterns of behavior and thought by teaching people with PTSD relaxation techniques and examining (and challenging) the mental processes that are causing the problem.

Psychodynamic psychotherapy focuses on helping the individual examine personal values and how behavior and experience during the traumatic event affected them.

Family therapy may also be recommended because the behavior of spouse and children may result from and affect the individual with PTSD.

Discussion groups or peer-counseling groups encourage survivors of similar traumatic events to share their experiences and reactions to them. Group members help one another realize that many people would have done the same thing and felt the same emotions.

Medication can help to control the symptoms of PTSD. The symptom relief that medication provides allows most patients to participate more effectively in psychotherapy when their condition may otherwise prohibit it. Antidepressant medications may be particularly helpful in treating the core symptoms of PTSD—especially intrusive symptoms.

Additional Information

American Psychiatric Association
1400 K Street, N.W.
Washington, DC 20005
Toll-Free: 888-357-7924
Tel: 202-682-6000
Fax: 202-682-6850
Website: www.psych.org
E-mail: apa@psych.org

Anxiety Disorders Association of America, Inc.
11900 Parklawn Drive
Suite 100
Rockville, MD 20852-2624
Tel: 301-231-9350
Website: www.adaa.org

International Society for Traumatic Stress Studies
60 Revere Drive
Suite 500
Northbrook, IL 60062
Tel: 877-507-7873
Website: www.istss.org

National Center for PTSD
VA Medical Center (116D)
White River Junction, VT 05009
Tel: 802-296-5132
Fax: 802-296-5135
Website: www.ncptsd.org
E-mail: ptsd@dartmouth.edu

National Institute of Mental Health Public Inquiries
6001 Executive Blvd.
Room 8184 MSC 9663
Bethesda, MD 20892-9663
Tel: 301-443-4513
TTY: 301-443-8431
Fax: 301-443-4279
Facts on Demand: 301-443-5158
Website: www.nimh.nih.gov
E-mail: nimhinfo@nih.gov

National Organization for Victim Assistance
1730 Park Road, N.W.
Washington, DC 20010
Tel: 202-232-6682
Fax: 202-462-2255
Website: www.try-nova.org

U.S. Veterans Administration
Mental Health and Behavioral Sciences Services
810 Vermont Avenue, N.W., Room 990
Washington, DC 20410
Tel: 202-273-8431
Website: www.va.gov

Chapter 27

Trauma Information for Parents

When It's Too Late to "Be Careful"

When I showed my mother the stitches on my head, she laid down the law: "From now on, wrap yourself up with pillows before you play basketball." We both laughed—but she really did wish she could protect me, from every bit of harm the world has to offer. Parents are like that.

Of course, even the best parents can't protect their children from every hurt. Nor would we want to. Part of growing up is learning to cope with skinned knees and lost games. On the other hand, we consider it a tragedy when a child is exposed to a severe trauma or loss. We read about such children in a Florida hurricane, a California earthquake, a Scotland school shooting, and say, "How awful! I'm glad my child wasn't there."

How could this be so common? We don't have earthquakes here! But we do have: car accidents, house fires, robberies, attacks by bullies, child abuse, divorce and abandonment, deaths of family members, friends, pets, etc. "Wait a minute," somebody always interrupts at this point, "You're just talking about life. Everyone has something like this. Are you saying this is all child trauma?"

Maybe. Let me explain what I mean by child trauma. There are two ways of handling an upsetting experience. Ideally, the child will go through the memories, thoughts, and feelings over and over, until

"When It's Too Late to 'Be Careful'," © Ricky Greenwald, Psy.D., 6/30/97, updated 10/13/99, reprinted with permission.

little by little, it is somehow mastered, and no longer disturbing. However, some experiences are so upsetting and overwhelming that instead of facing the memory the child tries to push it out of the way. This strategy may provide temporary relief, but when the memory is not worked through it keeps its disturbing power. In fact, the more the child avoids facing the memory, the more stuck he or she will be. And this can happen with many types of experiences, including loss as well as trauma.

When your child experiences a trauma or loss, you may notice some changes, perhaps in attitude, mood, or behavior. Children's natural feelings of sadness, fear, anger, guilt, and helplessness can be expressed in a variety of ways, some of which might not seem to make sense. One child may argue more, become clingy, have trouble getting to sleep, and have bad dreams. Another child might react completely differently, for example, by becoming quiet, withdrawn, anxious, and sad. Your child might have other symptoms you don't notice, for example, feeling at fault, thinking a lot about the memory, and being afraid that something like it will happen again.

Remember that these are normal reactions—your child's world has just been shaken-up. Such symptoms do not mean that there is something wrong with your child. If all goes well, the symptoms will gradually fade as the child works it out.

You can help your child get through this difficult time by being supportive and reassuring. Some parents try to protect their child after the fact, by not talking about the event. But this just gives the message that it is too scary even for a grown-up to face. The child needs to feel free to talk about it, to express thoughts and feelings at his or her own pace. And the child may need to hear, over and over again, that he or she is not to blame, is safe now, etc. This is also an important time for parents to be consistent in their discipline. After a trauma or loss, children often feel very insecure, and might test parents by trying to get special treatment or by acting up. Although you might be tempted to indulge your child, be careful. Being inconsistent can give your child the message that even you can't be counted on anymore.

Unfortunately, sometimes even your best effort might not be enough. You may be so upset yourself that it's just too hard to handle your child in the best way. Or your child may refuse to let you get through; the trauma or loss may be too severe. Then the child might get stuck. This can happen even when the acute symptoms subside, and the child "seems okay" again. Many children keep their distress to themselves, so as not to worry their parents or seem strange to their friends. Untreated, your child's response to trauma or loss can have long-term consequences. This can range from being more sensitive to similar wounds in the future, all the way to major problems such as long-term behavior problems, depression, anxiety, or post-traumatic stress disorder.

Remember, it will not go away by itself. Your child needs your help. If you feel that your child may be stuck, it is time to consult a child psychologist or other mental health professional. There is no shame in getting help for your family. As a parent, it is your job to handle the day-to-day problems, and to recognize when more help is needed. You wash a cut yourself, but a broken bone you bring to the doctor. Right? The principle here is the same, even if the wound is of a different sort.

There are many child therapists, and it is important to find one who is right for your family. First of all, try to find someone with a good reputation, who has training and experience in working with children like yours. Then schedule an appointment and see if you feel comfortable, if you trust this person to help your family. If you are not sure, you can express your concerns and see how the therapist responds. If you still have serious doubts, it is okay to try someone else. You are the customer and you have a right to choose.

The therapist should keep you involved and informed, even if the focus is on the child. This does not mean that you are told every detail about your child's session, but you should be generally aware of progress, and of what you can do to help. You can usually expect to see progress within a few weeks to a few months, depending on circumstances. You can help the therapist by being reliable, cooperative, and honest.

For better or worse, we can't wrap our children up in pillows, and they will get hurt sooner or later. Then it is up to us to help them through it, so that they can grow stronger from the experience, and not become crippled. Parents can help by being supportive, reassuring, and consistent. When the hurt is more severe, or when the child seems stuck, it can be very useful to consult a professional. The good news is that, even after the trauma or loss has happened, you can do a lot to help your child recover. And with recent advances in treatment, there is more reason for hope than ever before.

How Parents Can Help

Children who experience a trauma (such as a car accident) have reactions that may include denial, fear, anger, guilt, sadness, and confusion. These reactions are part of the normal recovery process. You can help your child by showing acceptance of her feelings, reassuring her that she is safe now, and by being consistent with your discipline and expectations, so that she will feel secure. You may observe some of the following behaviors:

1. **Sleep Disturbance.** Your child may sleep fitfully, talk in sleep, have nightmares, scream, cry out, etc. When he awakens, he might need consoling and reassurance. Even though he may not recall what he was dreaming, he was probably remembering and reliving the accident. This is normal, and how our minds resolve traumatic events. Reassure your child that he is safe; tell him that he just had a bad dream about the accident, but it's all over now. In the child's waking hours, encourage him to talk about the accident—tell the story over and over. If he doesn't remember, you can talk to him about it and tell him what happened. It's important to talk about this to help normalize it. Many parents do not know this and are afraid to make their child think about it as it is unpleasant. However, then the child is left to deal with his memories all alone. Get him to share it with you even if it is hard for you to hear.

2. **Guilt.** Some children think they have been bad and that is why the accident happened. Most children feel guilty about something they have done or thought about. Though unrelated, they think the accident is punishment. Tell your child that she is not a bad person, that she is not being punished. Reinforce this often.

3. **Acting Younger.** Some children become frightened and afraid to be alone. Some children regress—act younger than their age. This is also normal. Give your child love and reassurance, but do not change drastically how you treat him. Understand that he feels ill and may be younger acting, but do not let him "get away" with behaviors you normally would not tolerate. Otherwise, your child will get the message that you believe something is wrong with him.

4. **Fear.** Some children will continue to be afraid of things they associate with the accident, e.g., cars, the driver of the car. Gently, together, in small steps, increase their exposure to these things. Talk about each step along the way.

5. **Your Feelings.** Sometimes parents will feel guilty and responsible. Remember, it is not your fault either. Parents can
never watch their children at all times. Do not spend your energy feeling guilty and trying to make it up to your child. This
is the time to be focusing on your child's feelings, and helping
her recover. If your feelings persist, and get in the way of
helping your child, seek the support of another adult or a professional.

Common Reactions to Trauma

Here are some of the common reactions to experiencing a trauma.
You may notice one or more of these items following a traumatic event.
These reactions may begin immediately or after a delay.

1. Sleep Disturbance
    • Nightmares
    • Bad or scary dreams
    • Talk or yell in sleep
    • Fitful or restless sleep
    • Trouble getting to sleep
    • Afraid of sleeping
    • Bed wetting

2. Guilt
    • Blaming self for traumatic event
    • Blaming self for other things
    • Excessive "bad" behavior that requires punishment
    • Excessive "good" behavior that replaces usual level of ma-
      turity and playfulness

3. Acting Younger
    • Clinging
    • Not wanting to be left alone
    • Demanding attention
    • Demanding extra care or privileges
    • Acting "like a baby"

4. Fear
    • Fear of thing related to trauma (getting into a car after
      being in a car accident)

- Fear of loud noises, sudden moves, being touched, etc.
- Fear of being alone
- Fear of strangers
- Other fears or phobias

5. Parents' Reactions
   - Guilt
   - Anxious or over-protective
   - Sleep disturbances
   - Inconsistency with discipline or expectations
   - Over-indulging, letting child "get away with" things

While these reactions are normal, sometimes recovery does not seem to progress. If you feel that your child is stuck, you should feel free to call a child psychologist or other mental health professional. There is effective, non-drug treatment to help children and their families recover from emotional trauma.

Part Four

Emergency Care

Chapter 28

What to Do in an Emergency

- Knowing what to do ahead of time will potentially prevent an emergency, possibly even save a life.

- Every emergency can be handled by remembering four things: prevent, prepare, recognize, act. Quick action can save a life, and the initial minutes after an injury or medical crisis are frequently the most important. The key is knowing what to do, remaining calm, and making a decision to act. Calling 911 is one of the most important things you can do.

What Steps Can I Take to Prevent Emergencies?

Preventing emergencies means getting yearly doctor's exams and regular exercise. Protect your health by determining whether you're at risk for any life-threatening conditions, and follow your doctor's suggestions to reduce any risk factors that can be dangerous to your health. For example, if you don't smoke, don't start. If you do smoke, quit. We're all busy people, and there's never enough time, but is it easier to handle a heart attack in progress or to prevent it in the first place with regular exercise and visits to the doctor? If we don't prevent now, we'll pay later.

This chapter includes "What to Do in an Emergency," © June 1998, and "Seconds Save Lives in Medical Emergencies," © 1998, both reprinted with the permission of the American College of Emergency Physicians.

How Can I Prepare for an Emergency?

After doing everything we can to prevent an emergency, the next step is to prepare for one. While it may seem negative to prepare for the worst, preparation takes prevention one step further. It means that if an emergency does occur, we can handle it calmly, quickly, and effectively to minimize its impact.

Being prepared means keeping a list of emergency numbers by the phone. The police, fire department, poison control center, local hospital, ambulance service, and your family doctor's office should all be included. Being prepared means making a list of all the medications you and your family take and their dosages. In an emergency, you might not be able to speak for yourself, so carry it with you. This list could help prevent serious drug interactions.

Also make a list of allergies, especially drug allergies or those with severe reactions. This list will help ensure that the care you receive won't make matters worse.

Keep a well-stocked first-aid kit at home, at work, and in your car. A good first-aid kit will help you handle medical situations—from minor shaving cuts, blisters from roller skating, or sunburns, to sprains or severe cuts.

Take a first-aid class. A basic class will teach CPR and proper methods for treating burns, wrapping sprains, applying splints, and performing the Heimlich maneuver. First-aid classes also will help you learn how to remain calm and how to calm others in an emergency.

How Do I Recognize an Emergency?

Recognize the difference between a minor crisis and a life-threatening emergency. For example, upper abdominal pain can be indigestion, ulcers, or an early sign of a heart attack. A toddler who falls down in the yard unconscious may have tripped or he could have been stung by an insect and be having an allergic reaction.

Not every cut needs stitches, nor does every burn require advanced medical treatment. Part of handling an emergency is being able to evaluate warning signs and make a fast decision. But it's always best to err on the side of caution. In an emergency, always call 911 or the local hospital for assistance.

When should you call an ambulance instead of driving to the emergency department? Ask yourself the following questions:

- Is the victim's condition life-threatening?

- Could the victim's condition worsen and become life-threatening on the way to the hospital?

- Could moving the victim need the skills or equipment of paramedics or emergency medical technicians?

- Would distance or traffic conditions cause a delay in getting the victim to the hospital?

If the answer to any of these questions is yes, or if you are unsure, it's best to call an ambulance.

When Do I Decide to Act?

Being prepared and understanding the situation will increase the effectiveness of your actions in an emergency. But deciding to act is crucial. It means being ready, willing, and able to help someone until emergency service arrives, or the crisis has passed.

Action can mean anything from calling paramedics, applying direct pressure to a wound, performing CPR, or splinting an injury. Never perform a medical procedure if you are unsure of how to do it.

Handling an emergency can be scary. We feel powerless and unable to help loved ones at a time when they need it most. But if we all take preventative measures and prepare for the worst, we can defuse emergencies before they start.

Seconds Save Lives in Medical Emergencies

Do you know what to do in an emergency? The few minutes after an injury occurs or at the onset of a medical crisis are frequently the most important.

"The key is knowing what to do, remaining calm, and making a decision to act," said Dr. Kathleen Clem, M.D., of the American College of Emergency Physicians. "You can make a difference in critical moments by remembering four important steps: prevent, prepare, recognize, act."

Prepare for Emergencies

After doing everything you can to prevent emergencies, the next step is to prepare for one. Some basic steps are:

- Keep well-stocked first-aid kits at home, at work, and in your car.

- Learn how to recognize emergency warning signs.

- Organize family medical information.

- Make lists of medications (and dosages) taken by you and your family; include allergies.

- Identify and eliminate safety hazards in your home.

- Take a first-aid class.

- Post emergency numbers near the telephone.

Learn to Recognize Life-Threatening Emergencies

Not every cut needs stitches, nor does every burn require advanced medical treatment. If you think someone could suffer significant harm or die unless prompt care is received, that situation is an emergency, and call 911 or the local hospital for help. Get help fast when the following warning signs are seen:

- Chest pain lasting 2 minutes or more.

- Uncontrolled bleeding.

- Sudden or severe pain.

- Coughing or vomiting blood.

- Difficulty breathing, shortness of breath.

- Sudden dizziness, weakness, or change in vision.

- Severe or persistent vomiting or diarrhea.

- Change in mental status (e.g., confusion, difficulty arousing).

Decide to Act

Be ready, willing, and able to help someone until emergency services arrive. Action can mean anything from calling paramedics, applying direct pressure on a wound, performing CPR, or splinting an injury. Never perform a medical procedure if you're unsure about how to do it.

- Do not move anyone involved in a car accident, serious fall, or is found unconscious unless he or she is in immediate danger of further injury.

- Do not give the victim anything to eat or drink.

- Protect the victim by keeping him or her covered.

- If the victim is bleeding, apply a clean cloth or sterile bandage. If possible, elevate the injury and apply direct pressure on the wound.

- If the victim is not breathing or does not have a pulse, begin rescue breathing or CPR

Additional Information

American College of Emergency Physicians
National Headquarters
1125 Executive Circle
Irving, TX 75038-2522
Toll-Free: 800-798-1822
Tel: 972-550-0911
Fax: 972-580-2816
Website: www.acep.org

Washington, DC Office
2121 K Street, NW
Suite 325
Washington, DC 20037
Toll-Free: 800-320-0610
Tel: 202-728-0610
Fax: 202-728-0617
Website: www.acep.org

ACEP publishes fliers about what to include in a home first aid kit and a traveler's first-aid kit, and offers a free Home Organizer for Medical Emergencies which can be obtained by sending a self-addressed stamped envelope.

Chapter 29

What to Expect in the Emergency Room

What Will Happen?

Medical emergencies are unpredictable—people don't expect to have one. You can ease the anxiety of a visit to an emergency department by learning some basic facts.

"First, it's important to know that emergency medicine over the past 30 years has evolved into a state-of-the-art, technologically advanced, fully recognized medical specialty," said Dr. Russell Harris of the American College of Emergency Physicians. "Today's emergency physicians are highly educated and trained to handle all kinds of emergency situations and to provide the best possible care."

Arrival

If you arrive by ambulance or are unconscious you will be assigned a patient bed immediately and be treated. If someone else drives you to the emergency department, you will first enter the waiting room, where your medical condition will be assessed.

Triage

Most likely, a nurse will determine the severity of your condition, based on your symptoms, and check your vital signs, including

This chapter includes the following documents reprinted with the permission of the American College of Emergency Physicians: "The Emergency Department: What To Expect," © 1996-2001; "Emergency Care of Children," © June 2000; and "Emergency Department Waiting Times."

temperature, heart rate, and blood pressure. This process is called "triage."

Additional information will also be obtained, such as your name and address and medical history, and someone will prepare a chart. Anyone who comes to an emergency department will not be turned away, regardless of their ability to pay or insurance coverage.

"There are many reasons a trip to the emergency department can take longer than a visit to the doctor's office," said Dr. Harris. Unlike a doctor's office, where appointments are spread out, many emergency patients may arrive at once. Also unlike a doctor's office, patients often must wait for the results of x-rays or tests. You can help make the time pass more quickly and speed your treatment by planning ahead. If you have children, take along a book or toys for them. If possible, bring along someone to remain at your bedside. Also, bring any up-to-date medical records, including lists of medications and allergies, and any advance directives, such as a living will.

Examination

Once you are placed in an examination area, an emergency physician will examine you, possibly ordering tests (e.g., x-ray, blood, electrocardiogram) and your vital signs will be monitored. Nurses and other assistants will also assist you during your visit.

Treatment

If you are critically ill or require constant intravenous medications or fluids, you may be admitted to the hospital. Otherwise, an emergency physician will discuss your diagnosis and treatment plan with you before you are discharged. You may also receive written instructions regarding medications, medical restrictions, or symptoms that may require a return visit.

"Every year almost 100 million people seek care in the nation's emergency departments, making the ED American's health care safety net—available 24 hours a day, 7 days a week-treating patients from all walks of life—rich and poor, young and old, insured and uninsured," added Dr. Harris.

Emergency Care of Children

- Emergency care of children in the United States is the best in the world. It's better today than even 10 years ago. Emergency

departments are staffed by career emergency specialists trained
to provide the highest levels of care to patients of all ages.

* Emergency departments each year care for 30 million ill and injured children. They are staffed and equipped to provide life-
saving emergency care to these children.

* Emergency medicine residency programs provide comprehensive training in the care of children in emergency situations.

* The American College of Emergency Physicians (ACEP) was
among the first organizations to develop guidelines for pediatric
equipment, staffing, and training for both the emergency department and the emergency medical services (e.g., ambulance)
settings.

* Parents should talk with their child's pediatrician or family
physician to develop an emergency plan and be familiar with
their nearest local emergency departments.

* The most important thing parents can do to protect the health
of their children is to practice injury prevention. Preventable injuries are the leading cause of childhood death and permanent
injury.

What Is the Status of Emergency Care of Children in the United States?

More than 30 million children receive acute and life-saving care
in the nation's emergency departments each year. Today, emergency
departments are staffed by career emergency specialists trained to
provide the highest levels of care to patients of all ages.

Emergency medicine residency programs provide comprehensive
training in the care of children in emergency situations. Residents
generally receive 4 to 6 months of training in emergency care of children. Additionally, during the second and third year of their residen-
cies, they spend 6 months in emergency departments under the
supervision of attending emergency physicians. During that time, 20
to 30 percent of their patients are children.

Since the 1980s, the field of emergency medicine has focused substantial attention on the emergency care of children. As a result of
research, training, and standardization, emergency care of children
is far more advanced today than it was when we were children. Emergency physicians have been and continue to be responsible for the

development of new treatment techniques and the widespread availability of specialized pediatric equipment.

Why Do We Hear about Problems Related to Emergency Care of Children?

Isolated examples of tragic cases may make high-profile headlines, but they do not reflect the status of emergency care of children in the United States. Emergency care of children is better today than ever before, and emergency physicians have been leaders in raising the standards and quality of care in emergency departments and in the emergency medical services environment (e.g., ambulances).

Every recent study examining the care of significant numbers of children has consistently demonstrated that quality emergency care is being provided in emergency departments. Sometimes, sadly, even with the best of medical personnel, the best of training, and the best of equipment, some children (and adults) have such severe injuries or illness, they can't be saved.

Should I Ask for a Pediatrician to Treat My Child in the Emergency Department?

No. Emergency physicians are specialists in treating children in emergencies and apply the same principles as pediatricians. Both draw from the same information sources (medical courses and clinical training in medical school). In fact, emergency medicine residents receive more training in pediatric airway management and lifesaving techniques than pediatric residents. Emergency physicians also have additional expertise in treating critically ill or injured children and have done extensive research and published numerous studies on many pediatric topics, including airway management and resuscitation. Emergency staff may contact your child's pediatrician or family physician to obtain important information about your child's medical history.

Should I Insist My Child Be Treated at a Children's Hospital?

No. Parents should take their child to the nearest emergency department, unless directed by their child's physician to another nearby emergency department. They should also understand that an ambulance will take their child to the nearest emergency department, or if appropriate, to a nearby specialty center. If necessary, your child may be transferred after stabilization to a hospital with advanced pediatric capabilities. However, it's important for parents to plan in advance what they will do in an emergency situation by working with their child's regular physician during a routine office visit to develop an emergency care plan.

What Can I Do to Make Sure My Child Gets Good Treatment in an Emergency?

The most important factor in dealing with an emergency is to be prepared. This means talking with your child's pediatrician about emergency care to develop an emergency plan and being familiar with the closest emergency departments. Ask when you should go directly to an emergency department, when you should call an ambulance, and what to do when the physician's office is closed. If your child requires treatment in the emergency department, make sure all your questions and concerns are answered by the staff. If your child is left in someone else's care (including a relative), always leave a consent-to-treat form and a medical history form, which also can be obtained through ACEP.

What Advice Do You Have for Parents about Children's Medical Emergencies?

The most important thing parents can do to protect the health of their children is to practice injury prevention. Preventable injuries are the leading cause of childhood death and permanent injury. Child safety seats, bicycle helmets, poison prevention, safety caps on medicines, window guards, and sports safety gear are just a start. Parents should also learn to recognize the warning signs and symptoms of serious childhood illnesses and be familiar with life-saving techniques like the Heimlich maneuver and CPR (cardiopulmonary resuscitation). Remember that every child comes with an important safety feature—his or her parents.

How Can We Make Sure That All Children Get Quality Emergency Care?

Thanks to the efforts of emergency physicians and other medical professionals, most American children now have access to high-quality, life-saving emergency care. Parents, community leaders, and elected officials can make emergency care of children a priority by supporting adequate funding for emergency education, training, equipment, and research.

What Are Emergency Physicians Doing to Improve Emergency Care of Children?

Physicians who specialize in emergency medicine have devoted their careers to improving the emergency care system through research, training, policy, and public education. Until 30 years ago, there was little recognition among the public or the medical community that emergency care required unique training, equipment, and procedures. ACEP was among the first organizations to develop guidelines for pediatric emergency equipment, staffing, training, and procedures. In addition, the training curriculum for emergency physicians continually is updated to keep up with new developments. Some studies have shown that as many as 90 percent of communities now meet these guidelines. Emergency physicians have also developed innovative systems to improve treatment of pediatric patients, such as the Broselow tape, which color-codes pediatric equipment and medicines, according to a child's height and weight.

What Are Pediatric Emergency Specialists?

The American Board of Emergency Medicine (ABEM) and the American Board of Pediatrics (ABP) in 1992 Pediatrics developed a subspecialty in pediatric emergency medicine to further advance training and education for emergency care of children, and members from ACEP and the American Academy of Pediatrics who were board-certified, were appointed to help develop the exam. Identical exams for board certification are now given in this subspecialty. These physicians, called pediatric emergency specialists, have chosen to focus their practices on emergency care of children, including performing research and teaching in pediatric emergency medicine.

More than 1,000 doctors have become board certified in the pediatric subspecialty, the majority of which are pediatricians who want additional training and education in emergency care of children. These pediatric emergency specialists primarily staff emergency departments in the nation's children's hospitals.

Emergency Department Waiting Times

- Emergency physicians are committed to treating everyone in need of emergency care in a timely manner. Emergency departments are the foundation of America's health care safety net.

Everyone who comes to an emergency department will be seen, regardless of his or her ability to pay or insurance status.

- When you visit an emergency department, a quick examination, known as triage, will be conducted to determine whether you need immediate treatment. This means you may have to wait for treatment when more seriously ill or injured patients need to be seen first.

- Treatment delays can result from large patient volumes, waiting for x-ray and laboratory results, waiting for specialist care, and shortages of beds for patients needing hospital admission.

- Managed care restrictions have contributed to hospital closings, mergers, and consolidations at record rates, resulting in increased crowding and delays in emergency departments.

- Approximately 43 million Americans do not have health insurance, and when they need medical care, they turn to their nearest emergency department.

- Despite these problems, emergency departments have sought to improve customer service and decrease waiting times by registering patients at bedsides and streamlining processes for care.

- Emergency care is an essential public service. When a community loses its emergency department, everyone loses.

Why Do Patients Have to Wait for Treatment in the Emergency Department?

People wait in emergency departments for many reasons. These include:

- Waiting for the sickest patients to be seen first.

- Overcrowding due to epidemics (e.g., flu season) or ambulance diversion of patients from other crowded hospitals. Also, unlike a doctor's office, where appointments are spread out, many emergency patients may arrive at once.

- Waiting for x-ray and laboratory results.

- Waiting for specialist consultations.

- Shortages of inpatient beds.

- Shortages of nurses. Shortages may result from a national nursing shortage, the unpredictable demands on the nursing resource, or unrealistic financial constraints on hospitals.

- Increasing number of uninsured people in the United States.

Why Are Emergency Departments Crowded?

Overcrowding is a significant national problem, contributing to long waits in emergency departments. It also is a symptom of a failing health care system. Solutions may be complex and expensive, but they are essential to making sure the public can continue to rely on emergency departments for quality and timely emergency care. Treating the causes of overcrowding must become a national priority in order to guarantee emergency medical care for all. Causes of overcrowding include:

- Dramatic increases in the use of emergency departments; nearly 100 million people visit emergency departments each year.

- Many people lack access to any sources of regular medical care. This is especially true for the poor and uninsured.

- Hospitals may lack sufficient resources to provide appropriate care to patients requiring emergency hospitalization. When a hospital has no room to admit patients, seriously ill or injured patients must remain in the emergency department until a bed becomes available. When emergency physicians and nurses must care for critical patients for extended periods of time, it requires dedicated resources and time, which means other patients must wait longer.

- Hospitals are closing, merging, and consolidating at record rates nationwide. Between 1994 and 1996, more than 300 medical-surgical hospitals with licensed emergency services shut their doors, according to the American Hospital Association. Additionally, the growth of managed care, in addition to bringing cutbacks in reimbursements and restrictions on hospital admissions and lengths of stay, has limited the ability of providers to offset the expense of treating the uninsured.

How Much Time Should You Expect to Be in an Emergency Department?

If you have a minor illness or injury, and the emergency department isn't crowded, your visit may be as brief as 1 to 2 hours. If you require blood tests, x-rays, or other diagnostic tests, your visit may be longer because it will take time to obtain the test results. If the emergency medicine specialist consults another physician specialist, you may have to wait longer. Some patients who need to be hospitalized may have extensive waits for transfer from the emergency department to an inpatient bed because the hospital is full. Hospitals no longer enjoy a large reserve of empty beds, as they strive for maximal financial efficiency in a time of revenue constraints.

According to the Centers for Disease Control and Prevention (Advance Data No. 313, May 10, 2000), on average patients wait about 41 minutes to see a physician in emergency departments. The waiting time related to the patient's conditions. For example, patients with emergent conditions waited approximately 19.5 minutes (± 1.4 minutes) before seeing a physician. (Emergent conditions were defined as those the triage practitioner "determines must receive care immediately to combat danger to life or limb and where any delay would likely result in deterioration.") Patients with semiurgent and nonurgent conditions waited 59.7 minutes (± 2.7 minutes) and 60.1 minutes (± 3.8 minutes), respectively. (Semiurgent conditions were defined as those in which patients need treatment within 1 to 2 hours.)

According to the same survey, the distribution of visits in an emergency department was fairly constant between 8 a.m. and midnight, with a peak occurring during the late afternoon and early evening hours (4:00 p.m.-7:59 p.m.). Less than 7 percent of visits took place in the early morning hours (4:00 a.m.-7:59 a.m.). According to many emergency physicians, weekends and Mondays are the busiest days of the week.

What Is Triage?

Triage is the process used to sort patients in order of acuity—or the severity of their illness. Triage determines who needs to be seen first. In most emergency departments, a triage nurse will determine the severity of a patient's condition, based on symptoms. In addition, when a patient first comes to the emergency department, personal and medical history information will be obtained, and vital signs will be checked, including temperature, heart rate, and blood pressure. If you have a minor illness or injury, you may have to wait while sicker or more severely injured patients are seen first.

What Effect do Hospital Consolidations and Closings Have on Patient Waiting Times?

Hospitals are closing, merging, and consolidating at record rates nationwide. This means that those emergency departments which remain open may experience more overcrowding. If cutbacks are too severe, a community will be left unprepared for disasters, epidemics, or large volumes of patients.

Do Extensive Waiting Times Affect Treatment Outcomes?

Long waits can affect patient outcomes. Patients may get tired of waiting and leave, even though they need emergency medical care. Some patients may wait longer than optimal, but emergency departments work hard to make sure the sickest patients are seen first and that all patients are seen in a timely manner. However, when emergency departments are crowded, the quality of care may suffer.

What Steps Have Been Taken to Improve Customer Service in Emergency Departments?

The goal in emergency care is to be more responsive to patients and families. Many hospital emergency departments seek to improve customer service by decreasing waiting times by using such measures as registering people at bedsides, using pneumatic tube systems to speed specimens to the laboratory, computerizing tracking systems, and developing alternative systems for streamlining patient flow and processing laboratory tests. New technologies also have helped reduce emergency department crowding by using rapid tests to evaluate patients. A few emergency departments have even offered individualized services, valet parking, computer outlets, patient care advocates, and advertised that patients will be seen by doctors within specified amounts of time. However, these measures have not reduced emergency department crowding related to hospitals that are closing, merging, or consolidating; outbreaks of disease (e.g., flu); and major natural disasters (e.g., hurricanes, fires, etc.) or major multiple motor vehicle crashes.

The American College of Emergency Physicians (ACEP) supports hospital efforts to promote quality patient care through reduced emergency department waiting times.

Chapter 30

Childcare First Aid

Note: Wear disposable gloves if coming in contact with blood. Dispose of gloves in a sturdy leakproof plastic bag. Wash hands.

First Aid Measures

Condition: Action

Abdominal Pain

Abdominal Pain (Severe): Notify parents.

- If the child has been injured, or has severe vomiting, bloody vomiting, or is very pale, call 911.
- Bloody diarrhea accompanied by severe abdominal pain is a medical emergency. Call 911.
- Do not allow child to eat or drink.

Abrasions

Abrasions (Scrapes): Wash abrasion with soap and water.

- Allow to dry.

"The ABC's of Safe and Healthy Child Care," National Center for Injury Prevention and Control, January 1997, revised by David A. Cooke, M.D., October 29, 2001.

- Cover with a sterile nonstick band-aid or dressing.
- Notify parents.

Asphyxiation

Asphyxiation (Suffocation): Call 911.

- If the child is in a closed area filled with toxic fumes, move the child outside into the fresh air.
- Perform CPR if child is not breathing.
- If you are alone, perform CPR for one minute first, then call 911.

Asthma

Asthma Attack: Give prescribed medication, if any, as previously agreed to by parents. If attack does not stop after the child is given the medication, and the child is still having difficulty breathing, call 911.

- **If you have no medication** and the attack does not subside within a few minutes, call the parents and ask them to come immediately and take the child for medical care.
- If the child has difficulty breathing, call 911.

Bites and Stings

Animal: Wash the wound with soap and water.

- Notify parents to pick up the child and seek medical advice.
- If bite is from a bat, fox, raccoon, skunk, or unprovoked cat or dog, or any animal that may have rabies, call the health department, which will contact animal control to catch the animal and observe it for rabies. Do not try to capture the animal yourself. Make note of the description of the animal and any identifying characteristics (whether dog or cat had a collar, for example).

Human: Wash the wound with soap and water.

- Notify parents.
- If bite causes bleeding, contact the health department for advice.

Insect: Do not pull out stinger as it may break off; remove the stinger by scraping it out with a fingernail or credit card, then apply a cold cloth.

- Notify parents. Call 911 if hives, paleness, weakness, nausea, vomiting, difficult breathing, or collapse occurs.

Snake: Call local poison control center. Do not apply ice.

- Notify parents immediately, then the health department.
- If the child has difficulty breathing, call 911.

Ticks: Notify parents to seek preferences. If removal is desired, this is best done by a medical professional. Do not try to smother the tick with oil or to burn it.

Waterlife: For stingray or catfish stings, submerge affected area in warm water to deactivate the toxin. For other stings, such as from jellyfish, rinse with clean water. Call parents to seek medical care.

Bleeding

External: For small wounds, apply direct pressure with a gauze pad for 10-15 minutes. (Use gloves.)

- If bleeding continues or is serious, apply a large pressure dressing and call 911 immediately.

Internal: If child has been injured and vomits a large amount of blood or passes blood through the rectum, call 911. Otherwise, contact parents to seek medical care.

- If a child is a hemophiliac and has injured a joint through a minor bump or fall, call the parents. The child may need an injection of blood factor.

Bruises: Apply cold compresses to fresh bruises for the first 15 to 30 minutes.

- Note: A child with bruises in unusual locations should be evaluated for child abuse.

Burns and Scalds

Note: A child with burns and scalds should be evaluated for child abuse.

No blisters: Place burned extremity in cold water or cover burned area with cold, wet cloths until pain stops (at least 15 minutes).

With blisters: Same as for no blisters. Do not break blisters. Call parents to take child to get medical care.

Deep, extensive burns: Call 911.

- Do not apply cold water.

- Cover child with a clean sheet and then a blanket to keep the child warm.

Electrical: If possible, disconnect power by shutting off wall switch, throwing a breaker in the electrical box, or any other safe way.

- Do not directly touch child if power is still on. Use wood or thick dry cloth (non-conducting material) to pull child from power source.

- Call 911.

- Start CPR if necessary.

- Notify parents.

Croup and Epiglottitis

Croup: Call parents to pick up child and get medical care.

Epiglottitis: Similar to croup, but with high fever, severe sore throat, drooling, and difficulty breathing.

- Transport child in upright position to medical care.

- Call 911 for ambulance if child has severe breathing difficulty.

Dental Injuries

Braces (Broken): Remove appliance, if it can be done easily.

- If not, cover sharp or protruding portion with cotton balls, gauze, or chewing gum.

- If a wire is stuck in gums, cheek, or tongue, *do not* remove it. Call parent to pick up and take the child to the orthodontist immediately.

- If the appliance is not injuring the child, no immediate emergency attention is needed.

Cheek, Lip, Tongue (Cut/ Bitten): Apply ice to bruised areas.

- If bleeding, apply firm but gentle pressure with a clean gauze or cloth.

- If bleeding continues after 15 minutes, call the parent to pick up the child and get medical care.

Jaw Injury: Immobilize jaw by having child bite teeth together.

- Wrap a towel, necktie, or handkerchief around child's head under the chin.

- Call parent to pick up and take the child to the emergency room.

Tooth (Broken): Rinse dirt from the injured area with warm water.

- Place cold compresses over the face in the area of the injury.

- Locate and save any tooth fragments.

- Call the parent to pick up and take the child and tooth fragments to the dentist *immediately*.

Tooth (Knocked Out): Find the tooth. Handle tooth by the smooth, white portion (crown), not by the root. Rinse the tooth with water, but *do not* clean it.

- Place tooth in a cup of milk or water. Call the parent to pick up and take the child and tooth to the dentist *immediately*. (Time is critical.)

Tooth (Bleeding Due to Loss of Baby Tooth): Fold and pack clean gauze or cloth over bleeding area.

- Have child bite on gauze for 15 minutes.

- Repeat again. If bleeding persists, call parent to pick up and take the child to the dentist.

Sores (Cold/ Canker): Tell parent and request physician examination if sore persists for more than a week.

Eye Injuries

Eye Injuries: If a chemical is splashed in the eye, immediately flush eye with tepid water, with the eyelid held open. Then remove contact lens, if present, and rinse eye with tepid water for at least 15 minutes.

- Do not press on injured eye.
- Gently bandage both eyes shut to reduce eye movement.
- Call parent to pick up and take child to get medical care.

Fractures

Arm, Leg, Hand, Foot, Fingers, Toes: Do not move injured part if swollen, broken, or painful.

- Call parent to pick up and take child to get medical care.

Neck or Back: Do not move child; keep child still. Call 911 for ambulance.

Cold

Frostbite/Freezing: Warm arm, leg, hand, foot, fingers, or toes by holding them in your armpit.

- Warm ears and noses with a warm palm.
- For deeper freezing, hold extremity in warm water (105°-110° F) for 20 minutes. For severe frostbite, do not attempt to rewarm the extremity yourself. Transport the child to an emergency room.
- Do not rub frostbitten areas with snow. Protect involved area from further damage.
- Apply a sterile gauze and elevate injured area for 40 minutes.
- Call parents to pick up and take child to get medical care.
- If child is lethargic, call 911.

Frozen to Metal: Do not allow child to pull away from metal.

- Blow hot breath onto the stuck area or pour warm (not hot) water onto the object.
- Gently release child.

- If bleeding occurs, such as on the tongue, grasp tongue with folded sterile gauze and apply direct pressure. Call parents to pick up and take child to get medical care.

Head and Nose Injuries

Head Injuries

- Keep child lying down.
- Call parents
- Call 911 if the child is:
    - complaining of severe or persistent headache
    - less than 1 year old
    - oozing blood or fluid from ears or nose
    - twitching or convulsing
    - unable to move any body part
    - unconscious or drowsy
    - vomiting

Nosebleeds: Have child sit up and lean forward.

- Loosen tight clothing around neck.
- Pinch lower end of nose close to nostrils (not on bony part of nose).

Poisons

Poisons: Immediately, **before you do anything**, call the local poison control center, hospital emergency room, or physician.

- Call parents. If child needs to go to for medical evaluation, bring samples of what was ingested. Bring with you all containers, labels, boxes, and package inserts that came with the material that the child took in. Look carefully for extra containers around the immediate area where the incident occurred. Try to estimate the total amount of material the child might have taken in, and whether the material was swallowed, inhaled, injected, or spilled in the eyes or on the skin. If possible, also bring with you the child's health file, including consent forms and names and telephone numbers of parents/guardians.
- Do not make a child vomit unless instructed to do so by the Poison Control Center. Even if directed to make the child vomit, do not do so if:

- the child is unconscious or sleepy,

- the child has swallowed a corrosive product (acid/drain cleaner/oven cleaner), or

- the child has swallowed a petroleum product (furniture polish/kerosene/gasoline).

- If instructed by the poison control center to make the child vomit:

  - Use ipecac syrup:

  - Children 1 year to 10 years old: 1 tablespoon or 3 teaspoons of ipecac and 4 to 8 ounces of water

  - Children over 10 years old: 2 tablespoons of ipecac and 4 to 8 ounces of water

  - Follow with another 4 to 8 ounces of water. Repeat dose once if child has not vomited in 20 minutes.

- If a chemical is spilled on someone, dilute it with water and remove any contaminated clothing, using gloves if possible. Place all contaminated clothing and other items in an airtight bag and label the bag. If the chemical has been splashed in the eye, flush immediately with tepid water and follow instructions listed for "Eye Injuries."

- Some poisons have delayed effects, causing moderate or severe illness many hours or even some days after the child takes the poison. Ask whether the child will need to be observed afterward and for how long. Make sure the child's parents/guardians understand the instructions.

Seizures

Seizures: Remain calm.

- Protect child from injury.

- Lie child on his or her side or on his or her stomach.

- Loosen clothing.

- Do not put anything in the child's mouth.

- Call 911 if seizure lasts more than 5 minutes or if they are the result of a head injury.

- Notify parents.

Chapter 31

Emergency Wound Care

Doctors Urge Fast Aid First

A slip with a kitchen knife, a fall from a bicycle, or an accident on the playground may all cause serious lacerations that require an emergency physician's care. In fact, each year nearly 37 million people visit the emergency department due to an injury, including 11.5 million people who come to be treated for a serious laceration, according to the National Center for Health Statistics. Summer months bring on the year's peak of these injuries as people become more involved in outdoor activities. Yet physicians say that some people who sustain this type of injury wait too long to seek care, making it more difficult for doctors to close the wound, increasing the risk of infection and serious scarring. That is why the American College of Emergency Physicians (ACEP) is urging Americans to practice "Fast Aid First," and learn the basics of emergency wound care.

"I see many patients come into our emergency department with serious open wounds who have waited hours before coming to see us," says Dr. John Moorhead, president of ACEP. "Whether they delayed due to reluctance to appear foolish or simply not understanding how seriously they were injured, blood loss, increased risk of infection, and serious scarring may be the result."

"Emergency Physicians Want Americans to Know When to Seek Medical Care for Serious Cuts," © July 1, 1999, American College of Emergency Physicians, reprinted with permission; and "Fast Aid First, Understanding Emergency Wound Care," © 1996-2001, American College of Emergency Physicians, reprinted with permission.

Many lacerations, after only a few hours of delay, will contain enough bacteria that serious infections can occur if the wound is closed. Early treatment improves the chances of successful treatment in all lacerations.

How should you evaluate a wound to determine whether you need to seek immediate medical care? The following guidelines highlight the types of wounds that should prompt immediate treatment:

Wound Warning Signs

- Wounds still bleeding after 5 minutes of steady, firm pressure
- Wounds that appear particularly deep or "gaping" open
- Deep puncture wounds, such as those caused by stepping on a nail
- Wounds that have foreign materials, such as dirt, glass, or metal, embedded in them
- Any cut from animal bites and all human bites
- Any wound that shows signs of infection (e.g., fever, swelling, pain, bad smell, fluid draining from area, or increasing pain).
- Problems with movement or sensation after a laceration

According to the Centers for Disease Control and Prevention, injuries that require emergency care generally result from: falls, such as from playground equipment; accidental collisions with objects or people such as an in-line skating collision; accidents with a knife or other cutting or piercing instruments; and bicycle and pedestrian accidents. People may be more at risk for these types of injuries in the summer months.

Treatments Available

Emergency physicians now have a variety of effective treatments available to close serious wounds and get patients quickly on the road to recovery.

- Topical skin adhesive is one of the newest innovations in skin closure. The physician applies the adhesive on top of the skin while holding the edges of the wound together. For some wounds, the adhesive takes less time to apply than stitches and forms a strong, flexible bond over the top of the wound and does not require a bandage. In some cases, it also may not require an injection of local anesthetic and can be associated with less patient pain and anxiety than sutures. The topical skin adhesive sloughs off the wound as it heals, usually in five to ten days, and does not require a return visit to the physician for suture removal.

- Traditional stitches (or sutures) are often used to close cuts. This involves "sewing" the skin together with a needle and surgical thread. This procedure usually requires an injection of anesthetic. A bandage is generally applied to the wound. After the wound is sufficiently healed, a physician will remove the stitches from the wound. Sometimes, the sutures are absorbed.

- Staples may also be used to close cuts.

- Skin strips are adhesive bands placed on top of the closed wound to hold skin edges together as it heals. This type of treatment is only used on very minor, superficial cuts.

"There are several new treatments available for treating patients with serious lacerations," says Dr. Moorhead. "People shouldn't delay seeking treatment. We can close their wounds quickly and relatively painlessly. You can never know when an emergency is going to occur. Our goal is to remind people that during the summer, when these types of injuries increase, fast action is important."

Where Do Serious Wounds Occur?

"Open wound" is the leading diagnosis for injury-related visits to the emergency department. There are a wide variety of accidents that may cause a serious wound requiring medical treatment. Some common accidents are:

- In the Kitchen—cuts from knives, scissors, broken glass, and kitchen equipment

- Playing with Pets—animal bites and scratches, cuts from falls

- Playing Sports—cuts sustained during sports activities, such as bicycling or contact sports

- On the Playground—falls from playground equipment can cause serious cuts to the head, face, hands, knees, and other areas of the body

- At Work—almost any workplace has some equipment that may cause an injury

Risk of injury also increases when someone is intoxicated or impaired.

Do You Know How to Provide Proper First Aid for a Serious Cut?

If you or someone you were with sustained a serious wound, would you know what to do? The American College of Emergency Physicians recommends the following steps to ensure you provide "Fast Aid First:"

- Apply firm (but not heavy) direct pressure over a bleeding wound with a sterile bandage or clean cloth.

- While maintaining steady pressure on the wound, elevate the affected part of the body above the heart, if possible. (If you suspect a limb may be broken, do not move it.)

- If blood soaks through a bandage, do not remove it. Apply additional clean bandages on top of the soaked one.

- If possible, rinse the wound with tap water. Do not cleanse with soap or apply antiseptic to a deep wound. This could damage healthy tissue that is exposed due to the injury.

- Evaluate the wound to determine whether emergency medical care should be sought—see the Wound Warning Signs.

- If the wound is still bleeding after 5 minutes of steady pressure, or exhibits any other Wound Warning Signs, seek medical care immediately.

Be Wound Wise: Know the Wound Warning Signs

One of the oldest known medical texts, dated 2200 BC, established founding principles of wound care, which are still in use today. An injury with the following warning signs should prompt you to seek immediate treatment:

- Bleeding that doesn't stop after 5 minutes when direct, steady pressure is applied

- A wound that is 'gaping' open, a deep puncture, or one in which the skin is badly torn

- Wound edges that cannot be easily held together
- Problems with movement or sensation following an injury
- Almost any cut on the head, face, neck, or hand
- Any wound in which you can see tissue that appears to be fat or muscle
- Any wound that shows signs of infection (e.g., fever, swelling, redness, or bad smell, fluid draining from the area, or increasing pain)
- Any cut from animal bites and all human bites

If the Wound Meets Any of These Criteria, Get Medical Attention Immediately. Don't Delay!

Waiting can interfere with the physician's treatment of the wound. Waiting several hours also can result in an increased risk for infection or increasing scarring. Waiting too long may prevent physicians from being able to close the wound properly.

What Can You Expect in the Emergency Department?

You've evaluated you wound and determined that it exhibits one or more of the "Wound Warning Signs." Your doctor's office is closed, so you're headed to the Emergency Department. What can you expect there?

Most likely, a nurse will determine the severity of the wound and check your vital signs, including temperature, heart rate, and blood pressure. This process is called triage. Additional information will also be obtained, such as your name, address, and medical history, and someone will prepare a chart. If you have a traumatic wound that requires sutures, you will be treated in a timely manner.

You also may be asked about any allergies you have or any medications you are taking. Bring up-to-date medical records with you.

Once you are placed in an examination area, an emergency physician will examine you and treat the wound. Nurses and other assistants will also assist you during your visit.

You will be given instructions for caring for the wound during the healing process and then be on your way.

How Will the Doctor Treat the Wound?

First, the doctor or health care professional will thoroughly examine and clean the wound, removing dirt or other foreign objects. This is extremely important so the wound does not become infected. This process may be painful and therefore may require a local anesthetic — either a cream, gel, or an injection.

Once the cut has been completely cleaned, the physician has a variety of options available for closing it, depending on the type of laceration. If the wound requires stitches, the physician will use surgical thread to sew the wound together. Because a needle is being passed through the skin, it may require some sort of local anesthetic. Stapling of wounds is another option. This is fast and may not require an anesthetic.

Another option in skin closure is topical skin adhesive. A skin adhesive works like glue and is spread on top of the wound while a physician holds the skin edges together. The adhesive dries quickly and forms a strong, flexible covering for the cut. The adhesive does not require a bandage and you can get it wet in the course of normal activities. Showering is fine, although soaking or bathing is not advisable.

Skin strips, another option, are small tape-like devices that are placed on top of the skin to hold wound edges together. Generally, they are used for less serious cuts.

What Questions Should You Ask?

Although wound closure is a fairly straightforward procedure, there are a few questions you should ask, including:

What Method of Skin Closure Is Being Used and Why?

Wounds across areas of low skin tension, such as the face, upper arm, or torso, may be closed with topical skin adhesive. It is not as effective on joints, such as the knee or elbow, the scalp or other areas with hair. Care must be taken when a wound near the eye is closed with topical skin adhesive. The eye should be covered during application, and the patient should be positioned so that any adhesive that may "run off" does not get near the eye.

How Should the Wound Be Cared for as It Heals? Can You Get It Wet? Do Bandages Need to Be Changed?

Post-treatment care will depend on the method used to close the wound. If you are treated with topical skin adhesive, very little care may be required. You can get it wet during the course of normal activities (although you shouldn't soak it), and there is no need for a bandage because the adhesive forms its own protective covering. If you are treated with stitches, you'll likely put ointment on the wound and cover it with a bandage. You may be advised not to get it wet.

What Are the Warning Signs of a Wound That Is Getting Infected?

Warning signs for infection include swelling, warmth, redness, and fluid drainage. Be sure to ask your doctor what to watch for, because an infection can be serious.

How Long Should Healing Take?

Healing depends on the type of wound. Some wounds may heal in three days and some will be well on their way within two weeks. Topical skin adhesive will gradually slough off the wound as it heals, usually within five to ten days. For wounds treated with stitches or staples, you'll probably be asked to return to the doctor to have them removed, some stitches, however, are absorbed. As the wound heals, the appearance of the resulting scar will change. The scar will continue to change over a full year following the repair.

Do You Need to See Your Own Physician in a Week or Two for Follow-Up, Such as to Have Stitches Removed?

Almost all wounds treated with stitches or staples will require a follow-up visit to the doctor to have them removed. Those treated with topical skin adhesive may not require this type of visit. However, depending on the injury, your physician may want to see you for follow-up, so be sure to ask.

Can the Wound Be Exposed to Sunlight?

Patients should avoid exposing the wound to the sun as it heals, even after stitches are removed or skin adhesive flakes off. Exposing newly formed skin cells to sunlight may cause problems with pigmentation.

What Pain Medication Does the Physician Recommend?

Each physician will have his or her own recommendations about the type and dose of pain medication you should use if necessary. Be sure to ask his or her advice before leaving.

Most importantly, make sure you know how to care for the wound so that it will heal properly, and recognize the signs of infection.

Being Prepared for an Emergency

More than 90 million wounds are closed in the United States each year. Understanding proper wound management and evaluation is an important step in being prepared for an emergency. A few other items to make sure you're ready to provide "Fast Aid First:"

- Keep emergency telephone numbers posted by the phone. Know how to contact emergency medical services.

- Always know the location and shortest route to the nearest emergency department. Leave a map in an accessible place for guests or babysitters. Ask your regular physician for a hospital recommendation.

- Talk to your physician about how to handle emergencies in advance.

- Above all, trust your instincts. If you think your medical condition is life- or health-threatening, seek medical attention.

Part Five

Injury Prevention Strategies for the Community and Home

Chapter 32

Identifying Alcohol-Related Injury Risks

Early Drinking Onset Increases Lifetime Injury Risk

Ralph Hingson, Sc.D., and other researchers at the Boston University School of Public Health reported in the September 27, 2000 issue of the *Journal of the American Medical Association* that the younger people are when they begin drinking the more likely they are to be injured later in life when under the influence of alcohol. Those who start drinking before age 14 are 12 times more likely to be injured than those who begin drinking at or after age 21. After adjusting for history of alcoholism, family history of alcoholism, and other characteristics associated with early onset drinking, the researchers found that people who begin drinking before age 14 are about three times more likely than those who begin drinking at or after age 21 to be injured while drinking.

"This analysis shows that for each year under age 21 that drinking onset is delayed, risk for later life injury diminishes," said Enoch Gordis, M.D., Director, National Institute on Alcohol Abuse and Alcoholism. The NIAAA reported in 1998 that early drinking onset is associated with increased lifetime risk for the clinical disorders alcohol dependence (alcoholism) and alcohol abuse.

"Early Drinking Onset Increases Lifetime Injury Risk," News Advisory September 29, 2000, National Institute on Alcohol Abuse and Alcoholism (NIAAA); and *Alcohol Alert* No. 40, April 1998, National Institute on Alcohol Abuse and Alcoholism (NIAAA).

315

Finding the reasons for these associations is a focus of continuing NIAAA research. "What is clear now—and grows clearer with each new scientific report—is that young people and their parents need to be aware of both short- and long-term risks of adolescent drinking," said Dr. Gordis.

The source of the data for both the alcohol disorder and the injury-risk analyses was the National Longitudinal Alcohol Epidemiologic Survey (NLAES), conducted in 1992 for NIAAA by the U.S. Bureau of the Census to assess drinking practices and effects among adult Americans. The most comprehensive survey of alcohol use ever conducted, NLAES involved 42,862 face-to-face interviews of Americans 18 years of age and older. Reports from the NLAES data (published in 1998 as *Drinking in the United States*) continue to provide the epidemiologic basis that guides research and informs public policy formulation.

Dr. Hingson's analysis for the injury risk study was supported by the National Highway Traffic Safety Administration and used NLAES data. The NLAES will be repeated in 2002 as the *National Epidemiologic Survey of Alcohol-Related Conditions*.

About 66 percent of the 1992 NLAES sample reported having ever consumed alcohol, 49 percent had their first drink before age 21, and 3 percent had their first drink (defined as the first full drink of alcohol excluding tastes or small sips) before age 14. About 15 percent of the 27,081 NLAES respondents who had ever consumed alcohol reported having been at some time in their lives in a drinking situation that increased the risk of injury; 3 percent had been in such a situation in the past year. Of the respondents who had ever consumed alcohol, about 8 percent had been injured after or while drinking and about 3 percent had been injured during the past year.

Unintentional injury (including motor vehicle crashes, falls, drowning, burns, and unintended gunshot wounds) claimed 94,331 lives in 1998 and is the leading cause of death for persons aged 1-34 years. Approximately one-third of unintentional injuries are estimated to be alcohol-related.

"Our report shows that younger age of drinking onset is associated with frequent heavy drinking later in life—not only for persons who are alcohol dependent but also for other drinkers. This is part, but not all of the reason that early drinking heightens the injury risk for persons both above and below the legal drinking age," said Dr. Hingson. "These findings provide important information for physicians and other health care providers to share with their adolescent patients."

Combined Effects of Alcohol and Aging

Although many medical and other problems are associated with both aging and alcohol misuse, the extent to which these two factors may interact to contribute to disease is unclear. Some examples of potential alcohol-aging interactions include the following:

- The incidence of hip fractures in the elderly increases with alcohol consumption.[3,4] This increase can be explained by falls while intoxicated combined with a more pronounced decrease in bone density in elderly persons with alcoholism compared with elderly nonalcoholics.[1]

- Studies of the general population suggest that moderate alcohol consumption (up to two drinks per day for men and one drink per day for women) may confer some protection from heart disease.[5,6] (A standard drink is generally considered to be 12 ounces of beer, 5 ounces of wine, or 1.5 ounces of distilled spirits, each drink containing approximately 0.5 ounces of alcohol.) Although research on this issue is limited, evidence shows that moderate drinking also has a protective effect among those older than 65.[7] Because of age-related body changes in both men and women, NIAAA recommends that persons older than 65 consume no more than one drink per day.[8]

- Alcohol-involved traffic crashes are an important cause of trauma and death in all age groups. The elderly are the fastest growing segment of the driving population. A person's crash risk per mile increases starting at age 55, exceeding that of a young, beginning driver by age 80. In addition, older drivers tend to be more seriously injured than younger drivers in crashes of equivalent magnitude.[9] Age may interact with alcoholism to increase driving risk. For example, an elderly driver with alcoholism is more impaired than an elderly driver without alcoholism after consuming an equivalent dose of alcohol, and has a greater risk of a crash.[9]

- Long-term alcohol consumption activates enzymes that break down toxic substances, including alcohol. Upon activation, these enzymes may also break down some common prescription medications. The average person older than 65 takes two to seven prescription medications daily. Alcohol-medication interactions are especially common among the elderly, increasing the risk of negative health effects and potentially influencing the effectiveness of the medications.[10,11]

- Depressive disorders are more common among the elderly than among younger people and tend to co-occur with alcohol misuse.[2,12] Data from the *National Longitudinal Alcohol Epidemiologic Survey* demonstrate that, among persons older than 65, those with alcoholism are approximately three times more likely to exhibit a major depressive disorder than are those without alcoholism.[13] In one survey, 30 percent of 5,600 elderly patients with alcoholism were found to have concurrent psychiatric disorders.[14] Among persons older than 65, moderate and heavy drinkers are 16 times more likely than nondrinkers to die of suicide, which is commonly associated with depressive disorders.[15]

References

1. Council on Scientific Affairs, American Medical Association. Alcoholism in the elderly. *JAMA* 275(10):797-801, 1996.

2. Adams, W.L. Late life outcomes: Health services use and the clinical encounter. In: Gomberg, E.S.L.; Hegedus, A.M.; and Zucker, R.A. *Alcohol Problems and Aging.* NIAAA Research Monograph No. 33. NIH Pub. No. 98-4163. Bethesda, MD: NIAAA, 1998.

3. Bikle, D.D.; Stesin, A.; Halloran, B.; et al. Alcohol-induced bone disease: Relationship to age and parathyroid hormone levels. *Alcohol Clin Exp Res* 17(3):690-695, 1993.

4. Schnitzler, C.M.; Menashe, L.; Sutton, C.G.; et al. Serum biochemical and haematological markers of alcohol abuse in patients with femoral neck and intertrochanteric fractures. *Alcohol Alcohol* 23(2):127-132, 1988.

5. Klatsky, A.L.; Armstrong, M.A.; and Friedman, G.D. Alcohol and mortality. *Ann Intern Med* 117(8):646-654, 1992.

6. Thun, M.J.; Peto, R.; Lopez, A.D.; et al. Alcohol consumption and mortality among middle-aged and elderly U.S. adults. *New Engl J Med* 337(24):1705-1714, 1997.

7. Fried, L.P.; Kronmal, R.A.; Newman, A.B.; et al. Risk factors for 5-year mortality in older adults: The cardiovascular health study. *JAMA* 279(8):585-592, 1998.

8. Dufour, M.C.; Archer, L.; and Gordis, E. Alcohol and the elderly. *Clin Geriatr Med* 8(1):127-141, 1992.

9. Waller, P.F. Alcohol, aging, and driving. In: Gomberg, E.S.L.; Hegedus, A.M.; and Zucker, R.A. *Alcohol Problems and Aging*. NIAAA Research Monograph No. 33. NIH Pub. No. 98-4163. Bethesda, MD: NIAAA, 1998.

10. Korrapati, M.R., and Vestal, R.E. Alcohol and medications in the elderly: Complex interactions. In: Beresford, T., and Gomberg, E., eds. *Alcohol and Aging*. New York: Oxford University Press, 1995. pp. 42-55.

11. National Institute on Alcohol Abuse and Alcoholism. *Alcohol Alert*. No. 27: Alcohol-Medication Interactions. Bethesda, MD: the Institute, 1995.

12. Welte, J.W. Stress and elderly drinking. In: Gomberg, E.S.L.; Hegedus, A.M.; and Zucker, R.A. *Alcohol Problems and Aging*. NIAAA Research Monograph No. 33. NIH Pub. No. 98-4163. Bethesda, MD: NIAAA, 1998.

13. Grant, B.F., and Harford, T.C. Comorbidity between DSM-IV alcohol use disorders and major depression: Results of a national survey. *Drug Alcohol Depend* (39):197-206, 1995.

14. Moos, R.; Brennan, P.; and Schutte, K. Life context factors, treatment, and late-life drinking behavior. In: Gomberg, E.S.L.; Hegedus, A.M.; and Zucker, R.A. *Alcohol Problems and Aging*. NIAAA Research Monograph No. 33. NIH Pub. No. 98-4163. Bethesda, MD: NIAAA, 1998.

15. Grabbe, L.; Demi, A.; Camann, M.A.; et al. The health status of elderly persons in the last year of life: A comparison of deaths by suicide, injury, and natural causes. *Am J Public Health* 87(3):434-437, 1997.

Chapter 33

Avoiding Accidents in Your Home

Home safety is no accident. Tragically, more than 28,000 deaths and more than 6.8 million injuries occurred from injuries in the home in 1997. Accidental injuries also are the number 1 killer of children in the United States.

How safe is your home? Most homes probably could be safer, especially if children live there. "It's important to take steps to prevent emergencies," said Dr. Elaine Josephson of the American College of Emergency Physicians. "For example, keep emergency numbers on each telephone in your home and have a first aid kit on hand stocked with appropriate items, such as syrup of ipecac to induce vomiting in case of poisoning, bandages, gauze, antiseptic ointment, ice bags, and a first aid manual."

In addition, inspect your home using the following home safety checklist:

- Install smoke detectors and carbon monoxide detectors on each floor; replace batteries twice a year.

- Make sure your house number is clearly visible from the street so you easily can be located in an emergency.

- Have and rehearse an emergency evacuation plan in case of fire.

This chapter includes "Avoiding Accidents in Your Home," and "Avoiding Household Burns," © 1996-2001, American College of Emergency Physicians, reprinted with permission.

- Keep on hand and make sure family members know how to use lifesaving equipment, such as a fire extinguisher and an escape ladder (for two-story homes).

- Keep electrical cords out of children's reach.

- Set your hot water thermostat to no more than 125 degrees Fahrenheit.

- Put child-resistant safety latches on cabinets and drawers to prevent children from getting at harmful substances. Never store chemicals or medicines in food containers.

- Keep toys with small parts and other small objects out of reach of toddlers and young children.

- Don't depend on insect screens to keep small children from falling out of a window. Unguarded windows opened only five inches can pose a danger. Install window guards to keep children from falling out.

- If you have firearms, make sure they are unloaded, stored, and locked properly.

"After you do all you can to prevent an emergency, the next step is to prepare for one," Dr. Josephson added. "Take a CPR class and learn first aid. Know what to do until emergency help arrives when someone, for example, gets burned, breaks a bone, stops breathing, starts choking, or has an allergic reaction."

ACEP also is a partner with the U.S. Department of Housing and Urban Development in the Health Homes for Healthy Children campaign, distributing safety brochures throughout the nation designed to help protect children from health hazards in their homes.

Avoiding Household Burns

More than two million Americans suffer burn injuries each year, and about 70,000 of them require admission to the hospital.

"Burns are one of the leading causes of accidental injuries in childhood, and the greatest tragedy is that many of these could have been prevented," said Dr. David Wilcox of the American College of Emergency Physicians. "Fortunately, there are steps you can take to protect your family and avoid a trip to the emergency department."

- When cooking, keep pot handles turned toward the rear of the stove, and never leave the pans unattended.

- Do not leave hot cups of coffee on tables or counter edges.

- Do not carry hot liquids or food near your child or while holding your child.

- Always test food temperatures before serving a child, especially foods or liquids heated in a microwave.

- Keep matches and lighters out of children's reach in a locked cabinet. Use only child-resistant lighters.

- Prevent scalding by keeping your water heater set at 120° to 125° F; test bath water before putting a child in the bathtub.

- Cover unused electric outlets with safety caps, and replace damaged, frayed, or brittle electrical cords.

- Keep fire extinguishers on every floor of your house, especially in the kitchen, and know how to use them.

- Do not put water on a grease fire—it can spread the fire.

- Have a working smoke detector on every floor of your home. Check batteries at least once a year.

- Know what to do in case clothing catches fire: Stop (don't run), Drop (to the floor, immediately), and Roll (cover your face and hands while rolling over to smother the flames).

"For burns and other medical emergencies, it's important to know first aid," added Dr. Wilcox. "Get medical attention for any burns to the eyes, mouth, hands, and genital areas, even if mild. If the burn covers a large area, get medical attention immediately."

For minor burns, run cool—not cold—water over the burn or hold a clean, cold compress on it until the pain subsides. Do not use not butter or other types of grease. Do not use ice. Remove jewelry or tight clothing from around burned areas, and apply a clean, dry dressing.

For more serious burns, do not use water or break blisters. Do not remove clothing if it is stuck to the burned skin. Keep the victim warm and dry, and keep burned arms or legs raised to reduce swelling.

Get immediate medical attention if you have any of the following symptoms related to a burn:

- fever

- pus-like or foul-smelling drainage

- excessive swelling
- redness of the skin
- a blister filled with greenish or brownish fluid
- a burn that doesn't heal in 10 days to 2 weeks

Chapter 34

What You Can Do to Prevent Falls

Falls affect everyone. For younger children and older adults, however, falls are a special concern and fall-related injuries can be extremely serious. In 1997, 87 children age 9 and younger and 9,023 adults age 65 and older died as a result of fall-related injuries. Falls are also the most common cause of injury visits to the emergency department for young children and older adults. Each year, approximately 3,125,000 children visit emergency departments for fall-related injuries. Falls are responsible for more open wounds, fractures, and brain injuries than any other cause of injury.

Preventing Childhood Falls

Childhood falls account for an estimated 2 million Emergency Department visits each year and in 1997, fall-related injuries claimed the lives of 87 children under age 9. The majority of childhood fall-related injuries occur at home, particularly among younger children.

Adult supervision, home modification, and informed product selection can help reduce the likelihood of childhood falls and fall-related injuries. To help protect your children from fall-related injuries, follow these safety tips from the American Academy of Pediatrics, National

This chapter includes "Preventing Childhood Falls," Centers for Disease Control and Prevention, updated October 9, 2001; and information from the following National Center for Injury Prevention and Control documents: "Falls and Hip Fractures among Older Adults–Fact Sheet," reviewed November 13, 2000; "What You Can Do to Prevent Falls"; and "Check for Safety," October 1999.

Safety Council, HUD, and the Lowe's Home Safety Council. (Note: If your child falls and acts abnormally in any way, call your pediatrician immediately.)

Infants

Babies are particularly vulnerable to falls and need to be closely supervised at all times.

- Never leave babies alone on any furniture, including beds, tables, sofas, or cribs and changing tables with the guard rails down—even if they have never rolled over before. In just a few seconds, babies can wiggle or roll off furniture and potentially hurt themselves. Instead, put babies on the floor or in a crib with secured guardrails.

- When changing a baby's diaper in a crib or on a changing table, be sure the guard rails are up and latched securely. Some changing tables also come with safety straps that you can use to secure your baby. When you do not have access to a crib or changing table with guard rails or safety straps, be sure to keep at least one hand on your baby at all times.

Choosing Safe Baby Products

When purchasing baby products, buy items and equipment that meet current safety standards and be sure to follow instructions and use the equipment properly (e.g., use the straps on highchairs, strollers, and changing tables). Be particularly cautious when buying used cribs or furniture as certain safety standards or regulations may have changed since the time they were built. Refer to some of the safety resources listed below for more specific information about current standards and features.

Highchairs

- In one year, approximately 7,000 children were sent to the hospital for falls from highchairs.

- Buy a highchair that has important safety features like a wide base, a locking tray, and a restraining belt or safety strap. Look for a label on the chair certifying that it meets current safety standards.

- Always use safety straps to restrain children in their high chairs.

Cribs

When buying a crib, look for the following features:

- Certification that it meets safety standards.

- Corner posts that do not stick up more than 1/16 of an inch.

- Rail slats that are spaced less than 2 and 3/8 inches apart (to prevent strangulation from children getting their heads caught between the slats). If a soda can fits through the openings between slats, the slats are too wide.

- A snug-fitting mattress.

- As the baby gets older and learns to sit and pull himself up to a standing position, lower the mattress in the crib. You should stop using the crib as soon as the top rails are less than 3/4 of the child's height.

- Do not put toys or pillows in the crib that she could stand on or use to crawl out of the crib. (The Consumer Product Safety Commission recommends that you avoid putting any toys or soft bedding in infants' cribs as they may contribute to suffocation.

- When your child switches to a toddler bed, be sure to install guard rails on both sides of the bed. Check to make sure the mattress fits snugly into the frame.

- You might also consider installing soft flooring around your child's crib or bed to lessen the severity of a fall-related injury. Examples of such flooring include thick carpeting, a pad, or a gym mat.

Baby Walkers

- According to the American Academy of Pediatrics, baby walkers should not be used. In 1997, baby walker-related injuries resulted in more than 16,000 children receiving treatment in hospital emergency rooms. Most of the injuries occur when children in baby walkers fall down stairs (80%) or tip over (5%). And falls down stairs are associated with the most severe injuries and are more likely to result in head injury and hospitalization. Supervision is not enough to make these products safe—nearly 80% of the baby walker-related injuries occurred while infants were being supervised. Baby walkers enable children to be more mobile than they are ready to be developmentally. And baby walkers make it easier for infants to reach dangerous things on tables–things they would not be able to reach if they were crawling.

- A safer alternative to a baby walker is a "stationary walker"—a play table that has a turning seat.

Infants, Toddlers, and Older Children

Constant supervision is extremely important in preventing falls among children. Children are active, energetic, and fast moving and serious falls can occur in a matter of seconds. There are some steps you can take, however, to modify your home and reduce the likelihood of a fall occurring.

Modify Your Home to Make It Child-Friendly

- Crawl through each room and look at your house from a child's perspective. Look under the sofa cushions, cabinets, throw rugs, etc.

- Arrange furniture in such a way that you can see children from all parts of the room.

- Install padding on sharp corners to lessen the severity of fall-related injuries against them. Pay special attention to coffee tables, file cabinets, and other items that may be low to the ground.

- Lock doors and block access to any dangerous areas. Hide the keys from your children.

Floors

Look closely at your floor surfaces. Modify slippery surfaces and remove hazards whenever possible.

- Secure area rugs and throw rugs by using a nonskid backing (foam carpet backing, double-sided tape, and rubber pads can be found at many carpet and department stores.)

- If you have hard floors (e.g., wood, tile, linoleum), clean up spills immediately to avoid slipping. Avoid over-waxing.

- Use rubber mats or slip-resistant stickers on bathroom tiles and in the bathtub to prevent slips and falls. And never leave children alone in the tub—if they slip and falls, they may not be able to call for help.

- To prevent tripping on wires, route electrical and other cords behind furniture or along the walls, and tape or tack them down.

- Remove clutter from the floor—pick up toys, books, clothing, and any other items that may be on the floor.

- Make your stairs safer by keeping them well-lit and free of clutter. You can also install non-skid stair runners.

Safety Gates

- Use safety gates to prevent infants and toddlers from falling down stairs or entering dangerous rooms or areas (i.e., rooms with furniture that babies might climb on or hard edges against which they might fall).

- Properly install gates at the top and bottom of all staircases.

- Teach members of the family, including older children, to consistently latch the gate whenever they use it.

- Look for gates with vertical slats that are no more than 2 and 3/8 inches apart. If the gate has diamond-shaped openings, they should be less than 12 inches wide.

- Do not use accordion gates with large openings as a child's neck can get trapped.

Windows

- Install window guards on all windows above the first floor (excluding those that serve as fire emergency exits). Window guards that can be forcefully dislodged from the inside in case of fire are safest.

- When using double-hung windows, or windows that can open at the top or the bottom, open them from the top to prevent children from falling out. Install locks on all other types of windows.

- Keep furniture away from windows to prevent children from climbing out.

- Do not rely on insect screens to prevent falls. They are designed to keep insects out and are not strong enough to keep children in. Keep children away from all open windows—with or without screens.

Monitor Outdoor Play

- Select play equipment that is safe for children. For example, select tricycle models that keep children low to the ground.

- Discourage active play on outdoor decks, balconies, fire escapes, high porches, and roofs. When possible, remove climbing aids in yards or on balconies (e.g., woodpiles, tree branches, furniture near deck railings).

- Cover window wells to prevent children from falling in.

- Buy your children shoes that will reduce their chances of falling. A good example would be low-cut sneakers with rough, rubber soles.

How Serious Is the Problem of Fall-Related Injuries for Older Adults?

- In the United States, one of every three adults 65 years old or older falls each year.[1,2]

- Falls are the leading cause of injury deaths among people 65 years and older.[3]

- In 1998, about 9,600 people over the age of 65 died from fall-related injuries.[4]

- Of all fall deaths, more than 60% involve people who are 75 years or older.[3]

- Fall-related death rates are higher among men than women and differ by race. White men have the highest death rate, followed by white women, black men and black women.[3]

What Other Health Outcomes Are Linked with Falls?

- Among older adults, falls are the most common cause of injuries and hospital admissions for trauma.[5]

- Falls account for 87% of all fractures for people 65 years and older.[5] They are also the second leading cause of spinal cord and brain injury among older adults.[6]

- Each year in the United States, one person in 20 receives emergency department treatment because of a fall.[7] Advanced age greatly increases the chance of a hospital admission following a fall.

- Among older adults, fractures are the most serious health outcomes associated with falls. About 3% of all falls cause fractures.[8] The most common are fractures of the pelvis, hip, femur, vertebrae, humerus, hand, forearm, leg, and ankle.[9]

Where Are People Most Likely to Fall?

- For adults 65 years old or older, 60% of fatal falls happen at home, 30% occur in public places, and 10% occur in health care institutions.[10]

Falls are not just the result of getting older. Many falls can be prevented. Falls are usually caused by a number of things. By changing some of these things, you can lower your chances of falling.

You can reduce your chances of falling by doing these things.

1. Begin a regular exercise program.

Exercise is one of the most important ways to reduce your chances of falling. It makes you stronger and helps you feel better. Exercises that improve balance and coordination (like Tai Chi) are most helpful.

Lack of exercise leads to weakness and increases your chances of falling. Ask your doctor or health care worker about the best type of exercise program for you.

2. Make your home safer.

About half of all falls happen at home. To make your home safer:

- Remove things you can trip over (such as papers, books, clothes, and shoes) from stairs and places where you walk.

- Remove small throw rugs or use double-sided tape to keep the rugs from slipping.

- Keep items you use often in cabinets you can reach easily without using a step stool.

- Have grab bars put in next to your toilet and in the tub or shower.

- Use non-slip mats in the bathtub and on shower floors.

- Improve the lighting in your home. As you get older, you need brighter lights to see well. Lamp shades or frosted bulbs can reduce glare.

- Have handrails and lights put in on all staircases.

- Wear shoes that give good support and have thin non-slip soles. Avoid wearing slippers and athletic shoes with deep treads.

3. Have your health care provider review your medicines.

Have your doctor or pharmacist look at all the medicines you take (including ones that don't need prescriptions such as cold medicines). As you get older, the way some medicines work in your body can change. Some medicines, or combinations of medicines, can make you drowsy or light-headed which can lead to a fall.

4. Have your vision checked.

Have your eyes checked by an eye doctor. You may be wearing the wrong glasses or have a condition such as glaucoma or cataracts that limits your vision. Poor vision can increase your chances of falling.

5. A home fall prevention checklist for older adults.

Each year, thousands of older Americans fall at home. Many of them are seriously injured, and some are disabled. In 1996, more than 8,500 people over age 65 died because of falls.

Falls are often due to hazards that are easy to overlook but easy to fix. This checklist will help you find and fix those hazards in your home.

Table 34.1 asks about hazards found in each room of your home. For each hazard, the table tells you how to fix the problem.

Other Things You Can Do to Prevent Falls

- Keep emergency numbers in large print near each phone

- Put a phone near the floor in case you fall and cannot get up.

- Think about wearing an alarm device that will bring help in case you fall and cannot get up.

References

1. Tinetti ME, Speechley M, Ginter SF. Risk factors for falls among elderly persons living in the community. *New England Journal of Medicine* 1988;319(26):1701-7.

2. Sattin RW. Falls among older persons: A public health perspective. *Annual Review of Public Health* 1992;13:489-508.

3. Hoyert DL, Kochanek KD, Murphy SL. Deaths: Final Data for 1997. National vital statistics reports; vol. 47 no. 19. Hyattsville, Maryland: National Center for Health Statistics, 1999.

4. National Center for Health Statistics Vital Statistics System, 2000.

5. Fife D, Barancik JI. Northeastern Ohio Trauma Study III: Incidence of fractures. *Annals of Emergency Medicine* 1985; 14:244-8.

6. Kraus KF, Black MA, Hessol N et al. The incidence of acute brain injury and serious impairment in a defined population. *American Journal of Epidemiology 1984*;119:186-201.

7. Cummings SR, Kelsey JL, Nevitt MC et al. Epidemiology of osteoporosis and osteoporotic fractures. *Epidemiology Review* 7;1985:178-208.

8. Cooper C; Campion G; Melton LJ. Hip fractures in the elderly: a world-wide projection. *Osteoporosis International* 1992;2(6):285-9.

9. Scott JC. *Osteoporosis and hip fractures*. Rheumatic Diseases Clinics of North America 1990;16(3):717-40.

10. Sorock GS. Falls among the elderly: Epidemiology and prevention. *American Journal of Preventive Medicine* 1988;4(5):282-8.

Table 34.1. Home Fall Hazards and How to Fix Them

Question	Safety Response
Floors	
When you walk through a room, do you have to walk around furniture?	Ask someone to move the furniture so your path is clear.
Do you have throw rugs on the floor?	Remove the rugs or use double-sided tape or a non-slip backing so the rugs won't slip.
Are papers, magazines, books, shoes, boxes, blankets, towels, or other objects on the floor?	Pick up things that are on the floor. Always keep objects off the floor.
Do you have to walk over or around cords or wires (like cords from lamps, extension cords, or telephone cords)?	Coil or tape cords and wires next to the wall so you can't trip over them. Have an electrician put in another outlet.
Stairs and Steps	
Are papers, shoes, books, or other objects on the stairs?	Pick up things on the stairs. Always keep objects off the stairs.
Are some steps broken or uneven?	Fix loose or uneven steps.
Are you missing a light over the stairway?	Have a handyman or an electrician put in an overhead light at the top and bottom of the stairs.
Has the stairway light bulb burned out?	Have a friend or family member change the light bulb.
Do you have only one light switch for your stairs (only at the top or at the bottom of the stairs)?	Have a handyman or an electrician put in a light switch at the top and bottom of the stairs. You can get light switches that glow.
Are the handrails loose or broken? Is there a handrail on only one side of the stairs?	Fix loose handrails or put in new ones. Make sure handrails are on both sides of the stairs and are as long as the stairs.

Table 34.1. Home Fall Hazards and How to Fix Them, continued

Question	Safety Response
Stairs and Steps, continued	
Is the carpet on the steps loose or torn?	Make sure the carpet is firmly attached to every step or remove the carpet and attach non-slip rubber treads on the stairs.
Kitchen and Eating Areas	
Are the things you use often on high shelves?	Move items in your cabinets. Keep things you use often on the lower shelves (about waist high).
Is you step stool unsteady?	Get a new, steady step stool with a bar to hold on to. Never use a chair as a step stool.
Bedrooms	
Is the light near the bed hard to reach?	Place a lamp close to the bed where it is easy to reach.
Is the path from your bed to the bathroom dark?	Put in a nightlight so you can see where you're walking. Some nightlights go on by themselves after dark.
Bathrooms	
Is the tub or shower floor slippery?	Put a non-slip rubber mat or self-stick strips on the floor of the tub or shower.
Do you have some support when you get in and out of the tub or up from the toilet?	Have a handyman or a carpenter put in a grab bar inside the tub and next to the toilet.

Chapter 35

Preventing Choking, Strangulation, and Suffocation among Infants and Young Children

Many infants and children die each year from strangulation and suffocation. These deaths can often be prevented if parents and caregivers watch their children more closely; keep dangerous toys, foods, and household items out of their reach; and take steps to improve safety in the home, especially in sleeping areas.

Tips for Preventing Choking

If you are the parent or caregiver of an infant or child under 4 years old, follow these tips from the American Academy of Pediatrics, the American Red Cross, and the Centers for Disease Control and Prevention (CDC) to reduce the chances of choking.

At Mealtime

• Insist that your children eat at the table, or at least sitting down. Watch young children while they eat. Encourage them to eat slowly and chew their food well.

• Cut up foods that are firm and round and can get stuck in your child's airway, such as

---

"Preventing Strangulation and Suffocation among Infants and Young Children—SafeUSA," Centers for Disease Control and Prevention, updated October 9, 2001; and "Preventing Choking among Infants and Young Children," Centers for Disease Control and Prevention, updated October 9, 2001.

- hotdogs—always cut hotdogs length-wise and then into small pieces

- grapes—cut them into quarters

- raw vegetables—cut them into small strips or pieces that are not round

- Other foods that can pose a choking hazard include:
  - hard or sticky candy, like whole peppermints or caramels
  - nuts and seeds (don't give peanuts to children under age 7)
  - popcorn
  - spoonfuls of peanut butter

During Playtime

- Follow the age recommendations on toy packages. Any toy that is small enough to fit through a 1 and 1/4-inch circle or is smaller than 2 and 1/4 inches long is unsafe for children under 4 years old.

- Don't allow young children to play with toys designed for older children. Teach older children to put their toys away as soon as they finish playing so young siblings can't get them.

- Frequently check under furniture and between cushions for dangerous items young children could find, including:

  coins

  marbles

  watch batteries (the ones that look like buttons)

  pen or marker caps

  cars with small rubber wheels that come off

  small balls or foam balls that can be compressed to a size small enough to fit in a child's mouth

- Never let your child play with or chew on uninflated or broken latex balloons. Many young children have died from swallowing or inhaling them.

- Don't let your small child play on bean bag chairs made with small foam pellets. If the bag opens or rips, the child could inhale these tiny pieces.

If you're a parent, grandparent, or other caregiver, learn how to help a choking child and how to perform CPR in case of an emergency.

Who Is Affected?

More than 2,800 people die each year from choking; many of them are children. According to one study, nearly two-thirds of the children who choked to death during a 20-year period were 3 years old or younger.

The majority of choking deaths are caused by toys and household items. One study found that nearly 70 percent of choking deaths among children age 3 and under were caused by toys and other products made for children. According to CDC, balloons account for 7 to 10 deaths a year. And the U.S. Consumer Product Safety Commission has received reports of five deaths from bean bag chairs, resulting from children choking on the small foam pellets inside.

The most common cause of nonfatal choking incidents is food. In one study, nearly 70 percent of choking cases presented in the emergency department were caused by foods such as hotdogs, nuts, and vegetable and fruit pieces.

Tips for Preventing Strangulation and Suffocation

The American Academy of Pediatrics, Centers for Disease Control and Prevention (CDC), and U.S. Consumer Product Safety Commission have provided the following safety tips to reduce the chances of suffocation and strangulation among infants and young children in your care.

Reduce the Chances of Suffocation

At Bedtime

- Place babies to sleep on their backs on a firm, flat mattress.

- Do not use pillows or heavy comforters in your baby's crib.

- Make sure your baby's crib mattress is big enough for the crib. The space between the crib slats and the mattress should be smaller than the width of two adult fingers.

- Never let your baby sleep in bed with you. Babies have died when their breathing was blocked by pillows, bedding, and even their parents.

- Never let a baby sleep on a waterbed.

Around the House

- Keep plastic shopping, garbage, and dry cleaning bags away from babies and children. Never use a plastic shipping bag or other plastic film as a mattress cover.

- Choose a toy chest without a lid. If your child's toy chest has a lid, make sure it has a safety latch that stays open in any position. And make sure there are holes in the back or bottom of the chest to allow airflow, in case your child gets stuck inside.

- Lock your car—including the trunk—when it's not in use. Keep the car keys away from children. Children have died after climbing into car trunks and becoming trapped. Always supervise children around cars.

Reduce the Chances of Strangulation

In the Crib

- Check with the U.S. Consumer Product Safety Commission before buying a new or second-hand crib to make sure it hasn't been recalled.

- Make sure the slats on your crib are no more than 2 ³/₈ inches apart—this is really important for second-hand cribs that are a few years old. If slats are wider than 2 ³/₈ inches apart, babies can slide through the slats and strangle when their heads get stuck.

- Do not use a crib with cut-outs in the end panels or with corner posts more than 1/16 inch higher than the end panels. Strangulation can occur if a baby's clothing gets caught on a high corner post or if a baby's head gets caught in a cut-out.

- Remove your baby's bib before bedtime or nap time.

- Remove mobiles and crib gyms as soon as your baby is five months old or can push up on hands and knees.

Around the House

- Pull drapery and mini-blind cords out of children's reach and away from cribs. If the cords have a loop, cut the loop and attach separate tassels to avoid strangulation.

- If your child has a bunk bed, check the guard rails on the top bunk. There should be only a very small space between the rail and the mattress or bed frame so your child's body cannot slide through.

- Don't let your child lie in or play with a hammock that doesn't have spreader bars (wooden strips at the ends of the hammock that stop the netting from bunching up). Mini-hammocks, often used to store toys and stuffed animals, are also a hazard. Your child can get entangled in them.

- Remove hood cords and drawstrings from your child's clothing. These cords can get caught in playground equipment or on crib parts and strangle your child.

- Remove loose ribbons or strings on toys and stuffed animals.

- Never use a string or ribbon to tie a pacifier or toy to your baby.

Who Is Affected?

Each year, products that are thought safe for children—namely cribs and clothing—cause deaths from suffocation or strangulation. Approximately 50 babies suffocate or strangle each year when they become trapped between broken crib parts or between parts of an older crib with an unsafe design. Clothing with drawstrings also presents a hazard for children. Drawstrings can become entangled in playground equipment, fences, and furniture, causing strangulation. Such entanglements were associated with 17 deaths and 42 nonfatal incidents between 1985 and 1995.

Car trunks present a special risk for children. Between 1987 and 1998, nearly 20 children between 2 and 6 years old died from being trapped inside car trunks. The children had either climbed into trunks that were open or managed to open the trunks themselves, with or without keys. While hyperthermia (becoming too hot) was the most frequent cause of death, asphyxia (suffocation) was a contributing factor in half of the cases.

References

American Academy of Pediatrics. *Toy safety: Guidelines for parents.* Available at www.aap.org/family/toybroc.htm. Accessed July 15, 1999.

American Academy of Pediatrics. *Infants at increasing risk of suffocation death.* Press release, May 3, 1999. Available at www.aap.org/advocacy/releases/mayinf.htm. Accessed July 15, 1999.

American Academy of Pediatrics. *Choking prevention and first aid for infants: Guidelines for parents.* Available at www.aap.org/family/choking.htm. Accessed July 15, 1999.

American Red Cross. *Causes and signals of choking.* Available at www.redcross.org/tips/november/novtip98.html. Accessed July 26, 1999.

CALPIRG. CALPIRG joins Consumer Product Safety Commission to launch child safety campaign. Press release, April 16, 1997. Available at www.pirg.org/pirg/calpirg/consumer/products/recall97.htm. Accessed July 16, 1999.

CDC. Fatal car trunk entrapment involving children–United States, 1987-1998. *Morbidity and Mortality Weekly Report* 1998;47(47):1019-1022.

CDC. Toy-related injuries among children and teenagers-United States, 1996. *Morbidity and Mortality Weekly Report* 1997;46(5):1185-1189.

Juvenile Products Manufacturers Association. Safe & Sound for Baby: A guide to juvenile product safety, use and selection. *JPMA*, 1997. Available at www.jpma.org/public/safe-sound.html. Accessed July 26, 1999.

National Safety Council. *Baby-proofing your home.* Available at www.nsc.org/lrs/lib/fs/home/babyprf.htm. Accessed July 26, 1999.

Rimell F, Thome A, Stool S, Reilly J, Rider G, Stool D, et al. Characteristics of objects that cause choking in children. *JAMA*;274(22):1763-1766.

U.S. Consumer Product Safety Commission. *Guidelines for drawstrings on children's upper outerwear.* CPSC document #3006. November 1995. Available at www.cpsc.gov/cpscpub/pubs/strings.pdf. Accessed July 27, 1999.

U.S. Consumer Product Safety Commission. *Strings, cords, and necklaces can strangle infants:* Safety alert. CPSC document #5095. Available at www.cpsc.gov/cpscpub/pubs/5095.html. Accessed July 27, 1999.

U.S. Consumer Product Safety Commission. *Your used crib could be deadly: Safety alert.* CPSC document #5020. Available at www.cpsc.gov/cpscpub/pubs/5020g.html. Accessed August 31, 1999.

Additional Information

American Academy of Pediatrics
141 Northwest Point Boulevard
Elk Grove Village, IL 60007-1098
Tel: 847-434-4000
Fax: 847-434-8000
Website: www.aap.org
E-mail: kidsdocs@aap.org

The AAP offers toy safety guidelines for parents which include tips for preventing choking. They also offer a fact sheet on choking prevention and first aid.

American Red Cross
P.O. Box 37243
Washington, DC 20013
Tel: 202-639-3685
Website: www.redcross.org

U.S. Consumer Product Safety Commission
Washington, DC 20207-0001
Toll-Free: 800-638-2772
Toll-Free Teletypewriter: 800-638-8270
TTY: 800-638-8270
Website: www.cpsc.gov
E-mail: info@cpsc.gov

Juvenile Products Manufacturers Association
17000 Commerce Parkway, Suite C
Mt. Laurel, NJ 08054
Tel: 856-638-0420
Fax: 856-439-0525
E-mail: jpma@ahint.com
Website: www.jpma.org

Check out "Safe & Sound for Baby," (www.jpma.org/public/safesound.html) a publication of JPMA that shows parents how to properly use products made for children.

National Safety Council
1121 Spring Lake Drive
Itasca, IL 60143-3201
Tel: 630-285-1121
Fax: 630-285-1315
Website: www.nsc.org

Chapter 36

Prevention and Treatment of Burns

Fire in the United States

- The U.S. has one of the highest fire death rates in the industrialized world. For 1998, the U.S. fire death rate was 14.9 deaths per million population.

- Between 1994 and 1998, an average of 4,400 Americans lost their lives and another 25,100 were injured annually as the result of fire.

- About 100 firefighters are killed each year in duty-related incidents.

- Each year, fire kills more Americans than all natural disasters combined.

- Fire is the third leading cause of accidental death in the home; at least 80 percent of all fire deaths occur in residences.

- About 2 million fires are reported each year. Many others go unreported, causing additional injuries and property loss.

- Direct property loss due to fires is estimated at $8.6 billion annually.

"Facts on Fire," United States Fire Administration, updated March 10, 2000; "Let's Retire Fire: A Fact Sheet for Older Americans," United States Fire Administration, updated March 1999; "Hot Water Burns," National Ag Safety Database; and "Prevention and Treatment of Burns," National Ag Safety Database.

Where Fires Occur

- There were 1,755,000 fires in the United States in 1998. Of these:
  - 41% were Outside Fires
  - 29% were Structure Fires
  - 22% were Vehicle Fires
  - 8% were fires of other types

- Residential fires represent 22 percent of all fires and 74 percent of structure fires.

- Fires in 1-2 family dwellings most often start in the:
  1. Kitchen 23.5%
  2. Bedroom 12.7%
  3. Living Room 7.9%
  4. Chimney 7.1%
  5. Laundry Area 4.7%

- Apartment fires most often start in the:
  1. Kitchen 46.1%
  2. Bedroom 12.3%
  3. Living Room 6.2%
  4. Laundry Area 3.3%
  5. Bathroom 2.4%

- The South has the highest fire death rate per capita with 18.4 civilian deaths per million population.

- 80 percent of all fatalities occur in the home. Of those, approximately 85 percent occur in single-family homes and duplexes.

Causes of Fires and Fire Deaths

- Cooking is the leading cause of home fires in the U.S. It is also the leading cause of home fire injuries. Cooking fires often result from unattended cooking and human error, rather than mechanical failure of stoves or ovens.

- Careless smoking is the leading cause of fire deaths. Smoke alarms and smolder-resistant bedding and upholstered furniture are significant fire deterrents.

- Heating is the second leading cause of residential fires and the second leading cause of fire deaths. However, heating fires are a larger problem in single family homes than in apartments. Unlike apartments, the heating systems in single family homes are often not professionally maintained.

- Arson is both the third leading cause of residential fires and residential fire deaths. In commercial properties, arson is the major cause of deaths, injuries, and dollar loss.

Who Is Most at Risk

- Senior citizens age 70 and over and children under the age of 5 have the greatest risk of fire death.

- The fire death risk among seniors is more than double the average population.

- The fire death risk for children under age 5 is nearly double the risk of the average population.

- Children under the age of 10 accounted for an estimated 17 percent of all fire deaths in 1996.

- Men die or are injured in fires almost twice as often as women.

- African Americans and American Indians have significantly higher death rates per capita than the national average.

- Although African Americans comprise 13 percent of the population, they account for 26 percent of fire deaths.

What Saves Lives

- A working smoke alarm dramatically increases a person's chance of surviving a fire.

- Approximately 88 percent of U.S. homes have at least one smoke alarm. However, these alarms are not always properly maintained and as a result might not work in an emergency. There has been a disturbing increase over the last ten years in the number of fires that occur in homes with non-functioning alarms.

- It is estimated that over 40 percent of residential fires and three-fifths of residential fatalities occur in homes with no smoke alarms.

- Residential sprinklers have become more cost effective for homes. Currently, very few homes are protected by them.

Why Are Older People at Risk?

The facts speak for themselves: Americans over the age of 65 are one of the groups at greatest risk of dying in a fire. Every year over 1,200 Americans over age 65 die in fires. People over the age of 80 die in fires at a rate three times higher than the rest of the population. However, there are a number of precautionary steps older Americans can take to dramatically reduce their chances of becoming a fire casualty.

Older Americans are at risk for fire death and injuries for a number of reasons:

- They may be less able to take the quick action necessary in a fire emergency.

- They may be on medication that affects their ability to make quick decisions.

- Many older people live alone and when accidents happen others may not be around to help.

What Fire Hazards Affect Older People?

- Cooking accidents are the leading cause of fire-related injuries for older Americans. The kitchen is one of the most active and potentially dangerous rooms in the home.

- The unsafe use of smoking materials is the leading cause of fire deaths among older Americans.

- Heating equipment is responsible for a big share of fires in seniors' homes. Extra caution should be used with alternate heaters such as wood stoves or electric space heaters.

- Faulty wiring is another major cause of fires affecting the elderly. Older homes can have serious wiring problems, ranging from old appliances with bad wiring to overloaded sockets.

Safety Tips for Older Americans

- **Kitchen Fires.** Most kitchen fires occur because food is left unattended on the stove or in the oven. If you must leave the kitchen while cooking, take a spoon or potholder with you to remind you to return to the kitchen. Never cook with loose, dangling sleeves that can ignite easily. Heat cooking oils gradually and use extra caution when deep-frying. If a fire breaks out in a pan, put a lid on the pan. Never throw water on a grease fire. Never use a range or stove to heat your home.

- **Space Heaters.** Buy only Underwriter's Laboratory (UL) approved heaters. Use only the manufacturer's recommended fuel for each heater. Do not use electric space heaters in the bathroom or around other wet areas. Do not dry or store objects on top of your heater. Keep combustibles away from heat sources.

- **Smoking.** Don't leave smoking materials unattended. Use "safety ashtrays" with wide lips. Empty all ashtrays into the toilet or a metal container every night before going to bed. Never smoke in bed.

Finally, having a working smoke alarm dramatically increases your chances of surviving a fire. And remember to practice a home escape plan frequently with your family.

Make Your Hot Water Heater Safe

- Turn down the water heater to 120 degrees.

- Test bath water before putting a child in it. If the water feels hot to you, it will burn a child.

- Put the child in the bath with their back to the faucet so they cannot turn the water on.

- Get knob covers for the bathroom tub.

Causes of Hot Water Burns

- About 50 percent occur because parents put children in water that is too hot.

- Children turn the water faucet on or fall into a tub of hot water.

- Deliberate abuse by parents.

- Nearly 2 million people are treated for burns annually in the United States.

- About 100,000 will be hospitalized, and nearly 12,000 will die.

- About 112,000 of these burns are scald burns. According to Safe Kids Coalition, about 37,000 of these people are 14 or under, and about 18,000 are 5 or under.

- The United States has the highest rate of burns in the industrialized world, according to the National Safety Council.

- Burns are the second leading cause of death for young children ages 0 to 5.

- Children burn faster than adults because they have thinner skin.

- Everyday, 300 young children are taken to emergency rooms for burns caused by household water that was too hot. Annually, 3,000 of these children require hospitalization.

- Water heaters leave the factory set at 140 to 150 degrees Fahrenheit. It takes 2 seconds for a child to receive third degree burns from water at 150 degrees. It takes 5 seconds if the water is at 140 degrees, and 30 seconds at 130 degrees.

How to Test Your Water Heater's Temperature

- Check it in the early morning before anyone has used the hot water.

- Go into the kitchen and turn on the hot water tap and leave it running for two minutes.

- Hold an outdoor thermometer or candy thermometer in the stream of running water until the temperature stops rising.

- If the temperature is between 120 and 125, good.

- If higher, find the thermostat on the water heater and turn it down.

- Gas water heaters have an external thermostat, near the bottom.

- Electric water heaters have two panels screwed to the top and bottom of the tank or one panel on the side. Set it to "low" or "Energy Efficient."

- Wait 24 hours and then test the water temperature again to see it is in the safe range.

- Consult a professional if the temperature did not go down.

Prevent Accidental Burns in the Kitchen

Heating and cooking equipment are the number one cause of home fire injuries in the United States.

- Keep hot foods and drinks away from the edge of counters and tables. Don't set hot items on tablecloths because children could pull it onto themselves.

- Don't hold a child and something hot at the same time.

- Keep children away from the stove, turn pan handles in, and cook on the rear burners when possible.

- Do not allow children to use the microwave without supervision.

  - Children may not realize which dishes or containers are "microwave safe." Some plastics or paper can be over-heated in a microwave and catch on fire.

  - They may not reheat a leftover enough to kill the harmful bacteria growing in it.

  - Children may not realize how hot the bottom of the container "nuked" will be.

  - Steam burns to the face and hands are possible if the pop-corn or dish is opened too soon.

  - Burns to the mouth can occur due to unevenly heated foods.

  - Eggs, cooked in their shell, can explode, causing second degree burns.

Home Fires

During an average person's lifetime, households can expect to average two fires serious enough to alert the fire department.

- Each year in the United States, more than 400,000 residential fires account for approximately 3,600 deaths and 18,600 injuries. (Source: Karter, MF Jr. *Fire loss in the United States during 1995.* Quincy (MA): National Fire Protection Association, Fire Analysis and Research Division; 1996.)

- Older adults, children younger than 5 years old, and people in lower income groups are at the highest risk for fire and burn related deaths. (National Center for Health Statistics. *National summary of injury mortality data, 1995.*)

351

- Cooking is the primary cause of residential fires, and smoking is the leading cause of fire deaths. (Hall JR. *The U.S. fire problem and overview report. Leading causes and other patterns and trends.* Quincy (ma): National Fire Protection Assn. Fire Analysis & Research Division, 1998.)

- Approximately 59% of fatal residential fires occur in homes without smoke alarms. (Ahrens M. *US experience with smoke detectors and other fire detectors.* Quincy, MA: National Fire Protection Association, Fire Analysis and Research Division, 1997.)

- Most residential fires occur during the winter months (December-February.) (*Morbidity and Mortality Weekly Report* 1998, October 2; 47(38): 803-806.

- **Most of these residential deaths can be prevented.**

Critical burns need immediate medical attention because they can be life threatening. A burn is considered critical when any one of the following occurs:

- Victim has difficulty breathing.
- Burns cover more than one of the victim's body parts.
- Burns occur to the head, neck, hands, feet, or genitals.
- Victim is an infant, young child, or an elderly person (and the burn is other than a very minor one).
- Burns resulted from chemicals, explosions, or electricity.

Minor burns only affect the top layer of skin, leaving a red, dry patch of skin. Though painful, these burns will usually heal in 5 to 6 days.

1. Run cool water over the area for several minutes.
2. Wash the area with soap and water. If in doubt about the severity of the burns, treat them as critical and seek medical attention.

What You Can Do

- Install and maintain smoke detectors on each level of the home and outside each bedroom.

- Change the batteries when you change your clocks for daylight-saving time.

- Plan and practice two escape routes from every room in the home.

  - Teach children how to get out. Teach them to crawl to the door and test it before opening it. If the door or handle are hot or if smoke is coming in around the door, go out the other way. If they must go out through a window, make sure they know how to open it. Buy an approved chain ladder and teach children how to use it.

  - Set up a meeting place outside.

  - Phone the fire department from a neighbor's house. Teach children how to report a fire, give clear directions to the house, and to stay on the phone until the dispatcher says they are done.

  - Never go back into the house.

  - Teach children what to do if their clothes catch on fire. Stop, drop, roll, shout for help, cool the burns with cool water, not ice.

  - Make sure your children's sleepwear is not flammable. Clothing burn victims are more likely to die as a result of their injuries than people burned any other way. The clothing causes a deeper burn that affects a greater portion of the skin's surface.

Additional Information

The United States Fire Administration
Office of Fire Management Programs
16825 South Seton Avenue
Emmitsburg, MD 21727
Website: www.usfa.fema.gov
Kid's Web Page: www.usfa.fema.gov/kids

Chapter 37

Lock-Up Poison— Prevent Tragedy

- Poisonings happen every day. In 1998 alone, more than 2.2 million human poison exposures were reported to poison control centers in the United States,[1] and each year, nearly 900,000 visits to the emergency department occur because of poisonings.[2]

- Most poisonings happen in the home and involve children. In 1998, 92% of all poisonings occurred in the home, and 53% involved children under the age of six years.[1]

- Common household items are often the cause. The poisons usually involved are cleaning substances, pain relievers (analgesics), cosmetics, personal care products, plants, and cough and cold preparations.[1]

- Poison control centers help millions of people each year, ensuring that poisonings are treated rapidly and correctly. Poison control centers managed more than 2 million cases of poison exposure in 1998. Three-fourths of these cases were managed at home over the telephone with the help of specialists trained in providing poison information.[1]

- Poison control centers are extremely cost effective. For every $1 spent on poison control centers, an estimated $7 is saved in

"Facts about Poisoning," and "What Affect's a Child's Risk of Poisoning?" National Poison Prevention Week March 19-25, 2000, National Center for Injury Prevention and Control (NCIPC), 2000; and "Poisoning Prevention," SafeUSA.

medical care costs. By helping people manage emergencies at home, these centers prevent about 50,000 hospitalizations and 400,000 doctor's visits each year.[3]

References

1. Litovitz TL, Klein-Schwartz W, Caravati EM, Youniss J, Crouch B, Lee S. 1998 Annual Report of the American Association of Poison Control Centers Toxic Exposure Surveillance System. *American Journal of Emergency Medicine* 1999; 17(5):435-87.

2. Burt CW, Fingerhut LA. *Injury Visits to Hospital Emergency Departments: United States*, 1992-95. Vital Health Stat 13 (131). DHHS publication no. 98-1792. Hyattsville, MD: National Center for Health Statistics, 1998.

3. Miller TR, Lestina DC. Costs of Poisoning in the United States and Savings From Poison Control Centers: A Benefit-Cost Analysis. *Annals of Emergency Medicine* 1997;29(2):239-45.

What Affects a Child's Risk of Poisoning?

A host of risk factors affect a child's chances of being poisoned. Among children younger than 12, poisonings are slightly more common among boys than among girls, and very few cases are classified as suicide attempts. Among adolescents, more than half of poison exposures involve girls. In addition, about half of all poison exposures among teens are classified as suicide attempts. A number of developmental and environmental factors also come into play.

Babies and Toddlers

Because of their limited motor skills and the close supervision they receive from parents, young infants have less of a risk of poisoning than their older siblings. But when children are about to celebrate their first birthday, they become mobile enough to open cabinets under sinks and reach objects on counter tops, and they can often open unsecured caps, bring containers to their mouths, and grasp and ingest small objects such as pills. Babies and toddlers are curious and love to put things into their mouths, but they don't know what's poisonous and what's safe to eat.

Preschoolers

Like toddlers, preschoolers aren't aware of the danger of poisoning, and they are likely to spend increasing amounts of time out of their parents' line of sight and supervision. Various factors—such as motor skills, cognitive ability, and temperament—place some children at a greater risk of poisoning than others.

School-Age Children

These children are beginning to develop the ability to recognize danger and to develop self-control, so they are at less of a risk of unintentional poisoning than are younger kids. With this group of children, however, inadequate supervision when the child must take medications can lead to an inadvertent overdose.

Adolescents

Suicide attempts—by intentionally taking an overdose of medication—are a risk factor among teenagers, with girls being more likely than boys to take an overdose of pills. Unintentional overdoses are also a risk, because of peer pressure to take drugs, easy access to drugs, and many teens have a natural inclination to take risks.

Environmental Factors

Two environments that affect a child's risk of poisoning are the home and the community. In the home, toxic substances must be stored not only out of the reach and sight of children, but also in a well-secured cabinet with a lock or safety latch. In the community, factors such as access to drugs can increase an adolescent's risk of death from poisoning. Communities must look out for children at risk for substance abuse or suicide to ensure that they receive early intervention and counseling that could save their lives.

Source: Adapted from recommendations in Injury Prevention and Control for Children and Youth, written by the Committee on Injury and Poison Prevention of the American Academy of Pediatrics (Elk Grove Village, IL: American Academy of Pediatrics, 1997).

Poisoning Prevention

Millions of poisoning exposures occur each year in the United States, resulting in nearly 900,000 visits to emergency departments.

About 90% of poisonings happen in the home, and more than half of them involve children under age six. Many poisonings can be prevented if safety precautions are taken around the home. If a poisoning occurs, calling a poison control center can help ensure rapid, appropriate treatment.

Preventing Poisonings in the Home

The simple steps that follow, provided by the American Association of Poison Control Centers, can help you protect children from poisons:

- Post the telephone number for your poison control center near your phone, in a place where all family members would be able to find it quickly in an emergency.

- Remove all nonessential drugs and household products from your home. Discard them according to the manufacturer's instructions.

- If you have small children, avoid keeping highly toxic products, such as drain cleaners, in the home, garage, shed, or other place children can access.

- Buy medicines and household products in child-resistant packaging and be sure that caps are always on tight. Do not remove child-safety caps. Avoid keeping medicines, vitamins, or household products in anything but their original packaging.

- Store all of your medicines and household products in a locked closet or cabinet—including products and medicines with child-resistant containers.

- Crawl around your house, including inside your closets, to inspect it from a child's point of view. You'll likely find a poisoning hazard you hadn't noticed before.

- Never refer to medicine or vitamins as "candy."

- Make sure visiting grandparents, family friends, or other caregivers keep their medications away from children. For example, if Grandma keeps pills in her purse, make sure the purse is out of children's reach.

- Keep a bottle of syrup of ipecac in your home—this can be used to induce vomiting. Use it only when the poison control center tells you to.

- Avoid products such as cough syrup or mouth wash that contain alcohol—these are hazardous for young children. Look for alcohol-free alternatives.

- Keep cosmetics and beauty products out of children's reach. Remember that hair permanents and relaxers are toxins as well.

Additional Information

[Editor's Note: Please turn to Chapter 62, "Directory of Resources," to review an extensive listing of resources available for education about and prevention of poisoning.]

Chapter 38

Smoke Alarms and Natural Gas Detectors

Smoke Alarms

Smoke alarm technology has been around since the 1960s. But the single-station, battery-powered smoke alarm we know today became available to consumers in the 1970s. NFPA estimates that 94% of U.S. homes have at least one smoke alarm, and most states have laws requiring them in residential dwellings.

Facts & Figures*

- 15 of every 16 homes (94%) in the US have at least one smoke alarm.

- One-half of home fire deaths occur in the 6% of homes with no smoke alarms.

- Homes with smoke alarms (whether or not they are operational) typically have a death rate that is 40%–50% less than the rate for homes without alarms.

This chapter includes "Smoke Alarms," NFPA Fact Sheet, and "Alarm Age Fact Sheet: Replacing Smoke Alarms," Saturday, November 17, 2001, both reprinted from www.nfpa.org with permission, © 2001, National Fire Protection Association, Quincy, MA 02269, 2001; and "What You Need to Know about Natural Gas Detectors," National Institute on Deafness and Other Communication Disorders (NIDCD), 1995.

- In three of every 10 reported fires in homes equipped with smoke alarms, the devices did not work. Households with non-working smoke alarms now outnumber those with no smoke alarms.

- Why do smoke alarms fail? Most often because of missing, dead, or disconnected batteries.

*Source: NFPA's *U.S. Experience with Smoke Alarms and Other Fire Alarms*.

Safety Tips

- While smoke alarms alert people to fires, families still need to develop and practice home fire escape plans so that they can get out quickly.

- Install at least one smoke alarm on every floor of your home (including the basement) and outside each sleeping area. If you sleep with the door closed, NFPA recommends installing smoke alarms inside the room. In new homes, smoke alarms are required in all sleeping rooms, according to the National Fire Alarm Code.

- Because smoke rises, alarms should be mounted high on walls or ceilings. Wall-mounted alarms should be positioned between 4 and 12 inches from the ceiling; ceiling-mounted alarms should be positioned 4 inches away from the nearest wall. On vaulted ceilings, be sure to mount the alarm at the highest point of the ceiling.

- Smoke alarms should not be installed near a window, door, or forced-air register where drafts could interfere with their operation.

- Be sure that the smoke alarm you buy carries the label of an independent testing lab.

- Alarms that are hard-wired to the home's electrical system should be installed by a qualified electrician.

Smoke Alarm Maintenance

- Test smoke alarms at least once a month, in accordance with NFPA 72, National Fire Alarm Code, by using the alarm's "test button" or an approved smoke substitute, and clean the units in accordance with the manufacturer's instructions.

- Install new batteries in all smoke alarms at least once a year, for example, on the day you change your clocks or when the alarm chirps (warning that the battery is dying).

- Replace all smoke alarm batteries immediately upon moving into a new home.

- Keep batteries in smoke alarms; do not borrow them for other purposes. Nuisance activations can be addressed by moving an alarm farther away from kitchen smoke or bathroom steam and by more frequent cleaning. If the problem persists, replace the alarm.

- Replace smoke alarms every 10 years.

Why NFPA Recommends Home Smoke Alarms Be Replaced after 10 Years

Smoke alarms are one of the most important safety features of your home. Properly installed, working smoke alarms will give you the early warning you need to safely escape from a fire. But how do you make sure your alarms are working? One important way is to replace them after 10 years.

As electronic devices, alarms are subject to random failures. Product, installation, and maintenance standards are used to assure products work as designed despite this. Part of the technical basis for the first alarm product standard was an assessment of expected failure rate, estimated at four per million hours of operation or one every 30 years. Early field studies of alarm reliability, notably by Canada's Ontario Housing Corporation, confirmed the essential accuracy of this estimate, restated as a 3% failure rate per year. This means a very small fraction of home smoke alarms will fail almost immediately, and 3% will fail by the end of the first year. After 30 years, nearly all the alarms will have failed, most years earlier.

How soon should you replace your alarm? This is a value judgment. Only 3% of alarms are likely to fail in the first year, and annual replacement would be very expensive, so that doesn't make sense. At 15 years, the chances are better than 50/50 that your alarm has failed, and that seems too big a risk to take. Manufacturers' warranties for the early alarms typically ran out in 3-5 years. So, in ten years there is roughly a 30% probability of failure before replacement. This seemed to balance safety and cost in a way that made sense to the responsible technical committees.

If a 30% failure probability still seems too high, remember that replacement on a schedule is only a backup for replacement based on testing. A national study found home smoke alarms, when they fail, tend to fail totally, as opposed to hard-to-detect creeping failure, such as a loss of sensitivity.[1] Regular monthly testing will help discover alarm failure as well as a dead or missing battery. You can replace your alarm when it needs replacing.

The same study showed all the inoperable alarms tested in 1992 were at least 5 years old and predated a 1987 change in product standards that reduced sensitivity to reduce nuisance alarms. Changes in alarm chip design, among other improvements, make it likely that electronic failure now occurs at a rate much less than 4 times per million hours of operation.

Replacing alarms after 10 years protects against the accumulated chance of failure, but monthly testing is still your first, best means of making sure alarms work. Today's alarms are even less vulnerable than the original alarms. Regular maintenance of the more sophisticated systems used in larger buildings can keep them working very reliably for many decades.

Natural Gas Detectors

Although rare, a natural gas leak can have dangerous consequences. Your gas company and the gas institute work hard to provide adequate warning in the event of a gas leak. A smell which can easily be detected by most people is added to the gas. However, people with a diminished sense of smell cannot benefit from this safety mechanism. If you have a concern about your ability to detect gas leaks, a gas detector can be an important tool to help protect you and your family.

Selecting a Natural Gas Detector

Natural gas detector units vary greatly in price, features, and ease of installation. Some of them must be professionally installed and may be connected to your home security system. Other brands resemble smoke detectors and are easy for you to install. Regardless of which detector you choose, certain facts are important:

- **Alarm activation.** It is important that the natural gas detector will not be set off by other elements in your home, such as cigarette smoke or humidity level. Many detectors will, however, respond to other dangerous chemicals in addition to natural gas, such as propane (LP) or methane gas.

The LEL (Lower Explosive Limit) is the lowest amount of gas which will cause an explosion. Gas detectors vary in the level of gas which will set off an alarm (for example, 15% of the LEL, 20% of the LEL, etc.). You will be more quickly warned of the presence of natural gas by detectors which sense lower levels of gas.

- **Location of detector.** The distance between your gas detector and potential sources of gas leaks is important. Gas detectors are similar to smoke detectors, in that they need to be in the same general area as the gas appliances. Ask a sales person to find out how close the detector that you are interested in needs to be to a source of natural gas to safely warn you of a leak. If you have multiple sources of natural gas in your home, you might consider purchasing two gas detectors or one detector with dual sensors, especially if the gas sources are spaced far apart.

- **Type of alarm.** Some gas detectors use both a light and a sound to alert you to a gas leak. Some use only a sound. Regardless of which type of alarm you prefer, you should make certain that you will be alerted from any area of your home. An alarm which is not noticeable will not help you.

- **Gas detector maintenance.** Most gas detectors are either battery operated, or have a battery back-up system for 110 volt electrical power supply. Often, there is a "test" button on the gas detector which will allow you to make certain that the detector's alarm and batteries are working properly. Remember to check the batteries and the alarm regularly. Some gas detectors will also warn you if there is a power loss or other malfunction.

Gas detectors use sensors to find out if there are dangerous levels of natural gas nearby. Like batteries, sensors can wear out. When purchasing a gas detector, ask about the average life of the sensor, as well as if there is a warning when the sensor needs replacing. You may also want to know whether the sensor can be replaced if it wears out, and the price of a new sensor.

Some types of gas detectors must be calibrated in order to keep functioning properly. Ask if the gas detector model that you are interested in will require this service. If the answer is "yes," ask how often this will be required, as well as the name of a firm which can perform the calibration.

Consequences

According to the Consumer Product Safety Commission approximately 300 people die each year from natural gas poisoning associated with home fuel-burning heating equipment.

Medical Complications/Symptoms

Exposure to natural gas reduces the blood's ability to carry oxygen. Although there is no fever, the initial symptoms associated with dangerous levels of natural gas exposure are similar to flu-like illnesses. These symptoms include:

- dizziness
- fatigue
- nausea
- headache
- irregular breathing

Exposure at higher levels causes vomiting, loss of consciousness, or can be fatal.

Treatments

An individual exposed to natural gas poisoning needs to get fresh air immediately and medical attention as soon as possible. If the person is unconscious and not breathing, mouth-to-mouth resuscitation should be administered until help arrives.

Problems Associated with the Elderly

Smell sensitivity begins to decrease in the 7th decade of life. A large segment of the elderly population has difficulty detecting mercaptan, a foul-smelling chemical added as a warning agent to natural gas which is odorless. For individuals with a diminished sense of smell and taste, natural gas detectors can provide an early warning before gas builds to dangerous levels.

Sources of Natural Gas

- Gas Appliances
- Gas Heating Systems
- Gas Barbecue Grills

- Gas Hot Water Heaters
- Gas Furnaces and Fireplaces

Gas Detector Alerts

If your gas detector alerts you to a natural gas leak:

- Leave the house.

- Contact your local gas utility company (Don't call from your own home, as using the telephone could produce a spark, which could cause a fire or explosion).

- Do not re-enter the house until the source of the leak has been found and corrected.

References

1. Julie I. Shapiro, *Smoke Detector Operability Survey*, Washington: U.S. Consumer Product Safety Commission, October 1994 revised.

Additional Resources

NFPA
1 Batterymarch Park
Quincy, MA 02269-9101
Tel: 617-770-3000
Fax: 617-770-0700

NIDCD Information Clearinghouse
1 Communication Avenue
Bethesda, MD 20892-3456
Toll-Free: 800-241-1044
TTY: 800-241-1055
Website: www.nidcd.nih.gov
E-mail: nidcdinfo@nidcd.nih.gov

Indoor Air Quality Information Clearinghouse (IAQ INFO)
P.O. Box 37133
Washington, DC 20013-7133
Toll-Free: 800-438-4318
Tel: 703-356-4020
Website: www.epa.gov/iaq/iaqinfo.html
E-mail: iaqinfo@aol.com

U.S. Consumer Product Safety Commission
Washington, DC 20207-0001
Toll-Free: 800-638-CPSC
TTY: 800-638-8270
E-mail: info@cpsc.gov
Website: www.cpsc.gov

American Gas Association
400 N. Capitol Street, N.W.
Washington, DC 20001
Tel: 202-824-7000
Fax: 202-842-7115
Website: www.aga.org

The Chemosensory Disorders Group
The Smell and Taste Disorders Clinic
SUNY Health Science Center
750 East Adams Street
Syracuse, NY 13210
Tel: 315-464-5588
Fax: 315-464-7712
Website: www.upstate.edu/ent/smelltaste.shtml

National Institute on Deafness and Other Communication Disorders
National Institutes of Health
31 Center Drive, MSC 2320
Bethesda, MD 20892-2320
Tel: 301-496-7243
TTY: 301-402-0252
Website: www.nidcd.nih.gov

Chapter 39

Carbon Monoxide Risk at Home

In the past decade, people have become more aware of the risk of carbon monoxide (or CO) poisoning in the home.

What Is Carbon Monoxide?

Carbon monoxide (CO) is an invisible, odorless, colorless gas created when fuels (such as gasoline, wood, coal, natural gas, propane, oil, and methane) burn incompletely. In the home, heating and cooking equipment that burn fuel are possible sources of CO. Vehicles or generators running in an attached garage can also produce dangerous levels of CO.

However, consumers can protect themselves against CO poisoning by properly installing, using, venting, and maintaining their heating and cooking equipment; by installing CO alarms inside their homes; and by being cautious with vehicles or generators in attached garages.

What Is the Effect of Exposure to CO?

CO is poisonous and can kill cells of the body. CO also replaces oxygen in the bloodstream, leading to suffocation. Mild effects feel like the flu, while severe effects include difficulty breathing and even death.

Just how sick people get from CO exposure varies greatly from person to person, depending on age, overall health, concentration of exposure (measured in parts per million), and length of exposure. As with anything harmful that is inhaled, swallowed, or absorbed by the body, the severity of harm depends on the dose. The same dose of CO can be received through a long exposure to a low concentration or a brief exposure to a high concentration. Given time, the body will get rid of CO, unlike substances like lead or arsenic. Therefore, at the end of a long exposure to a low concentration, some of the initial CO may already have been expelled. That means that if the same amount of CO is received over a long period of time, its effect on the body may

Table 39.1. Effects of Exposure to CO*

Concentration (parts per million)	Symptoms
100	Threshold limit value for no adverse effects even with 6-8 hours exposure
200	Possible mild headache after 2-3 hours
400	Headache and nausea after 1-2 hours
800	Earache, nausea, and dizziness after 45 minutes; collapse and possible unconsciousness after 2 hours
1,000	Loss of consciousness after 1 hour
1,600	Headache, nausea, and dizziness after 20 minutes
3,200	Headache and dizziness after 5-10 minutes; unconsciousness after 30 minutes
6,400	Headache and dizziness after 1-2 minutes; unconsciousness and danger of death after 10-15 minutes
12,800	Immediate physiological effects; unconsciousness and danger of death after 1-3 minutes

Source: James H. Meidl, *Explosive and Toxic Hazardous Materials*, Glencoe Press, 1970, Table 28, p. 293.

* Just how sick people get from CO exposure varies greatly from person to person, depending on age, overall health, concentration of exposure (measured in parts per million), and length of exposure.

be less than if the same amount of CO had been received quickly, in high concentration. Table 39.1 shows typical symptoms, based on concentration and time of exposure.

When blood carries CO rather than oxygen, the CO-carrying cells are called carboxyhemoglobin (COHb), in contrast to normal oxygen-carrying hemoglobin. The percentage of the blood that is carboxyhemoglobin—also called carboxyhemoglobin saturation—measures how badly a person is affected by CO. A doctor can measure COHb in the blood but cannot measure CO in the body directly. The more CO in the body, the higher the COHb, and the sicker the person will be. Table 39.2 links typical symptoms to the level of COHb saturation.

Table 39.2. Effects of Carboxyhemoglobin (COHb) Saturation

COHb Saturation (%)	Symptoms
0–10	None
10–20	Tension in forehead, dilation of skin vessels
20–30	Headache and pulsating temples
30–40	Severe headache, weariness, dizziness, weakened sight, nausea, vomiting, prostration
40–50	Same as above, plus increased breathing and pulse rates, and asphyxiation
50–60	Same as above, plus coma, convulsions, Cheyne-Stokes respiration
60–70	Coma, convulsions, weak respiration and pulse; death is possible
70–80	Slowing and stopping of breathing; death within hours
80–90	Death in less than one hour
90–100	Death within a few minutes

Source: Gordon E. Hartzell, Ed., *Advances in Combustion Toxicology*, Volume One, Technomic Publishing, Inc., 1989, p. 23.

What Is Your Risk of CO Poisoning?

Deaths from unintentional poisoning by gas or vapors, chiefly CO— about 600 in 1998, including 500 in homes, according to the National Safety Council—are fairly rare, and the number has been declining somewhat steadily, down by half since the early 1980s. Of all the unintentional gas and vapor poisoning deaths in the U.S., more than one-third involve motor vehicle exhaust gas, and more than one-fourth involve heating or cooking equipment. The total reflects more than CO-related deaths; it also reflects deaths resulting from other gases, such as natural gas leaks from pipelines.(National Safety Council's *Accident Facts, 1981-99.*)

Deaths from unintentional CO poisoning have dropped in recent years, thanks to lower CO emissions from automobiles and safer heating and cooking appliances. Deaths from "smoke inhalation" (largely CO) in fires and suicides involving CO are both far more common causes of gas-related suffocation deaths.

According to the U.S. Consumer Product Safety Commission, 207 CO-related non-fire deaths were attributed to heating and cooking equipment in 1996—the latest year for which statistics are available at this level of detail. The specific types of equipment were:

- Gas-fueled space heaters (99 deaths)
- Gas-fueled furnaces (35 deaths)
- Liquid-fueled heating equipment (21 deaths)
- Charcoal grills (19 deaths)
- Gas-fueled ranges (15 deaths)
- Solid-fueled heating equipment (10 deaths)
- Gas-fueled water heaters (8 deaths)

Table 39.3. 1996 Deaths Involving CO and Related Gases

Cause	Number of Deaths
Smoke Inhalation in Fire Deaths	2,677
Unintentional CO and Other Gases Deaths	638
Suicide by Gas or Vapor	2,007

Source: Dr. John Hall, Jr., *Burns, Toxic Gases, and Other Hazards Associated With Fires*, Fire Analysis and Research Division, NFPA, November 1999

As with fire deaths, the risk of unintentional CO death is highest for the very young (ages 4 or under) and the very old (ages 75 or above).

How Can You Protect Yourself from CO Poisoning?

Install CO alarms inside your home to provide early warning of accumulating CO. However, a CO alarm is no substitute for safe practices.

The best defenses against CO poisoning are safe use of vehicles (particularly in attached garages) and proper installation, use, venting, and maintenance of household cooking and heating equipment.

What Are CO Alarms?

Household CO alarms measure how much CO has accumulated. Currently, CO alarms sound when the concentration of CO in the air corresponds to 10% COHb level in the blood. Since 10% COHb is at the very low end of CO poisoning, the alarm may sound before people feel particularly sick. Most CO alarms now have silence/reset buttons and must be immune to elevated ambient levels such as those found in urban areas.

Do I Need a CO Alarm?

NFPA 720, *Recommended Practice for the Installation of Household Carbon Monoxide (CO) Warning Equipment,* 1998 Edition, recommends installing a CO alarm in households containing a fuel-burning appliance, fireplace, or in those having an attached garage.

What Causes CO Nuisance Alarms?

Pollution and atmospheric conditions in some areas cause low levels of CO to be present for long periods of time. In fact, these "background" conditions may increase CO to over the 10% COHb equivalency level, causing older CO alarms to sound even though conditions inside the home are not truly hazardous. However, newer alarms have been designed to reduce sensitivities to compensate for these background conditions. Treat all CO alarm warning sounds as real, until it has been verified that there is no threat from equipment inside the dwelling.

Safety Tips

- If you need to warm up a vehicle, remove it from the garage immediately after starting it. Do not run a vehicle, generator, or other fueled engine or motor indoors, even if garage doors are open. CO from a running vehicle or generator inside an attached garage can get inside the house, even with the garage door open. Normal circulation does not provide enough fresh air to reliably prevent dangerous accumulations inside.

- If you have any symptoms of CO poisoning, have your vehicle inspected for exhaust leaks. Have fuel-burning household heating equipment (fireplaces, furnaces, water heaters, wood stoves, and space or portable heaters) checked every year before cold weather sets in.

- All chimneys and chimney connectors should be evaluated by a qualified technician to verify proper installation, and check for cracks, blockages, or leaks. Make needed repairs before using the equipment.

- Before enclosing central heating equipment in a smaller room, check with your fuel supplier to ensure that air for proper combustion is provided. NFPA 54, National Fuel Gas Code, provides requirements for openings to allow sufficient air for the proper combustion of gas.

- When using a fireplace, open the flue for adequate ventilation.

- Open a window slightly whenever using a kerosene or gas heater. (Kerosene heaters are illegal in many states. Always check with local authorities before buying or using one.) Only refuel outside, after the device has cooled.

- Only use barbecue grills—which can produce CO—outside. Never use them in the home or garage.

- When purchasing new heating and cooking equipment, select products tested and labeled by an independent testing laboratory. Do not accept damaged equipment. Hire a qualified technician (usually employed by the local oil or gas company) to install the equipment. Ask about—and insist that the technician follow—applicable fire safety and building codes.

- When purchasing an existing home, have a qualified technician evaluate the integrity of the heating and cooking systems, as well as the sealed spaces between the garage and house.

- When camping, remember to use battery-powered heaters and flashlights in tents, trailers, and motorhomes. Using fossil fuels inside these structures is extremely dangerous. NFPA 1192, Standard on Recreational Vehicles, requires the installation of CO detectors in recreational vehicles.

- Boat operators should be aware that CO is emitted from any boat's exhaust. When your boat is moored or anchored alongside others be aware of the effect your exhaust may have on those vessels and vice versa. The trim of the boat, as well as side curtains, can contribute to increased concentrations of CO by altering the airflow. Fuel burning appliances located in accommodation spaces need to be properly ventilated and maintained.

If You Buy CO Alarms

- Select alarms listed by a qualified, independent testing laboratory.

- Follow recommendations of NFPA 720 and manufacturer's recommendations for placement in your home.

- Install CO alarms in a central location outside each separate sleeping area in the immediate vicinity of the bedrooms. Each alarm should be installed on the wall, ceiling, or other location as specified by the manufacturer's instructions that accompany the unit.

- Call your local fire department's non-emergency telephone number. Tell the operator that you have purchased a CO alarm and ask what number to call if the CO alarm sounds. Clearly post that number by your telephone(s). Make sure everyone in the household knows the difference between the fire emergency and CO emergency numbers (if there is a difference).

- Test CO alarms at least once a month, following the manufacturer's instructions.

- Replace CO alarms according to the manufacturer's instructions.

- Follow manufacturer's instructions for battery replacement.

What to Do if Your CO Alarm Sounds

- Have everyone move to an area with fresh (outside) air. Open windows to ventilate.

- Report the CO alarm warning, following the instructions you received from the fire department when you bought the alarm.

- Be on the lookout for any symptoms of CO poisoning. Evacuate the home if symptoms are present. Get immediate medical attention if anyone shows signs of CO poisoning.

- Call a qualified technician to inspect all equipment.

Safety Checklist

- CO alarms are not substitutes for smoke alarms. Smoke alarms react to fire by-products, before CO alarms would sound. Smoke alarms give earlier warning of a fire, providing more time to escape.

- To guard against smoke and fire, be sure that your home has working smoke alarms on every level and directly outside and inside all sleeping rooms

- Know the difference between the sound of the smoke alarms and the sound of the CO alarms.

- Have a home escape plan for any home emergency and practice the plan with all members of the household regularly, at least twice a year.

Chapter 40

Preventing Dog Bite Attacks

In order to estimate the magnitude of the dog bite problem in the U.S., data on dog bites were gathered as part of a 1994 national telephone survey of 5,238 randomly dialed households. Data were weighted to provide national estimates. The results showed a weighted total number of dog bites at 4,494,083 (estimated incidence equal to 18 per 1,000 population); of these, 756,701 persons sustained bites necessitating medical attention (incidence rate equal to 3 per 1000 population). Children had 32 times higher medically attended bite rates than adults (64 per 1000 children vs. 2 per 1000 adults).

More attention and research needs to be devoted to the prevention of dog bites. Potential prevention strategies include: educational programs on canine behavior, especially directed at children; laws for regulating dangerous or vicious dogs; enhanced animal control programs; and educational programs regarding responsible dog ownership and training. Unfortunately, the relative or absolute effectiveness of any of these strategies has not been assessed. Continuing surveillance for dog bites will be needed if we are to better understand how to reduce the incidence of dog bites and evaluate prevention efforts.

"Dog Bites: How Big a Problem?" Abstract by Jeffrey J. Sacks, Marcie-jo Kresnow, and Barbara Houston, *Injury Prevention* 1996; 2:52-54, National Center for Injury Prevention and Control (NCIPC); and "Dog Bites: How to Teach Your Children to Be Safe," Reprinted with permission from http://www.familydoctor.org/handouts/668.html; 2001. Copyright © American Academy of Family Physicians. All Rights Reserved.

Dog Bites: How to Teach Your Children to Be Safe

Most dogs will never bite anyone. However, any dog may bite if it feels threatened. Children are the most common victims of dog bites. Infants and young children should never be left alone with a dog. This chapter tells you how to teach your children to avoid getting bitten.

What Should I Do if I Want a Dog for a Pet?

Take time to learn about the breed of dog you want. To learn about dog breeds, talk with a veterinarian, read books about dogs, and search the Internet. Don't get a dog only because of the way it looks. If you have an infant or young child, think about getting a puppy. Be especially careful if you have a baby in your house. Aggressive dog breeds aren't right for families with children. Neutered male dogs are generally less aggressive.

Consider taking your new dog to obedience school. Keep your dog's immunizations up to date. Have your dog checked regularly by a veterinarian.

What Do I Tell My Children about Dogs?

- Don't go near strange dogs.
- Never bother a dog that is eating, sleeping, or caring for puppies.
- Tell an adult about any stray dogs.
- Always have an adult with you when you play with a dog.
- Never tease a dog.
- Never pet a dog without first letting it smell you.

What Should I Tell My Children to Do When a Dog Approaches Them?

- Don't run away and scream.
- Stand very still, "like a tree."
- Avoid making direct eye contact with the dog.
- If you fall or are knocked down, act "like a log."
- When the dog understands that you are not a threat, it will probably walk away.

- If a dog bites you, tell an adult right away.

A dog is a wonderful addition to a family, but it can be a problem if you aren't careful. Always talk to children about how they should act when they're with a dog. Remember that dogs can feel threatened by new surroundings or strangers.

Chapter 41

Playground Injuries and Safety

Chapter Contents

Section 41.1

Playground Injuries

This section includes "Playground Injuries," National Center for
Injury Prevention and Control Publication (NCIPC), reviewed
January 27, 2000; and "Playground Safety," SafeUSA,
updated February 2001.

How Large Is the Problem of Playground-Related Injuries?

- Each year in the United States, 200,000 preschool and elementary school children visit emergency departments for care of injuries sustained on playground equipment (about 1 injury every 2½ minutes).[1]

- About 35% of all playground-related injuries are severe (e.g., fractures, internal injuries, concussions, dislocations, amputations, crushes).[1]

- Public playgrounds account for about 70% of injuries related to playground equipment.[1]

- In schools, most injuries to students between the ages of 5 and 14 years occur on playgrounds.[2]

Which Playground Equipment Causes the Most Injury?

- Most injuries occur when children fall off swings, monkey bars, climbers, or slides.[1]

- Falls off of playground equipment to the ground account for more than 60% of all playground-related injuries.[1, 3]

How Many Injuries Require Hospitalization?

- Slightly less than 3% of all playground injuries require hospitalization.[1]

How Many Children Die Each Year Because of Playground-Related Injuries?

- Each year, nearly 20 children die from playground-related injuries. More than half of these deaths result from strangulation and about one-third result from falls.[2]

What Costs Are Associated with Playground-Related Injury?

- In 1995, the costs were $1.2 billion for children younger than 15 years old.[2]

Playground Safety

Every two-and-a-half minutes a child is injured on a playground in the United States. Supervising children as they play on equipment and choosing playgrounds with cushioning materials under the equipment will reduce children's risk of injury.

Playground Safety Tips

You can help keep your child safe from injuries on the playground if you follow a few simple tips. These tips apply to backyard and fast-food restaurant playgrounds, as well as to public or school playgrounds.

Nearly all severe playground-related injuries are the result of children falling or jumping from climbing equipment, slides, and swings. Protective surfaces made of energy-absorbing (cushioning) materials under and around equipment can prevent and reduce the severity of injuries related to falling on the playground. Supervising children while they play on equipment is also extremely important.

- Supervise children at all times, especially when they are on climbing equipment, swings, and slides. Prevent behaviors like pushing, shoving, and crowding around equipment.

- Make sure that children play on playground equipment that is appropriate for their age. For example, don't let young children play on high climbing equipment such as monkey bars. Keep all children off equipment from which they might fall six or more feet.

- Check the surface under playground equipment. Avoid playgrounds with asphalt, concrete, grass, and soil surfaces under the equipment. Look for surfaces of hardwood fiber, mulch chips, pea gravel, fine sand, or shredded rubber—materials that can cushion a fall—with a depth of at least 4-6 inches. The deeper the cushioning material, the better.

- Remove or cut the hood and neck drawstrings from all children's outerwear to prevent entanglement and strangulation. Children have died when hood or neck drawstrings were caught on slides and other playground equipment.

- Make sure spaces that could trap children's heads, such as openings in guardrails or between ladder rungs, measure less than 3.5 inches (so children can't get their heads in) or more than 9 inches (so they can get out).

- Check playground equipment to make sure it is in good repair, without jagged edges or sharp points.

- Check for hot surfaces on metal playground equipment before allowing young children to play on it. Metal equipment can heat up in direct sunlight and cause burn injuries in a few seconds.

- Make sure there are no obvious hazards around the playground, such as broken glass.

- Make sure there is fencing between the playground and the street to prevent children from running in front of cars.

What Is CDC Doing to Prevent Playground-Related Injuries?

The National Center for Injury Prevention and Control, CDC, funds the National Program for Playground Safety (NPPS), which works to prevent playground-related injuries and the attendant suffering and costs. This program is based at the University of Northern Iowa in Cedar Falls, Iowa. The NPPS goals include:

- Implementing a national plan for the prevention of playground-related injuries.

- Maintaining a clearinghouse of materials on playground safety and making those materials available to anyone who requests them.

- Providing an information hotline on preventing playground-related injury.

- Holding training programs for teachers and playground safety inspectors.

- Researching the impact attenuation characteristics of playground surfaces under a variety of conditions.

References

1. Consumer Product Safety Commission (CPSC). National Electronic Injury Surveillance System 1990-94. Washington (DC): CPSC.

2. Office of Technology Assessment. *Risks to students in school.* Washington (DC): U.S. Government Printing Office, 1995.

3. U.S. Consumer Product Safety Commission (CPSC). *Handbook for public playground safety.* Washington, DC: author, 1997.

Additional Information

National Program for Playground Safety
School of Health, Physical Education & Leisure Services
WRC 205, University of Northern Iowa
Cedar Falls, IA 50614-0618
Toll-Free: 800-554-PLAY
Tel: 319-273-7308
Fax: 319-273-7308
Website: www.uni.edu/playground
E-mail: playground-safety@uni.edu

The National Program for Playground Safety has the following brochures available:

- Inspection Guide for Parents
- A Blueprint for Increasing Playground Safety
- Supervision Means...
- All Children Should Play on Age-Appropriate Equipment
- Falls to Surface Should Be Cushioned
- Equipment Should Be Safe
- Planning a Play Area for Children

- The National Action Plan for Playground Safety
- Funding Tips for Playgrounds
- SAFE Playground Resources
- Videos
- ABC's of Supervision (training for elementary school supervisors)
- America's Playgrounds—Make Them Safe (NPPS overview)
- Sammy's Playground (for grades K-3)
- SAFE Playgrounds—General Description of SAFE Playgrounds

Other Materials

- Summary Report for NPPS
- SAFE Playground Workbook
- SAFE Playground Handbook

SafeUSA

P.O. Box 8189
Silver Springs, MD 20907-9189
Toll-Free: 888-252-7751
Website: www.cdc.gov/safeusa
E-mail: sainfo@cdc.gov

U.S. Consumer Product Safety Commission

Washington, DC 20207-0001
Toll-Free: 800-638-2772
Toll-Free Teletypewriter: 800-638-8270
TTY: 800-638-8270
Website: www.cpsc.gov
E-mail: info@cpsc.gov

Tips for parents and community groups, standards for playground equipment, surfaces, etc.

National Center for Injury Prevention and Control

Mailstop K65
4770 Buford Highway N.E.
Atlanta, GA 30341-3724
Tel: 770-488-1506
Fax: 770-488-1667
Website: www.cdc.gov/ncipc/
E-mail: OHCINFO@cdc.gov

Section 41.2

Home Playground Safety Tips

"Home Playground Safety Tips," Consumer Product Safety Commission, CPSC Document #323.

Each year, about 200,000 children are treated in U.S. hospital emergency rooms for playground equipment-related injuries—an estimated 148,000 of these injuries involve public playground equipment and an estimated 51,000 involve home playground equipment. Also, about 15 children die each year as a result of playground equipment-related incidents. Most of the injuries are the result of falls. These are primarily falls to the ground below the equipment, but falls from one piece of equipment to another are also reported. Most of the deaths are due to strangulation, though some are due to falls.

Protective Surfacing

- Since almost 60% of all injuries are caused by falls to the ground, protective surfacing under and around all playground equipment can reduce the risk of serious head injury.

- Falls on asphalt and concrete can result in serious head injury and death. Do not place playground equipment over these surfaces. Also grass and turf lose their ability to absorb shock through wear and environmental conditions. Always use protective surfacing.

Table 41.1. Fall Height in Feet from which a Life Threatening Head Injury Would Not Be Expected

Type of Material	6" Depth	9" Depth	12" Depth
Double Shredded Bark Mulch	6 feet	10 feet	11 feet
Wood Chips	7 feet	10 feet	11 feet
Fine Sand	5 feet	5 feet	9 feet
Fine Gravel	6 feet	7 feet	10 feet

- Certain loose-fill surfacing materials are acceptable, such as the types and depths shown in the table.

- Certain manufactured synthetic surfaces also are acceptable; however, test data on shock absorbing performance should be requested from the manufacturer.

Use Zones

- A use zone, covered with a protective surfacing material, is essential under and around equipment where a child might fall. This area should be free of other equipment and obstacles onto which a child might fall.

- Stationary climbing equipment and slides should have a use zone extending a minimum of 6 feet in all directions from the perimeter of the equipment.

- Swings should have a use zone extending a minimum of 6 feet from the outer edge of the support structure on each side. The use zone in front and back of the swing should extend out a minimum distance of twice the height of the swing as measured from the ground to the swing hangers on support structure.

Swing Spacing

To prevent injuries from impact with moving swings, swings should not be too close together or too close to support structures. Swing spacing should be:

- At least 8 inches between suspended swings and between a swing and the support frame.

- At least 16 inches from swing support frame to a pendulum seesaw.

- Minimum clearance between the ground and underside of swing seat should be 8 inches.

- Swing sets should be securely anchored.

Elevated Surfaces

Platforms more than 30" above the ground should have guardrails to prevent falls.

Potential Head Entrapment Hazards

In general, openings that are closed on all sides, should be less than 3.5 inches or greater than 9 inches. Openings that are between 3.5 inches and 9 inches present a head entrapment hazard because they are large enough to permit a child's body to go through, but are too small to permit the head to go through. When children enter such openings, feet first, they may become entrapped by the head and strangle.

Potential Entrapment and Strangulation Hazards

Open "S" hooks, especially on swings, and any protrusions or equipment component/hardware which may act as hooks or catch-points can entangle with children's clothing and cause strangulation incidents. Close "S" hooks as tightly as possible and eliminate protrusions or catch-points on playground equipment.

Pinch or Crush Points

There should be no exposed moving parts which may present a pinching or crushing hazard.

Playground Maintenance

Playgrounds should be inspected on a regular basis. Inspect protective surfacing especially mulch, and maintain the proper depth. If any of the following conditions are noted, they should be removed, corrected, or repaired immediately to prevent injuries:

- Hardware is loose or worn, or that has protrusions or projections.

- Ropes, and items with cords placed around the neck can get caught on playground equipment and strangle a child. Many children have died when a rope they were wearing got caught on playground equipment, or they became entangled in a rope.

- Supervise, and teach your child safe play. Teach your child not to walk or play close to a moving swing, and not to tie ropes to playground equipment.

- Exposed equipment footings.

- Scattered debris, litter, rocks, or tree roots.

- Rust and chipped paint on metal components.

- Splinters, large cracks, and decayed wood components.

- Deterioration and corrosion on structural components which connect to the ground.

- Missing or damaged equipment components, such as handholds, guardrails, swing seats.

The U.S. Consumer Product Safety Commission protects the public from the unreasonable risk of injury or death from 15,000 types of consumer products under the agency's jurisdiction. To report a dangerous product or a product-related injury contact:

U.S. Consumer Product Safety Commission
Washington, DC 20207-0001
Toll-Free: 800-638-2772
Toll-Free Teletypewriter: 800-638-8270
TTY: 800-638-8270
E-mail: info@cpsc.gov
Website: www.cpsc.gov

Section 41.3

Public Playground Safety Checklist

"Public Playground Safety Checklist," Consumer Product Safety Commission, CPSC Document #327.

Is Your Public Playground a Safe Place to Play

Each year, more than 200,000 children go to U.S. hospital emergency rooms with inuries associated with playground equipment. Most injuries occur when a child falls from the equipment onto the ground.

Use this simple checklist to help make sure your local community or school playground is a safe place to play.

Public Playground Safety Checklist

1. Make sure surfaces around playground equipment have at least 12 inches of wood chips, mulch, sand, or pea gravel, or are mats made of safety-tested rubber or rubber-like materials.

2. Check that protective surfacing extends at least 6 feet in all directions from play equipment. For swings, be sure surfacing extends, in back and front, twice the height of the suspending bar.

3. Make sure play structures more than 30 inches high are spaced at least 9 feet apart.

4. Check for dangerous hardware, like open "S" hooks or protruding bolt ends.

5. Make sure spaces that could trap children, such as openings in guardrails or between ladder rungs, measure less than 3.5 inches or more than 9 inches.

6. Check for sharp points or edges in equipment.

7. Look out for tripping hazards, like exposed concrete footings, tree stumps, and rocks.

391

8. Make sure elevated surfaces, like platforms and ramps, have guardrails to prevent falls.

9. Check playgrounds regularly to see that equipment and surfacing are in good condition.

10. Carefully supervise children on playgrounds to make sure they're safe.

Part Six

Work-Related Injuries

Chapter 42

Incidence Rates of Injury by Occupation

A total of 5.7 million injuries and illnesses were reported in private industry workplaces during 1999, resulting in a rate of 6.3 cases per 100 equivalent full-time workers, according to a survey by the Bureau of Labor Statistics, U.S. Department of Labor. Employers reported a 4 percent drop in the number of cases and a 2 percent increase in the hours worked compared with 1998, reducing the case rate from 6.7 in 1998 to 6.3 in 1999. The rate for 1999 was the lowest since the Bureau began reporting this information in the early 1970s.

Among goods-producing industries, manufacturing had the highest incidence rate in 1999 (9.2 cases per 100 full-time workers). (See Table 42.2.) Within the service-producing sector, the highest incidence rate was reported for transportation and public utilities (7.3 cases per

Table 42.1. Incidence Rates Decline for Injuries and Illnesses Per 100 Full-Time Workers Since 1994.

	1994	1995	1996	1997	1998	1999
Private industry	8.4	8.1	7.4	7.1	6.7	6.3
Goods-producing	11.9	11.2	10.2	9.9	9.3	8.9
Service-producing	6.9	6.7	6.2	5.9	5.6	5.3

"Workplace Injuries and Illnesses in 1999," News Release December 12, 2000, Bureau of Labor Statistics, Occupational Safety and Health Administration (OSHA).

100 full-time workers), followed by wholesale and retail trade (6.1 cases per 100 workers).

This release is the second in a series of three releases covering 1999 from the BLS safety and health statistical series. The first release, in August 2000, covered work-related fatalities from the 1999 National Census of Fatal Occupational Injuries. In April 2001, a third release provided details on the more seriously injured and ill workers (occupation, age, gender, race, and length of service) and on the circumstances of their injuries and illnesses (nature of the disabling condition, part of body affected, event or exposure, and primary source producing the disability). "More seriously" is defined in this survey as involving days away from work.

Case Types

Of the 5.7 million total injuries and illnesses reported in 1999, about 2.7 million were lost workday cases, that is, they required recuperation away from work or restricted duties at work, or both. The remaining 3 million were cases without lost workdays. The incidence rate for both types of cases declined from 1998 to 1999. For lost workday cases, the rate declined from 3.1 cases per 100 workers to 3.0 cases per 100 workers, and, for cases without lost workdays, the rate decreased from 3.5 cases per 100 workers to 3.3 cases per 100 workers.

Lost workday cases are comprised of two case types, those requiring at least one day away from work, with or without restricted work activity, and those requiring restricted activity only. The latter type of case may involve shortened hours, a temporary job change, or temporary restrictions on certain duties (for example, no heavy lifting) of a worker's regular job. At 1.9 cases per 100 workers in 1999, the rate for cases with days away from work declined from 2.0 in 1998 and was the lowest on record. In contrast to the decreases posted by all the other major case types in 1999, the rate for cases involving restricted activity only remained at its 1998 level, 1.2 cases per 100 employees. In 1999, the rate in manufacturing for "restricted activity only"cases (2.4) was higher than the rate for "days away from work" cases (2.2). In all other divisions, the rate for "days away from work" cases was higher than the rate for "restricted activity only" cases.

Injuries and Illnesses

Injuries. Of the 5.7 million nonfatal occupational injuries and illnesses in 1999, 5.3 million were injuries. Injury rates generally are higher for mid-size establishments (those employing 50 to 249 workers) than for smaller or larger establishments, although this pattern does not hold within certain industry divisions. Nine industries, each having at least 100,000 injuries, accounted for about 1.6 million injuries, or 30 percent of the 5.3 million total. (See Table 42.4.) All but one of these industries were in the service-producing sector.

Illnesses. There were about 372,000 newly reported cases of occupational illnesses in private industry in 1999. Manufacturing accounted for three-fifths of these cases. Disorders associated with repeated trauma, such as carpal tunnel syndrome and noise-induced hearing loss, accounted for 4 percent of the 5.7 million total workplace injuries and illnesses. They were, however, the dominant type of illness reported, making up 66 percent of the 372,000 total illness cases. Seventy percent of the repeated trauma cases were in manufacturing industries.

The survey measures the number of new work-related illness cases that are recognized, diagnosed, and reported during the year. Some conditions (for example, long-term latent illnesses caused by exposure to carcinogens) often are difficult to relate to the workplace and are not adequately recognized and reported. These long-term latent illnesses are believed to be understated in the survey's illness measures. In contrast, the overwhelming majority of the reported new illnesses are those that are easier to directly relate to workplace activity (for example, contact dermatitis or carpal tunnel syndrome).

Background of the Survey

The Survey of Occupational Injuries and Illnesses is a Federal/State program in which employer reports are collected from about 174,000 private industry establishments and processed by state agencies cooperating with the Bureau of Labor Statistics. Occupational injury and illness data for coal, metal, nonmetal mining, and for railroad activities were provided by the Department of Labor's Mine Safety and Health Administration and the Department of Transportation's Federal Railroad Administration. The survey measures nonfatal injuries and illnesses only. The survey excludes the self-employed; farms with fewer than 11 employees; private households; federal government agencies; and, for national estimates, employees in State and local government agencies.

The annual survey provides estimates of the number and frequency (incidence rates) of workplace injuries and illnesses based on logs kept by private industry employers during the year. These records reflect not only the year's injury and illness experience, but also the employer's understanding of which cases are work-related under current record keeping guidelines of the U.S. Department of Labor. The number of injuries and illnesses reported in any given year also can be influenced by the level of economic activity, working conditions and work practices, worker experience and training, and the number of hours worked.

Establishments are classified in industry categories based on the 1987 Standard Industrial Classification (SIC) Manual, as defined by the Office of Management and Budget. The survey estimates of occupational injuries and illnesses are based on a scientifically selected probability sample, rather than a census of the entire population. Because the data are based on a sample survey, the injury and illness estimates probably differ from the figures that would be obtained from all units covered by the survey. To determine the precision of each estimate, a standard error was calculated. The standard error defines a range (confidence interval) around the estimate. The approximate 95-percent confidence interval is the estimate plus or minus twice the standard error. The standard error also can be expressed as a percent of the estimate, or the relative standard error. For example, the 95-percent confidence interval for an incidence rate of 6.5 per 100 full-time workers with a relative standard error of 1.0 percent would be 6.5 plus or minus 2 percent (2 times 1.0 percent) or 6.37 to 6.63. One can be 95-percent confident that the "true" incidence rate falls within the confidence interval. The 1999 incidence rate for all occupational injuries and illnesses of 6.3 per 100 full-time workers in private industry has an estimated relative standard error of about 0.6 percent.

The data also are subject to nonsampling error. The inability to obtain information about all cases in the sample, mistakes in recording or coding the data, and definition difficulties are examples of nonsampling error in the survey. Nonsampling errors are not measured. However, BLS has implemented quality assurance procedures to minimize nonsampling error in the survey.

Sector and Industry Divisions

The goods-producing sector consists of the following industry divisions: agriculture, forestry, and fishing; mining; construction; and manufacturing. The service-producing sector includes the following industry divisions: transportation and public utilities; trade; finance, insurance, and real estate; and services. BLS has generated estimates of injuries and illnesses combined and of injuries alone for nearly all 2-, 3-, and, for manufacturing, 4-digit private sector industries as defined in the 1987 edition of the Standard Industrial Classification Manual. Because of space limitations, a complete listing of these estimates is not possible in this chapter. The information is available from BLS staff at 202-691-6179 and from the BLS Internet site at http://stats.bls.gov/iif.

Statistical Tables 42.2–42.4 begin on the next page.

Table 42.2. Incidence Rates[1] of Nonfatal Occupational Injuries and Illnesses by Selected Industries and Case Types, 1999

Industry[2]	SIC code[3]	1999 Annual average employment[4] (000s)	Injuries and illnesses				Injuries			
			Total cases	Lost workday cases Total[5]	Lost workday cases With days away from work[6]	Cases without lost workdays	Total cases	Lost workday cases Total[5]	Lost workday cases With days away from work[6]	Cases without lost workdays
Private industry[7]		107,611.8	6.3	3.0	1.9	3.3	5.9	2.8	1.8	3.1
Agriculture, forestry, and fishing[7]		1,860.7	7.3	3.4	2.4	3.9	7.0	3.3	2.4	3.7
Agricultural production[7]	01-02	770.7	7.7	3.6	2.5	4.1	7.4	3.5	2.4	3.8
Agricultural production-crops[7]	01	578.2	7.0	3.1	2.1	3.9	6.6	3.0	2.0	3.6
Agricultural production-livestock[7]	02	192.4	10.0	5.2	3.5	4.9	9.5	5.0	3.4	4.5
Agricultural services	07	1,051.6	7.1	3.3	2.4	3.8	6.8	3.2	2.4	3.6
Forestry	08	27.1	6.1	2.9	2.2	3.2	5.6	2.7	2.0	2.9
Fishing, hunting, and trapping	09	11.4	6.9	4.5	3.0	2.4	6.3	4.0	2.9	2.3
Mining[8]		535.4	4.4	2.7	2.0	1.7	4.1	2.5	1.9	1.6
Metal mining[8]	10	43.5	5.0	2.9	1.7	2.1	4.7	2.7	1.6	2.0
Coal mining[8]	12	85.6	7.4	5.5	5.2	1.9	6.8	5.2	4.9	1.7
Oil and gas extraction	13	294.6	3.5	1.8	1.2	1.7	3.3	1.7	1.1	1.7
Nonmetallic minerals, except fuels[8]	14	111.8	4.3	2.8	2.0	1.4	4.1	2.8	2.0	1.4
Construction		6,337.3	8.6	4.2	3.3	4.4	8.4	4.1	3.3	4.3
General building contractors	15	1,453.3	8.0	3.7	2.9	4.3	7.9	3.6	2.9	4.3
Heavy construction, except building	16	860.0	7.8	3.8	2.8	4.0	7.6	3.7	2.7	3.9
Special trade contractors	17	4,024.1	8.9	4.4	3.6	4.5	8.8	4.4	3.5	4.4

Industry	Code	Employment								
Manufacturing		18,538.4	9.2	4.6	2.2	4.6	8.0	4.0	2.0	4.0
Durable goods		11,102.3	10.1	4.8	2.4	5.3	8.8	4.2	2.1	4.6
Lumber and wood products	24	831.9	13.0	6.7	3.9	6.3	12.5	6.4	3.8	6.0
Furniture and fixtures	25	547.0	11.5	5.9	2.5	5.7	10.3	5.2	2.2	5.1
Stone, clay, and glass products	32	566.6	10.7	5.4	3.0	5.3	10.1	5.2	2.9	4.9
Primary metal industries	33	698.8	12.9	6.3	3.1	6.7	11.9	5.9	2.9	6.0
Fabricated metal products	34	1,521.9	12.6	6.0	3.1	6.6	11.6	5.6	2.9	6.1
Industrial machinery and equipment	35	2,132.8	8.5	3.7	2.0	4.8	7.8	3.4	1.8	4.4
Electronic and other electric equipment	36	1,666.1	5.7	2.8	1.2	2.9	4.6	2.2	1.0	2.4
Transportation equipment	37	1,891.8	13.7	6.4	2.7	7.3	10.5	5.2	2.2	5.3
Instruments and related products	38	852.6	4.0	1.8	.9	2.2	3.1	1.4	.7	1.8
Miscellaneous manufacturing industries	39	392.9	8.4	4.0	1.9	4.4	7.7	3.5	1.7	4.1
Nondurable goods		7,436.1	7.8	4.2	1.9	3.6	6.8	3.7	1.7	3.1
Food and kindred products	20	1,686.2	12.7	7.3	2.8	5.3	10.4	6.0	2.5	4.4
Tobacco products	21	36.7	5.5	2.2	1.7	3.3	5.2	2.1	1.6	3.1
Textile mill products	22	557.2	6.4	3.2	1.2	3.2	5.7	2.9	1.1	2.8
Apparel and other textile products	23	689.9	5.8	2.8	1.4	3.0	4.5	2.2	1.1	2.3
Paper and allied products	26	667.8	7.0	3.7	1.8	3.3	6.5	3.5	1.7	3.0
Printing and publishing	27	1,545.7	5.0	2.6	1.6	2.4	4.6	2.4	1.5	2.2
Chemicals and allied products	28	1,035.0	4.4	2.3	1.1	2.2	3.8	2.0	1.0	1.8
Petroleum and coal products	29	132.0	4.1	1.8	1.0	2.3	3.9	1.8	1.0	2.1
Rubber and miscellaneous plastics products	30	1,008.6	10.1	5.5	2.8	4.7	9.3	5.0	2.5	4.3
Leather and leather products	31	76.9	10.3	5.0	1.6	5.3	7.5	3.8	1.3	3.7
Transportation and public utilities[8]		6,578.1	7.3	4.4	3.1	2.8	7.0	4.3	3.0	2.7
Railroad transportation[8]	40		3.6	2.8	2.4	.8	3.5	2.7	2.3	.8
Local and interurban passenger transit	41	463.3	9.1	4.7	3.5	4.4	8.9	4.7	3.5	4.3
Trucking and warehousing	42	1,804.1	8.7	5.1	3.6	3.6	8.6	5.0	3.5	3.6

Table 42.2. Incidence Rates[1] of Nonfatal Occupational Injuries and Illnesses by Selected Industries and Case Types, 1999 (continued from previous page)

Industry[2]	SIC code[3]	1999 Annual average employment[4] (000s)	Injuries and illnesses				Injuries			
			Total cases	Lost workday cases		Cases without lost work-days	Total cases	Lost workday cases		Cases without lost work-days
				Total[5]	With days away from work[6]			Total[5]	With days away from work[6]	
Transportation and public utilities[8] (continued)										
Water transportation	44	187.2	8.0	4.4	3.8	3.6	7.6	4.3	3.7	3.3
Transportation by air	45	1,243.1	13.3	9.4	6.6	3.9	12.8	9.1	6.3	3.7
Pipelines, except natural gas	46	13.2	5.1	2.6	2.2	2.5	5.1	2.6	2.2	2.5
Transportation services	47	457.5	3.8	2.2	1.3	1.6	3.5	2.1	1.3	1.5
Communications	48	1,548.5	3.1	1.7	1.2	1.4	2.6	1.5	1.0	1.2
Electric, gas, and sanitary services	49	859.6	6.1	3.3	1.7	2.9	5.7	3.2	1.7	2.6
Wholesale and retail trade		29,715.7	6.1	2.7	1.8	3.4	6.0	2.7	1.7	3.3
Wholesale trade		6,903.0	6.3	3.3	2.0	3.0	6.1	3.2	2.0	2.9
Wholesale trade–durable goods	50	4,102.2	5.6	2.6	1.7	2.9	5.4	2.6	1.6	2.9
Wholesale trade–nondurable goods	51	2,800.8	7.3	4.2	2.6	3.1	7.1	4.1	2.5	3.0
Retail trade		22,812.7	6.1	2.5	1.7	3.6	6.0	2.5	1.7	3.5
Building materials and garden supplies	52	989.1	8.3	3.8	2.4	4.5	8.2	3.8	2.4	4.4
General merchandise stores	53	2,782.6	8.5	4.6	2.4	3.9	8.4	4.5	2.3	3.9
Food stores	54	3,490.5	7.9	3.4	2.4	4.5	7.7	3.2	2.3	4.4
Automotive dealers and service stations	55	2,375.7	5.7	2.1	1.6	3.6	5.6	2.1	1.6	3.5
Apparel and accessory stores	56	1,174.2	3.2	1.4	.9	1.8	3.1	1.3	.9	1.8
Furniture and home furnishings stores	57	1,082.2	4.7	2.4	1.6	2.4	4.7	2.3	1.6	2.3

Occupation		Employment								
Eating and drinking places	58	7,954.4	5.6	1.8	1.4	3.8	5.5	1.8	1.4	3.8
Miscellaneous retail	59	2,963.9	4.1	1.8	1.1	2.3	3.9	1.7	1.1	2.2
Finance, insurance, and real estate										
Depository institutions	60	7,399.5	1.8	.8	.6	1.1	1.6	.7	.5	.9
Nondepository institutions	61	2,044.8	1.5	.6	.4	1.0	1.3	.5	.4	.8
Security and commodity brokers	62	707.1	1.0	.3	.3	.6	.8	.3	.2	.5
Insurance carriers	63	688.0	.6	.3	.3	.3	.5	.3	.2	.3
Insurance agents, brokers, and service	64	1,477.4	1.9	.7	.5	1.2	1.4	.5	.4	.9
Real estate	65	754.0	.9	.3	.2	.6	.8	.3	.2	.6
Holding and other investment offices	67	1,493.5	3.9	1.9	1.4	2.0	3.8	1.9	1.4	1.9
		234.7	1.4	.4	.3	1.0	1.3	.4	.2	.9
Services										
Hotels and other lodging places	70	36,374.0	4.9	2.2	1.5	2.6	4.6	2.1	1.4	2.5
Personal services	72	1,835.8	7.8	3.7	2.1	4.1	7.5	3.6	2.0	3.9
Business services	73	1,226.1	3.0	1.6	1.0	1.4	2.8	1.5	1.0	1.3
Auto repair, services, and parking	75	9,248.0	3.0	1.4	.9	1.6	2.8	1.3	.9	1.6
Miscellaneous repair services	76	1,192.9	6.1	2.9	2.3	3.2	5.9	2.8	2.3	3.1
Motion pictures	78	375.7	5.2	2.6	1.8	2.6	5.1	2.5	1.8	2.5
Amusement and recreation services	79	599.4	2.9	.8	.5	2.1	2.8	.8	.5	2.0
Health services	80	1,706.5	6.7	3.0	1.7	3.8	6.4	2.8	1.6	3.6
Legal services	81	9,946.9	7.5	3.4	2.2	4.0	7.0	3.3	2.1	3.7
Educational services	82	995.3	1.0	.4	.3	.6	.8	.3	.3	.5
Social services	83	1,667.0	2.9	1.1	.8	1.8	2.7	1.0	.8	1.7
Museums, botanical, zoological gardens	84	2,674.9	5.6	2.7	1.9	2.9	5.4	2.6	1.9	2.8
Membership organizations	86	99.7	7.0	2.5	1.7	4.5	6.6	2.4	1.5	4.2
Engineering and management services	87	1,060.6	3.1	1.2	0.9	1.9	3.0	1.2	0.8	1.8
Services, not elsewhere classified	89	3,262.9	1.7	.7	.5	1.0	1.6	.6	.4	.9
		50.4	1.8	.6	.4	1.2	1.7	.5	.4	1.2

Notes to Table are are on next page.

Table 42.2. Incidence Rates[1] of Nonfatal Occupational Injuries and Illnesses by Selected Industries and Case Types, 1999 (continued from previous pages)

Notes:

1. The incidence rates represent the number of injuries and illnesses per 100 full-time workers and were calculated as: (N/EH) x 200,000, where

    N = number of injuries and illnesses

    EH = total hours worked by all employees during the calendar year

    200,000 = base for 100 equivalent full-time workers (working 40 hours per week, 50 weeks per year)

2. Totals include data for industries not shown separately.

3. *Standard Industrial Classification Manual*, 1987 Edition.

4. Employment is expressed as an annual average and is derived primarily from the BLS-State Covered Employment and Wages program.

5. Total lost workday cases involve days away from work, days of restricted work activity, or both.

6. "Days away from work" cases include those which result in days away from work with or without restricted work activity.

7. Excludes farms with fewer than 11 employees.

8. Data conforming to OSHA definitions for mining operators in coal, metal, and nonmetal mining, and for employers in railroad transportation are provided to BLS by the Mine Safety and Health Administration, U.S. Department of Labor, and the Federal Railroad Administration, U.S. Department of Transportation. Independent mining contractors are excluded from the coal, metal, and non-metal mining industries.

Note: Because of rounding, components may not add to totals. Blank space indicates data not available.

Source: Bureau of Labor Statistics, U.S. Department of Labor

Table 42.3. Highest Incidence Rates[1] of Nonfatal Occupational Injury Cases Involving Days Away from Work,[2] Private Industry, 1999.

Industry[3]	SIC rate	1999 Annual average employment[5] (000s)	Incidence rate 1998	Incidence rate 1999
Air transportation, scheduled	451	1,058.7	8.2[6]	7.1[6]
Prefabricated wood buildings	2452	24.4	4.7	6.6
Wood pallets and skids	2448	45.8	5.5	6.0
Metal heat treating	3398	19.1	3.2[6]	5.6[6]
Structural wood members, not classified elsewhere	2439	46.9	4.3	5.4
Prefabricated metal buildings	3448	32.8	3.2[6]	5.4[6]
Roofing, siding, and sheet metal work	176	244.8	4.4	5.3
Aluminum foundries	3365	26.5	6.2	5.3
Prepared flour mixes and doughs	2045	14.6	4.9	5.2
Water well drilling	178	23.8	2.4	5.1
Bituminous coal and lignite mining	122	79.8	5.3	4.9
Steel foundries, not classified elsewhere	3325	27.8	5.3	4.9
Fabricated pipe and fittings	3498	30.1	4.1	4.9
Fluid milk	2026	60.8	5.2	4.8
Logging	241	78.4	5.2	4.7
Anthracite mining	123	1.2	5.7	4.6
Truck and bus bodies	3713	47.7	4.8	4.5
Water transportation services	449	122.8	4.2	4.5
Dimension stone	141	5.8	4.2	4.4
Concrete block and brick	3271	20.2	6.1	4.4
Nursing and personal care facilities	805	1,782.1	4.3	4.4
Masonry, stonework, and plastering	174	535.5	4.1	4.3
Concrete products, not classified elsewhere	3272	82.1	4.5	4.3

Table 42.3. Highest Incidence Rates[1] of Nonfatal Occupational Injury Cases Involving Days Away from Work,[2] Private Industry, 1999 (continued from previous page).

Industry[3]	SIC rate	1999 Annual average employment[5] (000s)	Incidence rate 1998	1999
Cold finishing of steel shapes	3316	20.3	4.4	4.3
Water transportation of freight, not classified elsewhere	444	14.3	2.6	4.3
Private industry[7]		107611.8	1.9[6]	1.8[6]

Notes:

1. The incidence rates represent the number of injuries per 100 full-time workers and were calculated as: (N/EH) x 200,000, where

    N = number of injuries

    EH = total hours worked by all employees during the calendar year

    200,000 = base for 100 equivalent full-time workers (working 40 hours per week, 50 weeks per year)

2. "Days away from work" cases include those which result in days away from work with or without restricted work activity.

3. High rate industries were those having the 15 highest cases with days away from work incidence rates for injuries at the most detailed or lowest SIC level at which rates are calculated and published. Generally, manufacturing industries were calculated at the 4-digit code level and the remaining industries at the 3-digit level based on *the Standard Industrial Classification Manual,* 1987 Edition.

4. *Standard Industrial Classification Manual,* 1987 Edition.

5. Employment is expressed as an annual average and is derived primarily from the BLS-State Covered Employment and Wages program.

6. A statistical significance test indicates that the difference between the 1999 incidence rate and the 1998 rate is statistically significant at the 95 percent confidence level.

7. Excludes farms with fewer than 11 employees.

Note: Data conforming to OSHA definitions for coal and lignite mining operators (SIC 12) and nonmetal mining operators (SIC 14) are provided to BLS by the Mine Safety and Health Administration, U.S. Department of Labor. BLS does not calculate relative standard errors for the estimates in SIC 12 and in SIC 14, therefore, differences in these estimates were not tested for statistical significance.

Source: Bureau of Labor Statistics, U.S. Department of Labor

Table 42.4. Number of Cases and Incidence Rates[1] of Nonfatal Occupational Injuries for Private Sector Industries with 100,000 or More Cases, 1999.

Industry[2]	SIC code[3]	Total cases (In thousands)	Incidence rate
Eating and drinking places	581	299.8	5.5
Hospitals	806	271.7	8.5
Nursing and personal care facilities	805	188.6	13.2
Grocery stores	541	182.3	8.1
Department stores	531	159.7	8.7
Trucking and courier services, except air	421	140.1	8.6
Motor vehicles and equipment	371	129.2	12.2
Air transportation, scheduled	451	119.7	13.9
Hotels and motels	701	108.3	7.6

Notes:

1. The incidence rates represent the number of injuries per 100 full-time workers and were calculated as: (N/EH) x 200,000, where

   N = number of injuries

   EH = total hours worked by all employees during the calendar year

   200,000 = base for 100 equivalent full-time workers (working 40 hours per week, 50 weeks per year)

2. Industries with 100,000 or more cases were determined by analysis of the number of cases at the 3-digit SIC code level.

3. *Standard Industrial Classification Manual,* 1987 Edition.

Source: Bureau of Labor Statistics, U.S. Department of Labor

Chapter 43

Musculoskeletal Disorders and Workplace Factors

What Are Musculoskeletal Disorders?

Musculoskeletal disorders include a group of conditions that involve the nerves, tendons, muscles, and supporting structures such as intervertebral discs. They represent a wide range of disorders, which can differ in severity from mild periodic symptoms to severe chronic and debilitating conditions. Examples include carpal tunnel syndrome, tenosynovitis, tension neck syndrome, and low back pain.

What Are Work-Related Musculoskeletal Disorders (WMSDs)?

Work-Related Musculoskeletal Disorders (WMSDs) are musculoskeletal disorders caused or made worse by the work environment. WMSDs can cause severe and debilitating symptoms such as pain, numbness, and tingling; reduced worker productivity; lost time from work; temporary or permanent disability; inability to perform job tasks; and an increase in workers compensation costs.

This chapter includes the following documents from the National Institute for Occupational Safety and Health (NIOSH): "Work-Related Musculoskeletal Disorders," Fact Sheet, Document #705005, July 1997; "Carpal Tunnel Syndrome," Document #705001, June 1997; Summaries for Chapters 4 and 6 of *Musculoskeletal Disorders (MSDs) and Workplace Factors A Critical Review of Epidemiologic Evidence for Work-Related Musculoskeletal Disorders of the Neck, Upper Extremity, and Low Back,* July 1997; and "Preventing Work-Related Musculoskeletal Disorders," from the Occupational Safety & Health Administration (OSHA).

Musculoskeletal disorders are often confused with ergonomics. Ergonomics is the science of fitting workplace conditions and job demands to the capabilities of workers. In other words, musculoskeletal disorders are the problem and ergonomics is a solution.

What Are the Risk Factors for WMSDs?

Repetitive, forceful, or prolonged exertions of the hands; frequent or heavy lifting, pushing, pulling, or carrying of heavy objects; prolonged awkward postures; and vibration contribute to WMSDs. Jobs or working conditions that combine risk factors will increase the risk for musculoskeletal problems. The level of risk depends on how long a worker is exposed to these conditions, how often they are exposed, and the level of exposure.

Why Are WMSDs a Problem?

In 1996, more than 647,000 American workers experienced serious injuries due to overexertion or repetitive motion on the job. These work-related musculoskeletal disorders (WMSDs) account for 34 percent of lost workday injuries. WMSDs cost employers an estimated $15 to $20 billion in workers' compensation costs in 1995 and $45 to $60 billion more in indirect costs.

WMSDs are not a comfort issue; they may result in crippling disability. Severely injured workers may never be able to return to their jobs or be able to handle simple, everyday tasks like combing their hair, picking up a baby, or reaching for a book on a high shelf.

Work-related musculoskeletal disorders occur when there is a mismatch between the physical requirements of the job and the physical capacity of the human body. More than 100 different injuries can result from repetitive motions that produce wear and tear on the body. Back pain, wrist tendinitis, and carpal tunnel syndrome may all stem from work-related overuse. Specific risk factors associated with WMSDs include repetitive motion, heavy lifting, forceful exertion, contact stress, vibration, awkward posture, and rapid hand and wrist movement.

What Can Be Done about WMSDs?

The good news is that for almost every job, there are different ways to do the work that can reduce the risk of injury. Simple, inexpensive solutions often can prevent these painful disorders.

The science of fitting the job to the worker is called ergonomics. Designing the work and the work environment properly can prevent WMSDs. Employers that have implemented ergonomics programs have had great success in avoiding WMSDs, keeping workers on the job, and boosting productivity and workplace morale.

Are MSDs Clearly Linked to Work?

Yes, often they are. In 1998, the National Institute for Occupational Safety and Health (NIOSH) reviewed more than 2,000 studies of work-related musculoskeletal disorders. The agency's in-depth analysis of 600 epidemiologic studies from this group of studies was further evaluated by a panel of 27 scientists and ergonomists from academia, government, and private practice. NIOSH concluded that "compelling scientific evidence shows a consistent relationship between musculoskeletal disorders and certain work-related physical factors, especially at higher exposure levels." NIOSH's effort produced the most comprehensive compilation to date of credible epidemiological research, and the research pinpointed, in many cases, a strong link between risk factors on the job and WMSDs.

In recent years, reports of repetitive motion injuries have risen dramatically in workplaces across the country. These problems, frequently termed "Cumulative Trauma Disorders" are being reported at alarming rates in all types of workplaces—from meatpacking plants to newspaper pressrooms. According to the Bureau of Labor Statistics, "disorders associated with repeated trauma" account for about 60% of all occupational illnesses. Of all these disorders, carpal tunnel syndrome is the condition most frequently reported.

What Is Carpal Tunnel Syndrome (CTS)?

The carpal tunnel receives its name from the 8 bones in the wrist, called carpals, that form a tunnel-like structure. The tunnel is filled with flexor tendons which control finger movement. It also provides a pathway for the median nerve to reach sensory cells in the hand. Repetitive flexing and extension of the wrist may cause a thickening of the protective sheaths which surround each of the tendons. The swollen tendon sheaths, or tenosynovitis, apply increased pressure on the median nerve and produce Carpal Tunnel Syndrome (CTS).

What Are the Symptoms of CTS?

The symptoms of CTS often first appear as painful tingling in one or both hands during the night, frequently painful enough to disturb sleep. Accompanying this is a feeling of uselessness in the fingers, which are sometimes described as feeling swollen, even though little or no swelling is apparent. As symptoms increase, tingling may develop during the day, commonly in the thumb, index, and ring fingers. A decreased ability and power to squeeze things may follow. In advanced cases, the thenar muscle at the base of the thumb atrophies, and strength is lost.

Many patients with CTS are unable to differentiate hot from cold by touch, and experience an apparent loss of strength in their fingers. They appear clumsy in that they have trouble performing simple tasks such as tying their shoes or picking up small objects.

What Causes CTS?

As stated earlier, swelling of the tendons that line the carpal tunnel causes CTS. Although there are many reasons for developing this swelling of the tendon, it can result from repetitive and forceful movements of the wrist during work and leisure activities. Research conducted by the National Institute for Occupational Safety and Health (NIOSH) indicates that job tasks involving highly repetitive manual acts, or necessitating wrist bending or other stressful wrist postures, are connected with incidents of CTS or related problems. The use of vibrating tools also may contribute to CTS. Moreover, it is apparent that this hazard is not confined to a single industry or job but occurs in many occupations especially those in the manufacturing sector. Indeed, jobs involving cutting, small parts assembly, finishing, sewing, and cleaning seem predominantly associated with the syndrome. The factor common in these jobs is the repetitive use of small hand tools.

How Large a Problem Is CTS?

In the past ten years, more and more cases of workers afflicted with CTS have been reported in medical literature. One reason for this increase may be that automation and job specialization have fragmented workers' tasks to the point where a given job may involve only a few manipulations performed thousands of times per workday. Increased awareness of work-related risk factors in the onset of CTS is reflected in the growing number of requests for health hazard evaluations (HHEs) received by NIOSH to investigate such suspected problems. NIOSH received about three times as many HHE requests related to hand and wrist pain in 1992 as compared to 1982.

Prevention

NIOSH recommendations for controlling carpal tunnel syndrome have focused on ways to relieve awkward wrist positions and repetitive hand movements, and to reduce vibration from hand tools. NIOSH recommends redesigning tools or tool handles to enable the user's wrist to maintain a more natural position during work. Other recommendations have involved modified layouts of work stations. Still other approaches include altering the existing method for performing the job task, providing more frequent rest breaks, and rotating workers across jobs. As a means of prevention, tool and process redesign are preferable to administrative means such as job rotation.

The frequency and severity of CTS can be minimized through training programs that increase worker awareness of symptoms and prevention methods. Proper medical management of injured workers also minimizes the frequency and severity of CTS.

Treatment

Treatment of CTS may involve surgery to release the compression on the median nerve and/or use of anti-inflammatory drugs and handsplints to reduce tendon swelling in the carpal tunnel. Such medical interventions have met with mixed success, especially when an affected person must return to the same working conditions.

Low-Back Musculoskeletal Disorders: Evidence for Work-Relatedness

Over 40 articles provided evidence regarding the relationship between low-back disorder and the five physical workplace factors that were considered in this review. These included (1) heavy physical work, (2) lifting and forceful movements, (3) bending and twisting (awkward postures), (4) whole-body vibration (WBV), and (5) static work postures. Many of the studies addressed multiple work-related factors. All articles that addressed a particular workplace factor contributed to the information used to draw conclusions about that risk factor, regardless of whether results were positive or negative.

The review provided evidence for a positive relationship between back disorder and heavy physical work, although risk estimates were more moderate than for lifting/forceful movements, awkward postures, and WBV. This was perhaps due to subjective and imprecise characterization of exposures. Evidence for dose-response was equivocal for this risk factor.

There is strong evidence that low-back disorders are associated with work-related lifting and forceful movements. Of 18 epidemiologic studies that were reviewed, 13 were consistent in demonstrating positive relationships. Several studies suggested that both lifting and awkward postures were important contributors to the risk of low-back disorder. The observed relationships are consistent with biomechanical and other laboratory evidence regarding the effects of lifting and dynamic motion on back tissues.

The review provided evidence that work-related awkward postures are associated with low-back disorders. Results were consistent in showing positive associations, with several risk estimates above three. Exposure-response relationships were demonstrated. Many of the studies adjusted for potential covariates and a few examined the simultaneous effects of other work-related physical factors. Again, it appeared that lifting and awkward postures both contribute to risk of low-back disorder.

There is strong evidence of an association between exposure to WBV and low-back disorder. Of 19 studies reviewed for this document, 15 studies were consistent in demonstrating positive associations, with risk estimates ranging from 1.2 to 5.7 for those using subjective exposure measures, and from 1.4 to 39.5 for those using objective assessment methods. Most of the studies that examined relationships in high-exposure groups using detailed quantitative exposure measures found strong positive associations and exposure-response relationships between WBV and low back disorders. These relationships were observed after adjusting for covariates.

Both experimental and epidemiologic evidence suggest that WBV may act in combination with other work-related factors, such as prolonged sitting, lifting, and awkward postures, to cause increased risk of back disorder. It is possible that effects of WBV may depend on the source of exposure (type of vehicle).

With regard to static work postures and low-back disorder, results from the studies that were reviewed provided insufficient evidence that a relationship exists. Few investigations examined effects of static work postures, and exposure characterizations were limited.

Elbow Musculoskeletal Disorders (Epicondylitis): Evidence for Work-Relatedness

Epicondylitis is an uncommon disorder, with the overall prevalence in the general population reported to be from 1% to 5%. There are fewer epidemiologic studies addressing workplace risk factors for elbow MSDs than for other MSDs. Most of these studies compare the prevalence of epicondylitis in workers in jobs known to have highly repetitive, forceful tasks (such as meat processing) to workers in less repetitive, forceful work (such as office jobs); the majority of these studies were not designed to identify individual workplace risk factors.

Over 20 epidemiologic studies have examined physical workplace factors and their relationship to epicondylitis. The majority of studies involved study populations exposed to some combination of work factors, but among these studies were also those that assessed specific work factors. Each of the studies examined (those with negative, positive, or equivocal findings) contributed to the overall pool of data to make our decision on the strength of work-relatedness. Using epidemiologic criteria to examine these studies, and taking into account issues of confounding, bias, and strengths and limitations of the studies, we conclude the following:

- There is insufficient evidence for support of an association between repetitive work and elbow musculoskeletal disorders (MSDs) based on currently available epidemiologic data. No studies having repetitive work as the dominant exposure factor met the four epidemiologic criteria. There is evidence for the association with forceful work and epicondylitis. Studies that base exposure assessment on quantitative or semiquantitative data tended to show a stronger relationship for epicondylitis and force. Eight studies fulfilling at least one criteria showed statistically significant relationships.

- There is insufficient evidence to draw conclusions about the relationship of postural factors alone and epicondylitis at this time.

- There is strong evidence for a relationship between exposure to a combination of risk factors (e.g., force and repetition, force and posture) and epicondylitis. Based on the epidemiologic studies reviewed, especially those with some quantitative evaluation of the risk factors, the evidence is clear that an exposure to a combination of exposures, especially at higher exposure levels (as can be seen in, for example, meatpacking or construction work) increases risk for epicondylitis. The one prospective study which had a combination of exposure factors had a particularly high incidence rate (IR=6.7), and illustrated a temporal relationship between physical exposure factors and epicondylitis. The strong evidence for a combination of factors is consistent

415

with evidence found in the sports and biomechanical literature. Studies outside the field of epidemiology also suggest that forceful and repetitive contraction of the elbow flexors or extensors (which can be caused by flexion and extension of the wrist) increases the risk of epicondylitis.

- Epidemiologic surveillance data, both nationally and internationally, have consistently reported that the highest incidence of epicondylitis occurs in occupations and job tasks which are manually intensive and require high work demands in dynamic environments—for example, in mechanics, butchers, construction workers, and boilermakers.

- Epicondylar tenderness has also been found to be associated with a combination of higher levels of forceful exertions, repetition, and extreme postures of the elbow. This distinction may not be a true demarcation of different disease processes, but part of a continuum. Some data indicate that a high percentage of individuals with severe elbow pain are not able to do their jobs, and they have a higher rate of sick leave than individuals with other upper extremity disorders.

What Is OSHA Doing about WMSDs?

Standard Setting

The Occupational Safety and Health Administration (OSHA) is developing a program-based ergonomics standard to help employers reduce the risk of work-related musculoskeletal disorders in their workplaces. For the first phase of its efforts, OSHA is focusing on manufacturing operations and manual handling and sites that experience one or more WMSDs.

OSHA met with various stakeholders in Washington in February 1998 to discuss its plan to require an ergonomics program rather than adherence to a specific list of requirements. A second series of meetings was held in July and September 1998 to seek individual stakeholder input on steps employers who would be covered under an ergonomics standard should take to protect their workers, what action levels should be used to trigger further action, how to determine when controls are adequate for a problem job, and what employers should be covered by the standard. Currently the agency is considering the following major elements for an ergonomics program: management leadership and employee participation, hazard awareness

416

and employee training, medical management, job hazard analysis, hazard prevention and control, program evaluation and documentation.

Do Ergonomics Programs Really Work?

Yes! Thousands of employers have already instituted ergonomics programs that include elements OSHA is considering for its proposal. For example:

- Red Wing Shoes in Minnesota modified work stations and gave its employees adjustable chairs. Even though the company added two new plants, workers' comp costs dropped 75 percent over four years.

- Fieldcrest-Cannon in Columbus, Georgia, cut MSDs from 121 in 1993 to 21 in 1996. They credit their success to worker involvement in designing systems to limit the need for workers to bend and reach.

- In North Carolina, Perdue Farms started an ergonomics program in 1991. It was so effective, the company expanded it to all its plants. Although the average lost workday injury and illness rate for poultry processing is about 12 per 100 full-time workers, six Perdue plants had no lost time injuries in 1996.

- Lunt Silversmiths in Massachusetts bought lifts so workers would no longer need to carry dies for silver casting by hand. The result—no more back injuries in the machine room.

- Woodpro Cabinetry in Cabool, Missouri, saved $42,000 in worker's compensation costs by bringing its injury rates down when it added conveyors to limit lifting. This is a significant amount for a company with about 100 workers.

What Can I Do to Prevent WMSDs?

Employers and employees can work together effectively to reduce WMSDs. Here are some ways:

- Look at injury and illness records to find jobs where problems have occurred.

- Talk with workers to identify specific tasks that contribute to pain and lost workdays.

- Ask workers what changes they think will make a difference.

- Encourage workers to report WMSD symptoms and establish a medical management system to detect problems early.

- Find ways to reduce repeated motions, forceful hand exertions, prolonged bending or working above shoulder height.

- Reduce or eliminate vibration and sharp edges or handles that dig into the skin.

- Rely on equipment—not backs—for heavy or repetitive lifting.

Simple solutions often work best. Workplace changes to reduce pain and cut the risk of disability need not cost a fortune. For example:

- Change the height or orientation of the product or give poultry processors knives with curved handles so they won't have to bend their wrists unnaturally to cut the birds apart.

- Provide lifting equipment so nursing home workers won't strain their backs lifting patients by themselves.

- Offer workers involved in intensive keyboarding more frequent short breaks to rest muscles.

- Vary tasks of assembly line workers to avoid repeated stress for the same muscles.

Current NIOSH Research

NIOSH continues to investigate musculoskeletal disorders, including cumulative trauma disorders (CTDs) such as CTS, in many work environments and will make its research information available as investigations are finalized.

Additional Information

National Institute for Occupational Safety and Health (NIOSH)
Occupational Safety and Health Administration (OSHA)
U.S. Department of Labor
200 Constitution Avenue, N.W.
Washington, D.C. 20210
Toll-Free: 800-356-4674

Fax: 513-533-8573
Fax on Demand: 888-232-3299
Website: www.cdc.gov/niosh
E-mail: eidtechinfo@cdc.gov

The agency also has developed a video profiling how four firms instituted ergonomics programs that worked to prevent injury and save money. "Ergonomics Programs that Work" can be purchased from the National Audiovisual Center for $55.

National Audiovisual Center
U.S. Department of Commerce Technology Administration
National Technical Information Service
5285 Port Royal Road
Springfield, VA 22161
Tel: 703-605-6000
Website: www.ntis.gov

Chapter 44

Work-Related Hearing Loss

Work-related hearing loss continues to be a critical workplace safety and health issue. The National Institute for Occupational Safety and Health (NIOSH) and the occupational safety and health community named hearing loss one of the 21 priority areas for research in the next century. Noise-induced hearing loss is 100 percent preventable but once acquired, hearing loss is permanent and irreversible. Therefore, prevention measures must be taken by employers and workers to ensure the protection of workers' hearing.

Magnitude

- Approximately 30 million workers are exposed to hazardous noise on the job and an additional nine million are at risk for hearing loss from other agents such as solvents and metals.

- Noise-induced hearing loss is one of the most common occupational diseases and the second most self-reported occupational illness or injury. Industry specific studies reveal:

  - 44% of carpenters and 48% of plumbers reported that they had a perceived hearing loss.

"Work Related Hearing Loss," National Institute for Occupational Safety and Health (NIOSH); "Ten Ways to Recognize Hearing Loss," National Institute on Deafness and Other Communication Disorders (NIDCD; and excerpts from Chapters 2 and 6 of *Occupational Noise Exposure, Recommendations for a Noise Standard*, National Institute for Occupational Safety and Health (NIOSH), 1998.

- 90% of coal miners will have a hearing impairment by age 52 (compared to 9% of the general population); 70% of male, metal/nonmetal miners will experience a hearing impairment by age 60.

- While any worker can be at risk for noise-induced hearing loss in the workplace, workers in many industries have higher exposures to dangerous levels of noise. Industries with high numbers of exposed workers include: agriculture; mining; construction; manufacturing and utilities; transportation; and military.

Costs

There is no national surveillance or injury reporting system for hearing loss. As such, comprehensive data on the economic impact of hearing loss are not available. Some estimates find that occupational hearing loss compensation costs alone are in the hundreds of millions of dollars per year. The following examples provide an indication of the economic burden of occupational hearing loss. Washington State workers' compensation disability settlements for hearing-related conditions cost $4.8 million in 1991. This figure does not include medical costs or personal costs which can include approximately $1,500 for a hearing aid and around $300 per year for batteries. Moreover, workers' compensation data are an underestimate of the true frequency of occupational illness, representing only the tip of the iceberg.

In British Columbia, in the five-year period from 1994 to 1998, the workers' compensation board paid $18 million in permanent disability awards to 3,207 workers suffering hearing loss. An additional $36 million was paid out for hearing aids.

Through their hearing conservation program, the U.S. Army saved $504.3 million by reducing hearing loss among combat arms personnel between 1974 and 1994. Between 1987 and 1997, as a result of military efforts to reduce civilian hearing loss, the Department of Veterans Affairs saved $220.8 million and the Army an additional $149 million.

Ten Ways to Recognize Hearing Loss

The following questions will help you determine if you need to have your hearing evaluated by a medical professional:

- Do you have a problem hearing over the telephone?

- Do you have trouble following the conversation when two or more people are talking at the same time?
- Do people complain that you turn the TV volume up too high?
- Do you have to strain to understand conversation?
- Do you have trouble hearing in a noisy background?
- Do you find yourself asking people to repeat themselves?
- Do many people you talk to seem to mumble (or not speak clearly)?
- Do you misunderstand what others are saying and respond inappropriately?
- Do you have trouble understanding the speech of women and children?
- Do people get annoyed because you misunderstand what they say?

If you answered "yes" to three or more of these questions, you may want to see an otolaryngologist (an ear, nose, and throat specialist) or an audiologist for a hearing evaluation. The material on this page is for general information only and is not intended for diagnostic or treatment purposes. A doctor or other health care professional must be consulted for diagnostic information and advice regarding treatment.

Recognition of Noise as a Health Hazard

Noise, which is essentially any unwanted or undesirable sound, is not a new hazard. Indeed, noise-induced hearing loss (NIHL) has been observed for centuries. Before the industrial revolution, however, comparatively few people were exposed to high levels of workplace noise. The advent of steam power in connection with the industrial revolution first brought general attention to noise as an occupational hazard. Workers who fabricated steam boilers developed hearing loss in such numbers that the malady was dubbed "boilermakers disease." Increasing mechanization in all industries and most trades has since proliferated the noise problem.

Noise-Induced Hearing Loss (NIHL)

NIHL is caused by exposure to sound levels or durations that damage the hair cells of the cochlea. Initially, the noise exposure may cause a temporary threshold shift—that is, a decrease in hearing sensitivity that typically returns to its former level within a few minutes to a few hours. Repeated exposures lead to a permanent threshold shift, which is an irreversible sensorineural hearing loss.

Hearing loss has causes other than occupational noise exposure. Hearing loss caused by exposure to nonoccupational noise is collectively called sociocusis. It includes recreational and environmental noises (e.g., loud music, guns, power tools, and household appliances) that affect the ear the same as occupational noise. Combined exposures to noise and certain physical or chemical agents (e.g., vibration, organic solvents, carbon monoxide, ototoxic drugs, and certain metals) appear to have synergistic effects on hearing loss [Hamernik and Henderson 1976; Brown et al. 1978; Gannon et al. 1979; Brown et al. 1980; Hamernik et al. 1980; Pryor et al. 1983; Rebert et al. 1983; Humes 1984; Boettcher et al. 1987; Young et al. 1987; Byrne et al. 1988; Fechter et al. 1988; Johnson et al. 1988; Morata et al. 1993; Franks and Morata 1996]. Some sensorineural hearing loss occurs naturally because of aging; this loss is called presbycusis. Conductive hearing losses, as opposed to sensorineural hearing losses, are usually traceable to diseases of the outer and middle ear.

Noise exposure is also associated with nonauditory effects such as psychological stress and disruption of job performance [Cohen 1973; EPA 1973; Taylor 1984; Öhrström et al. 1988; Suter 1989] and possibly hypertension [Parvizpoor 1976; Jonsson and Hansson 1977; Takala et al. 1977; Lees and Roberts 1979; Malchaire and Mullier 1979; Manninen and Aro 1979; Singh et al. 1982; Belli et al. 1984; Delin 1984; Talbott et al. 1985; Verbeek et al. 1987; Wu et al. 1987; Talbott et al. 1990]. Noise may also be a contributing factor in industrial accidents [Cohen 1976; Schmidt et al. 1980; Wilkins and Acton 1982; Moll van Charante and Mulder 1990]. Nevertheless, data are insufficient to endorse specific damage risk criteria for these nonauditory effects.

Physical Properties of Sound

The effects of sound on a person depend on three physical characteristics of sound: amplitude, frequency, and duration. Sound pressure level (SPL), expressed in decibels, is a measure of the amplitude of the pressure change that produces sound. This amplitude is perceived by the listener as loudness. In sound-measuring instruments, weighting networks are used to modify the SPL. Exposure limits are commonly measured in dBA. When used without a weighted network suffix, the expression should be dB SPL.

The frequency of a sound, expressed in Hz, represents the number of cycles occurring in 1 sec and determines the pitch perceived by the listener. Humans with normal hearing can hear a frequency range of about 20 Hz to 20 kilohertz (kHz). Exposures to frequency ranges that are considered infrasonic (below 20 Hz), upper sonic (10 to 20 kHz), and ultrasonic (above 20 kHz) are not addressed in this chapter.

Although no uniformly standard definitions exist, noise exposure durations can be broadly classified as continuous-type or impulsive. All nonimpulsive noises (i.e., continuous, varying, and intermittent) are collectively referred to as "continuous-type noise." Impact and impulse noises are collectively referred to as "impulsive noise." Impulsive noise is distinguished from continuous-type noise by a steep rise in the sound level to a high peak followed by a rapid decay. In many workplaces, the exposures are often a mixture of continuous-type and impulsive sounds.

Number of Noise-Exposed Workers in the United States

In 1981, OSHA estimated that 7.9 million U.S. workers in the manufacturing sector were occupationally exposed to daily noise levels at or above 80 dBA [46 Fed. Reg.* 4078 (1981a)]. In the same year, the U.S. Environmental Protection Agency (EPA) estimated that more than 9 million U.S. workers were occupationally exposed to daily noise levels above 85 dBA [see Table 44.1].

Prevention

Removing hazardous noise from the workplace through engineering controls (e.g. installing a muffler or building an acoustic barrier) is the most effective way to prevent noise-induced hearing loss. Hearing protectors such as ear plugs and ear muffs should be used when it is not feasible to otherwise reduce noise to a safe level. NIOSH recommends hearing loss prevention programs for all workplaces with hazardous levels of noise. These programs should include noise assessments, engineering controls, audiometric monitoring of workers' hearing, appropriate use of hearing protectors, worker education, record keeping, and program evaluation.

The best hearing protection for any worker is the removal of hazardous noise from the workplace. Until that happens, the best hearing protector for a worker is the one he or she will wear willingly and consistently. The following factors are extremely important determinants of worker acceptance of hearing protectors and the likelihood that workers will wear them consistently:

- Convenience and availability
- Belief that the device can be worn correctly
- Belief that the device will prevent hearing loss
- Belief that the device will not impair a workers ability to hear important sounds
- Comfort
- Adequate noise reduction
- Ease of fit
- Compatibility with other personal protective equipment

Table 44.1. Noise-Exposed Workers in the United States

Major group	Number of workers
Agriculture	323,000
Mining	255,000
Construction	513,000
Manufacturing and utilities	5,124,000
Transportation	1,934,000
Military	976,000
Total	9,125,000

Note: More than half of these workers were engaged in manufacturing and utilities [EPA 1981].

Exposure to Noise That Is Greater Than or Equal to 85 Decibels May Cause Hearing Loss.

Table 44.2. Estimate of Work-Related Noise

Sound	Decibels (dB)	Sound	Decibels (dB)
Whisper	30dB	Spray Painter	105dB
Normal conversation	60dB	Continuous miner	108dB
Ringing telephone	80dB	Chain saw	110dB
Hair dryer/Power		Hammer drill	114dB
lawn mower	90dB	Pneumatic percussion drill	119dB
Belt sander	93dB	Ambulance siren	120dB
Tractor	96dB	Jet engine at takeoff	140dB
Hand drill	98dB	12-guage shotgun	165dB
Impact Wrench	103dB	Rocket launch	180dB
Bulldozer	105dB	Loudest possible tone	194dB

Chapter 45

Construction Safety and Health

Protecting construction workers from injury and disease is among the greatest challenges in occupational safety and health.

- More than 7 million persons work in the construction industry, representing 6% of the labor force. Approximately 1.5 million of these workers are self-employed.

- Of approximately 600,000 construction companies, 90% employ fewer than 20 workers. Few have formal safety and health programs.

- From 1980-1993, an average of 1,079 construction workers were killed on the job each year, more fatal injuries than in any other industry.

- Falls caused 3,859 construction worker fatalities (25.6%) between 1980 and 1993.

- 15% of workers' compensation costs are spent on construction injuries.

- Assuring safety and health in construction is complex, involving short-term work sites, changing hazards, and multiple operations and crews working in close proximity.

"Construction Safety and Health," National Institute for Occupational Safety and Health (NIOSH), Document #705011, 1997.

- In 1990, Congress directed NIOSH to undertake research and training to reduce diseases and injuries among construction workers in the United States. Under this mandate, NIOSH funds both intramural and extramural research projects.

NIOSH Makes a Difference in the Health of Construction Workers

NIOSH and construction industry partners are collaborating to develop new strategies to reduce worker exposures to potentially hazardous substances. Examples of some successful collaborations include:

Controlling Lead Toxicity in Bridge Workers

Each year, 58,000 persons work in bridge, tunnel, and elevated highway construction and demolition jobs. About 90,000 bridges are coated with paint containing lead, creating the potential for dangerously high lead exposure to workers engaged in the maintenance, repainting, or demolition of bridges.

With funding from NIOSH, Connecticut state agencies and Yale University initiated the Connecticut Road Industry Surveillance Project (CRISP) to reduce lead toxicity in bridge workers. CRISP provides medical examinations and procedures to monitor and reduce occupational lead exposures at bridge sites; on-site technical assistance to overcome problems in reducing lead exposures; and a centralized, statewide surveillance system to monitor blood lead levels in workers.

CRISP saves Connecticut $2.5 million each year in workers' compensation costs. With CRISP, blood lead levels have decreased by 50%. Efforts are underway to implement this approach in other states.

Controlling Asphalt Fume Exposures during Paving

500,000 workers are exposed to asphalt fumes while paving roads, roofing, and waterproofing. Molten asphalt generates fumes that can cause skin diseases and eye and respiratory tract irritation. NIOSH laboratory studies found that fumes from asphalt roofing materials have potential cancer-causing and mutagenic properties.

The Department of Transportation and NIOSH are evaluating industry developed technology to control exposures to asphalt fumes in road paving. NIOSH's involvement was requested by the National Asphalt Pavement Association (NAPA), a trade organization of asphalt paving contractors, asphalt material manufacturers, and asphalt paving equipment manufacturers. Manufacturers developed and NIOSH evaluated prototype systems that reduce exposures by capturing fume emissions from paving equipment. NIOSH researchers are assisting the manufacturers in redesign efforts to reduce emissions. Preliminary results suggest these control systems will capture a significant amount of the asphalt fumes generated during the paving process.

A voluntary agreement signed by NAPA, the Occupational Safety and Health Administration (OSHA), the Federal Highway Administration, six equipment manufacturers, the Laborers' Health and Safety Fund of North America, and the International Union of Operating Engineers called for all highway-class asphalt pavers manufactured after July 12, 1997 to incorporate the engineering controls and be certified using the NIOSH test procedure.

NIOSH Makes a Difference in the Safety of Construction Workers

Each day, construction workers face trench cave-ins, falls, machinery accidents, electrocutions, and motor vehicle incidents. NIOSH researchers identify causes of and develop programs to prevent injuries and fatalities in construction. Examples include:

Preventing Injuries and Deaths Caused by Falls

Falls are the leading cause of fatal injury in the construction industry—in fact, half of all work-related fatal falls in the United States occur in the construction industry. Buildings and structures, scaffolds, and ladders are the primary locations from which fatal falls occur in the construction industry. NIOSH researchers have investigated 88 fall incidents, 75 of which were in construction. Specific prevention recommendations have included site-specific evaluation of potential fall hazards; implementation of fall protection programs; proper erection, maintenance, and use of access equipment (e.g., scaffolds and ladders); installation and maintenance of appropriate barriers (e.g., guard rails and/or covers on floor openings); and proper selection and use of fall restraint and fall arrest systems in situations where exposure to falls cannot be eliminated.

Preventing Electrocutions of Crane Operators and Crew Members

Each year, electrocutions represent 7% of injury-related fatalities. NIOSH onsite investigators found that 13% of work-related electrocutions involved crane contact with overhead power lines.

NIOSH Research Solves Safety and Health Problems in Construction

From October 1993 through March 1996, NIOSH researchers conducted 43 health hazard evaluations for construction industries and responded to 171 construction-related calls on the NIOSH 800-number. Since 1985, NIOSH researchers have developed recommendations for preventing fatal injuries based on over 425 field evaluations of fatal events in the construction industries. These evaluations were conducted as part of the NIOSH Fatality Assessment and Control Evaluation (FACE) Program. The recommendations are disseminated through NIOSH Alerts, and monographs.

Chapter 46

Employment May Be Hazardous for Adolescent Workers

Each year, more than 3 million teens under 18 will work at summer jobs. For the majority of teens, work will be a rewarding experience. However, a sizable number of teens will risk being injured or killed on the job. Statistics show that each year:

- 70 teens are killed on the job, about one every 5 days.

- 210,000 working teens are injured; 70,000 teens are injured seriously enough to require hospital emergency room treatment.

Adolescent workers are protected by two laws enforced by the Department of Labor, the Fair Labor Standards Act (FLSA) and the Occupational Safety and Health Act. However, enforcement efforts can only go so far. Many teen injuries and fatalities, though tragic, are not the result of labor law violations.

Where Teens Work/How They Are Hurt

Most teens (51 percent) work in the retail industry, which includes fast-food outlets and food stores. An additional 34 percent work in the service industry, including health, education, and entertainment/recreation.

This chapter includes "Protecting Working Teens," U.S. Department of Labor; "Most Teen Worker Injuries in Restaurants Occur in Fast Food, NIOSH Study Finds," National Institute for Occupational Safety and Health (NIOSH), December 22, 1999; and "Are You a Working Teen?" National Institute for Occupational Safety and Health (NIOSH), Pub. No. 97-132, 1997.

Fifty-four percent of teen occupational injuries occur in the retail industry, followed by the service industry (20 percent), agriculture (7 percent), and manufacturing (4 percent). Some tasks and tools associated with a large number of injuries include:

- driving a car
- driving heavy equipment, especially tractors
- using power tools, especially meat slicers

Teens are killed at work, most often, while driving or traveling as passengers in motor vehicles. Machine-related accidents, electrocution, homicide, and falls also account for many deaths. A NIOSH study has determined that the risk of injury death for workers age 16 and 17 was 5.1 per 100,000 full-time equivalent workers, compared with 6.0 for adult workers over age 18. This is of particular concern when you take into consideration the fact that as a whole, teens work fewer hours than adult employees.

Adolescent Workers Injured in Fast Food Establishments

Adolescent workers injured on the job in the restaurant industry are most likely to be working in fast food establishments, a study by the National Institute for Occupational Safety and Health (NIOSH) found.

Studying data from a national sample of hospitals over a two-year period, NIOSH estimated that approximately 44,800 occupational injuries to teen restaurant industry workers (age 14 to 17) were treated in hospital emergency departments across the U.S. during that time. Of these injuries, an estimated 28,000 or 63 percent occurred in hamburger, pizza, and other fast food establishments.

Adolescents working in the restaurant industry in general were at six times greater risk of sustaining a work-related burn injury than teens working in any other industry, the study found. Overall, during the period studied, emergency departments treated an estimated 108,000 work-related injuries to teens in all industries.

"As young people prepare to take temporary employment or work extra hours over the winter holidays, it is important to be aware that adolescents are injured on the job far too often," said NIOSH Director Linda Rosenstock, M.D., M.P.H. "All of us have key roles in preventing these injuries, now and throughout the year."

In general, the restaurant industry and other retail businesses rank high among U.S. industries for risk of adolescent worker injuries. The retail trades employ many of the nation's working adolescents.

Because statistics are not available on the number of adolescents working specifically in the fast food industry, researchers lack key data for determining if these teens are at higher risk proportionally than their counterparts in other segments of the restaurant industry. Even in the absence of those measures, the findings from the new study show a need for better training and other steps to protect young workers, NIOSH said.

The study, "Adolescent Occupational Injuries in Fast Food Restaurants: An Examination of the Problem from a National Perspective," was published in the December 1999 issue of the *Journal of Occupational and Environmental Medicine.*

The NIOSH study also found that for teens working in fast food establishments:

- Although males and females had similar injury rates, risks for injury by task and location differed by gender. Adolescent male employees were more likely to suffer burns, lacerations, and other injuries while performing tasks associated with cooking, while adolescent female employees were more likely to suffer contusions, strains, sprains, and other injuries while completing tasks related to cashiering and servicing tables.

- Nearly half of all burn injuries involved hot grease. Such injuries can be prevented by providing handles on scrapers and other cleaning tools, providing appropriate gloves, allowing grease to cool before it is moved, and training employees in safe work practices, among other precautions, NIOSH suggested.

- More than half of all fall injuries were related to wet or greasy floors. It is important to use slip-resistant floor materials and to keep floors dry and well-maintained, NIOSH said.

- By age, 17-year-olds suffered the highest proportion of injuries among teens working in fast food (55 percent), followed by 16-year-olds (38 percent).

- The majority of injuries to teen workers in fast food restaurants occurred in hamburger restaurants (52.6 percent), followed by pizza restaurants (12.6 percent), and chicken/fish restaurants (11.7 percent).

What Working Teens Should Know about Safety and Health on the Job

Could I Get Hurt or Sick on the Job?

Every year about 70 teens die from work injuries in the United States. Another 70,000 get hurt badly enough that they go to a hospital emergency room. Here are the stories of three teens:

- 18-year-old Sylvia caught her hand in an electric cabbage shredder at a fast food restaurant. Her hand is permanently disfigured and she'll never have full use of it again.

- 17-year-old Joe lost his life while working as a construction helper. An electric shock killed him when he climbed a metal ladder to hand an electric drill to another worker.

- 16-year-old Donna was assaulted and robbed at gunpoint at a sandwich shop. She was working alone after 11 p.m.

Why do injuries like these occur? Teens are often injured on the job due to unsafe equipment, stressful conditions, and speed-up. Also teens may not receive adequate safety training and supervision. As a teen, you are much more likely to be injured when working on jobs that you are not allowed to do by law.

What Are My Rights on the Job?

By law, your employer must provide:

- A safe and healthful workplace.

- Safety and health training, in many situations, including providing information on chemicals that could be harmful to your health.

- For many jobs, payment for medical care if you get hurt or sick because of your job. You may also be entitled to lost wages.

- At least the Federal minimum wage to most teens, after their first 90 days on the job. Many states have minimum wages which may be higher than the Federal wage, and lower wages may be allowed when workers receive tips from customers. (Call your state Department of Labor listed in the blue pages of your phone book for information on minimum wages in your state).

You also have a right to:

- Report safety problems to OSHA.

- Work without racial or sexual harassment.

- Refuse to work if the job is immediately dangerous to your life or health.

- Join or organize a union.

Table 46.1. Hazards to Watch Out For

Type of Work	Examples of Hazards
Janitor/Clean-up	Toxic chemicals in cleaning products
	Blood on discarded needles
Food Service	Slippery floors
	Hot cooking equipment
	Sharp objects
Retail/Sales	Violent crimes
	Heavy lifting
Office/Clerical	Stress
	Harassment
	Poor computer work station design

Is It Okay to Do Any Kind of Work?

No! There are laws that protect teens from doing dangerous work. No worker under 18 may:

- Drive a motor vehicle as a regular part of the job or operate a forklift at any time.

- Operate many types of powered equipment like a circular saw, box crusher, meat slicer, or bakery machine.

- Work in wrecking, demolition, excavation, or roofing.

- Work in mining, logging, or a sawmill.

- Work in meat-packing or slaughtering.

435

- Work where there is exposure to radiation.
- Work where explosives are manufactured or stored.

Also, no one 14 or 15 years old may:

- Bake or cook on the job (except at a serving counter).
- Operate power-driven machinery, except certain types which pose little hazard such as those used in offices.
- Work on a ladder or scaffold.
- Work in warehouses.
- Work in construction, building, or manufacturing.
- Load or unload a truck, railroad car, or conveyor.

Are There Other Things I Can't Do?

Yes! There are many other restrictions regarding the type of work you can and cannot do.

- If you are under 14, there are even stricter laws to protect your health and safety.
- States have their own child labor laws which may be stricter than the federal laws.
- Check with your school counselor, job placement coordinator, or state Department of Labor to make sure the job you are doing is allowed.

What Are My Safety Responsibilities on the Job?

To work safely you should:

- Follow all safety rules and instructions.
- Use safety equipment and protective clothing when needed.
- Look out for co-workers.
- Keep work areas clean and neat.
- Know what to do in an emergency.
- Report any health and safety hazard to your supervisor.

What If I Need Help?

- Talk to your boss about the problem.

- Talk to your parents or teachers.

- You have a right to speak up! It is illegal for your employer to fire or punish you for reporting a workplace problem.

- If necessary contact one of these government agencies. The phone numbers can be found under "Department of Labor" in the blue pages of your local telephone book.

  - **OSHA**—to make a health or safety complaint.

  - Wage and Hour—to make a complaint about wages, work hours, or illegal work by youth less than 18 years of age.

  - **Equal Employment Opportunities Commission**—to make a complaint about sexual harassment or discrimination.

Safety Protections for Working Teens

Child labor laws and regulations govern the ages and types of jobs children under 18 may work and the hours they may work. In June 1994, the Labor Department increased penalties for death or serious injury of minors employed in violation of child labor laws as a deterrent to employers. The new penalties allow a fine of up to $10,000 for each violation that leads to the serious injury or death of a child. The former penalty was a fine of up to $10,000 for each minor seriously injured or killed.

From October 1, 1995, through September 30, 1996, Department of Labor investigators found more than 7,000 young people working in violation of child labor laws and regulations, and assessed $6.8 million in civil money penalties for violations involving 1,341 establishments.

Virtually all workers, including teenagers, are protected by safety and health standards set by the Occupational Safety and Health Administration. These standards cover fire and electrical safety, chemical hazards, machine guarding, and many other on-the-job risks. Employers with 10 or more employees in more hazardous industries must keep records of injuries and illnesses that occur at their sites. All employers must report to OSHA incidents in which one or more workers are killed or three are more are hospitalized.

OSHA enforces its standards through inspections targeted toward high hazard industries or conducted in response to worker complaints. Penalties can range up to $7,000 for serious violations or $70,000 for willful violations of safety and health standards.

The agency strongly encourages employers to evaluate their work sites for potential hazards and to develop effective safety and health programs that actively involve all employees at the company. Part of an effective program is employee safety and health training, and many OSHA standards require specific training to ensure that employees can work safely amid potentially hazardous situations. OSHA provides assistance in establishing safety and health programs through free state consultation programs. Further, the agency is developing a standard covering safety and health programs and has revised on a pilot basis its penalty policies to significantly reduce penalties for companies that have excellent programs in place.

NIOSH works closely with diverse partners in industry, education, public health, communities, and other sectors to prevent adolescent worker injuries. For example, NIOSH issued "Promoting Safe Work for Young Workers," DHHS (NIOSH) Publication No. 99-141, a guide for working with community partners to prevent adolescent worker injuries and illnesses. The publication is based on results from three NIOSH-funded community-based projects.

Chapter 47

Workplace Violence

Every few days, there is another story on the news. One day, it may be a convenience store shooting; the next, a sexual assault in a company parking lot; a few days later, it's a disgruntled employee holding workers hostage, or a student attacking a teacher. Not surprisingly, the incidents of workplace violence that make the news are only the tip of the iceberg. What its victims all have in common is that they were at work, going about the business of earning a living, but something about their workplace environment—often something foreseeable and preventable—exposed them to attack by a customer, a co-worker, an acquaintance, or even a complete stranger.

Some 2 million American workers are victims of workplace violence each year. It is estimated that costs of workplace violence to employers is in the billions of dollars. Unfortunately, research into the prevention of violence in the workplace is still in its infancy.

In April 2000, The University of Iowa Injury Prevention Research Center took an important first step to meet this need by sponsoring the Workplace Violence Intervention Research Workshop in Washington, DC. The goal of this workshop was to examine issues related to violence in the workplace and to develop recommended research strategies to address this public health problem. The workshop brought together 37 invited participants representing diverse constituencies within industry, organized labor, municipal, state, and federal governments, and academia. The following is a summary of the problem

"Workplace Violence, a Report to the Nation," © February 2001, Injury Prevention Research Center, University of Iowa, reprinted with permission.

of workplace violence and the recommendations identified by participants at the workshop.

The Extent of the Problem

Workplace violence is receiving increased attention thanks to a growing awareness of the toll that violence takes on workers and workplaces. Despite existing research, there remain significant gaps in our knowledge of its causes and potential solutions. Even the extent of violence in the workplace and the number of victims are not well understood.

In 1999, the Bureau of Labor Statistics recorded 645 homicides in workplaces in the United States. Although this figure represents a decline from a high of 1,080 in 1994, homicide remains the third leading cause of fatal occupational injuries for all workers and the second leading cause of fatal occupational injuries for women. The number of non-fatal assaults is less clear. The National Crime Victimization Survey, a weighted annual survey of 46,000 households, estimates that an additional 2 million people are victims of non-fatal injuries due to violence while they are at work.

Addressing this problem is complicated because workplace violence has many sources. To better understand its causes and possible solutions, researchers have divided workplace violence into four categories. Most incidents fall into one of these categories.

Criminal Intent (Type I)

The perpetrator has no legitimate relationship to the business or its employees, and is usually committing a crime in conjunction with the violence. These crimes can include robbery, shoplifting, and trespassing. The vast majority of workplace homicides (85%) fall into this category.

In May 2000, two men entered a Wendy's in Flushing, NY, with the intent to rob the fast-food restaurant. They left with $2,400 in cash after shooting seven employees. Five of the employees died and two others were seriously injured.

This is an extreme example of Type I workplace violence: violence committed during a robbery or similar crime in the workplace. Type I is the most common source of worker homicide. Eighty-five percent of all workplace homicides fall into this category. Although the shootings in Flushing drew a great deal of media attention, the vast majority of these incidents barely make the news. Convenience store clerks, taxi drivers, security guards, and proprietors of "mom-and-pop" stores are all examples of the kinds of workers who are at higher risk for Type I workplace violence. In Type I incidents:

- The perpetrator does not have any legitimate business relationship with the establishment;

- The primary motive is usually theft;

- A deadly weapon is often involved, increasing the risk of fatal injury;

- Workers who exchange cash with customers as part of the job, work late night hours, and/or work alone are at greatest risk.

Customer/Client (Type II)

The perpetrator has a legitimate relationship with the business and becomes violent while being served by the business. This category includes customers, clients, patients, students, inmates, and any other group for which the business provides services. It is believed that a large proportion of customer/client incidents occur in the health care industry, in settings such as nursing homes or psychiatric facilities; the victims are often patient caregivers. Police officers, prison staff, flight attendants, and teachers are some other examples of workers who may be exposed to this kind of workplace violence.

Rhonda Bedow, a nurse who works in a state-operated psychiatric facility in Buffalo, NY, was attacked by an angry patient who had a history of threatening behavior, particularly against female staff. He slammed Bedow's head down onto a counter after learning that he had missed the chance to go outside with a group of other patients. Bedow suffered a concussion, a bilaterally dislocated jaw, an eye injury, and permanent scarring on her face from the assault. She still suffers from short-term memory problems resulting from the attack. When she returned to work after recuperating, the perpetrator was still on her ward, and resumed his threats against her.

In Type II incidents, the perpetrator is generally a customer or client who becomes violent during the course of a normal transaction. Service providers, including health care workers, schoolteachers, social workers, and bus and train operators, are among the most common targets of Type II violence. Attacks from "unwilling" clients, such as prison inmates on guards or crime suspects on police officers, are also included in this category. In Type II incidents:

- The perpetrator is a "customer" or a client of the worker;

- The violent act generally occurs in conjunction with the worker's normal duties;

- The risk of violence to some workers in this category (e.g., mental health workers, police) may be constant, even routine.

Worker-on-Worker (Type III)

The perpetrator is an employee or past employee of the business who attacks or threatens another employee(s) or past employee(s) in the workplace. Worker-on-worker fatalities account for approximately 7% of all workplace violence homicides.

Type III violence occurs when an employee assaults or attacks his or her co-workers. In some cases, these incidents can take place after a series of increasingly hostile behaviors from the perpetrator.

Worker-on-worker assault is often the first type of workplace violence that comes to mind for many people, possibly because some of these incidents receive intensive media coverage, leading the public to assume that most workplace violence falls into this category. For example, the phrase "going postal," referring to the scenario of a postal worker attacking co-workers, is sometimes used to describe Type III workplace violence. However, the U. S. Postal Service is no more likely than any other industry to be affected by this type of violence.

Type III violence accounts for about 7% of all workplace homicides. There do not appear to be any kinds of occupations or industries that are more or less prone to Type III violence. Because some of these incidents appear to be motivated by disputes, managers and others who supervise workers may be at greater risk of being victimized. In Type III incidents:

- The perpetrator is an employee or former employee;

- The motivating factor is often one or a series of interpersonal or work-related disputes.

Personal Relationship (Type IV)

The perpetrator usually does not have a relationship with the business but has a personal relationship with the intended victim. This category includes victims of domestic violence assaulted or threatened while at work.

Pamela Henry, an employee of Protocall, an answering service in San Antonio, had decided in the summer of 1997 to move out of the area. The abusive behavior of her ex-boyfriend, Charles Lee White, had spilled over from her home to her workplace, where he appeared one day in July and assaulted her. She obtained and then withdrew a protective order against White, citing her plans to leave the county. On October 17, 1997, White again appeared at Protocall. This time he opened fire with a rifle, killing Henry and another female employee before killing himself.

Because of the insidious nature of domestic violence, it is given a category all its own in the typology of workplace violence. Victims are overwhelmingly, but not exclusively, female. The effects of domestic violence on the workplace are many. They can appear as high absenteeism and low productivity on the part of a worker who is enduring abuse or threats, or the sudden, prolonged absence of an employee fleeing abuse. Occasionally, the abuser—who usually has no working relationship to the victim's employer—will appear at the workplace to engage in hostile behavior.

In some cases, a domestic violence situation can arise between individuals in the same workplace. These situations can have a substantial effect on the workplace even if one of the parties leaves or is fired. Type IV violence:

- Is the spillover of domestic violence into the workplace;

- Generally refers to perpetrators who are not employees or former employees of the affected workplace;

- Targets women significantly more often than me, although both male and female co-workers and supervisors are often affected.

These categories can be very helpful in the design of strategies to prevent workplace violence, since each type of violence requires a different approach for prevention, and some workplaces may be at higher risk for certain types of violence.

How often does workplace violence occur? An essential problem with efforts to reduce workplace violence is that data are scattered and sketchy, making it very difficult to study what works and what doesn't work to reduce violence in the workplace. The best data available cover fatal events. There is less information available concerning injuries from non-fatal events, economic impact on businesses affected, lost productivity, and other costs. Various data collection systems have different ways of defining "at work," especially when there are ambiguities such as commuting and travel, volunteers or students in a workplace, or workplaces that are also residences, such as farms or home offices. Sources of information such as police, physician, workers' compensation, or employee reports may capture only one element—the violent incident, or the injury, or the lost work time, or the setting (at work)—but not the whole picture of the trauma resulting from violence in the workplace. Finally, many non-fatal incidents, especially threats, simply go unreported, in part because there is no coordinated data-collection system to process this information.

Prevention

There are three general approaches to preventing workplace violence:

- **Environmental:** adjusting lighting, entrances and exits, security hardware, and other engineering controls to discourage would-be assailants;

- **Organizational/Administrative:** developing programs, policies, and work practices aimed at maintaining a safe working environment;

- **Behavioral/Interpersonal:** training staff to anticipate, recognize, and respond to conflict and potential violence in the workplace.

There has not been adequate research, however, into the effectiveness of these approaches for all types (I-IV) of workplace violence. For example, most research to date on criminal intent (Type I) violence in retail settings has focused only on environmental approaches. Although there have been some promising initial findings, more research is needed to help businesses properly protect their employees. Very little research has been conducted on behavioral/interpersonal or organizational/administrative approaches to prevention.

The Occupational Safety and Health Administration (OSHA) has developed voluntary guidelines for the prevention of workplace violence, including guidelines for specific industries such as late-night retail, health care and social service, and community workers. However, the effectiveness of these recommendations has yet to be fully evaluated. Funding is urgently needed to evaluate these guidelines.

The most troubling problem with existing research is that very little of it has been conducted using rigorous scientific methods. One of the papers prepared for this workshop (Peek-Asa, Runyan, and Zwerling; see "Resources") describes a comprehensive review of research to date. The authors raised a variety of concerns with a large proportion of the research, including sample sizes that were too small, a lack of appropriate control groups, publication without peer review, and other problems. This lack of good research severely hampers efforts to address the problem of violence in the workplace.

Victims of Violence, 1992-1996

Table 47.1. All Victimizations

Violent Action	Percent of Violent Actions
Rape and sexual assault	4.3%
Homicide	0.2%
Robbery	11.7%
Aggravated assault	21.7%
Simple assault	62%

Source: National Crime Victimization Study, July 1998

Table 47.2. Victimization in the Workplace

Violent Action in the Workplace	Percent of Violent Actions in the Workplace
Rape and sexual assault	2. 5%
Homicide	0.05%
Robbery	4.2%
Aggravated assault	19.7%
Simple assault	73.6%

Source: National Crime Victimization Study, July 1998

Laws and Regulations

Federal: There is no national legislation nor are there any federal regulations specifically addressing the prevention of workplace violence. OSHA has published voluntary guidelines for workers in late-night retail, health care, and taxicab businesses, but employers are not legally obligated to follow these guidelines.

State: To date, several states have passed legislation or enacted regulations aimed at reducing workplace violence in specific industries. California and Washington have enacted regulations aimed at reducing patient-employee (Type II) violence in health care settings. At least three states (Florida, Virginia, and Washington) have laws or regulations intended to prevent robbery-related homicides (Type I) in late-night retail establishments such as convenience stores. The Florida law is the most comprehensive. Many convenience stores in Florida have found it easier to simply close for business during the late-night hours (11 p.m. to 5 a.m.) rather than make the changes required by the law. Neither the legal changes nor the store closings have been evaluated as strategies to prevent workplace violence.

State OSHA regulations: The states of California and Washington both enforce regulations requiring comprehensive safety programs in all workplaces, including the prevention of "reasonably foreseeable" assault on employees.

Local: Taxi drivers appear to have by far the highest risk of fatal assault of any occupation. Safety ordinances, such as those requiring bullet-proof barriers in taxicabs, have appeared in several U.S. cities, including Los Angeles, Chicago, New York City, Baltimore, Boston, Albany (NY), and Oakland (CA). More study is needed to assess these approaches.

Industry

Some employers have responded to the problem of workplace violence by implementing measures to reduce the risk to their employees. Different industries have different kinds of risks depending on a multitude of factors, including the type of business, populations served, management, employees, location of the workplace, layout of the work area, and the relationship of that business with the community.

Employers have attempted to increase safety by various means, including:

- Physical security enhancements, such as lighting and cash handling procedures, that make it more difficult to carry out a violent assault (All Types);

- Threat management procedures, such as a team-oriented plan of action in the case of a violent incident (All Types);

- Employee Assistance Programs (EAPs), to provide intervention for at-risk employees (Type III and IV);

- "Zero tolerance" policies related to threatening or harassing behavior (Type III);

- Employee training, to promote recognition of hazards and appropriate responses to incidents of violence (All Types);

- Screening, to identify potentially high-risk employees (Type III);

- Company policies and training to facilitate employee comfort in reporting threatening behaviors (All Types) and timely management response to the employee reports;

- Hiring of security firms that specialize in prevention of workplace violence (All Types).

In workplaces that have only infrequent incidents of violence, many employers find it difficult to decide which safety measures are most appropriate. This is especially true when faced with very expensive or labor-intensive interventions. Private security services and consultants abound, but there is limited scientific information on which strategies work best for the various types of workplace violence. In addition, businesses are often reluctant to make their security methods public, not wanting to alarm customers or tip-off potential perpetrators, which makes it difficult to evaluate those methods.

Employers are often in a difficult position when it comes to responding appropriately to the problem of workplace violence. They must avoid over-reacting, under-reacting, or reacting in a way that exacerbates the problem. In addition, businesses may face serious legal implications with some security measures. For example, some kinds of pre-employment screening may be viewed as discriminatory, but an employer could also face a "negligent hiring" lawsuit if an applicant with a past history of violence is hired.

Labor

In the past decade, representatives of organized labor have pushed for the recognition of workplace violence as an occupational hazard, not just a criminal justice issue. Of particular concern is the high rate of violent incidents targeting health care workers (Type II violence). On some psychiatric units, for example, assault rates on staff are greater than 100 cases per 100 workers per year. Unions representing workers in the health care industry suspect that "short-staffing" may play a role in this problem, but there is little research into this issue to date.

Organized labor professionals or representatives have also expressed concerns about workplace violence interventions that target employee behavior, such as "zero tolerance" policies and "worker profiling" designed to identify employees or potential employees at risk for violent behavior. There is concern that zero tolerance policies may be unevenly enforced and that they fail to address some of the root causes of violence, such as stress or situations leading to conflict. Profiling based on personal characteristics, say its critics, is not an effective predictor of potentially violent behavior and may raise discrimination issues.

In general, labor unions favor an increase in voluntary implementation of workplace violence intervention by employers, coupled with some mandatory provisions such as state legislation or a mandatory OSHA standard. Labor also recognizes the need for more research to determine which current OSHA guidelines and other types of interventions are most effective in preventing violent incidents in the workplace.

Table 47.3. Average Annual Number of Violent Non-Fatal Victimizations in the Workplace, 1992-96 By Selected Occupations

Occupation	Average Number
Retail sales	285,000
Law enforcement	240,000
Teaching	135,000
Medical	130,000
Mental health	80,000
Transportation	75,000
Private security	65,000

Source: National Crime Victimization Study, July 1998

Table 47.4. Percent of Work-Related Homicides by Type, United States, 1997

Type	Percent
Type I: Criminal intent	85%
Type II: Customer/Client	3%
Type III: Co/Past Worker	7%
Type IV: Personal relationship	85%
Total number of homicides = 860	

Source: Census of Fatal Occupational Injuries, BLS

Conclusion

Workplace violence affects us all. Its burden is borne not only by victims of violence, but by their co-workers, their families, their employers, and by every worker at risk of violent assault—in other words, virtually all of us. Although we know that each year workplace violence results in hundreds of deaths, more than 2 million injuries, and billions of dollars in costs, our understanding of workplace violence is still in its infancy. Much remains to be done in the area of research, particularly in data collection and in intervention. Without basic information on who is most affected and which prevention measures are effective in what settings, we can expect only limited success in addressing this problem.

The first steps have been taken. With the help of a broad coalition, a number of key issues have been identified for future research. However, research funding focused on a much broader understanding of the scope and impact of workplace violence is urgently needed to reduce the human and financial burden of this significant public health problem.

Resources

Five review papers, each addressing a specific aspect of workplace violence, were prepared in conjunction with the workshop. They appeared in the February 2001 issue of the *American Journal of Preventive Medicine*, at www. elsevier.com/locate/ajpmonline. The papers are:

Barish RC. *Legislation and Regulations Addressing Workplace Violence in the U. S. and British Columbia.*

Peek-Asa C, Runyan CW, Zwerling C. *The Role of Surveillance and Evaluation Research in the Reduction of Violence Against Workers.*

Rosen J. *A Labor Perspective of Workplace Violence Prevention: Identifying Research Needs.*

Runyan CW. *Moving Forward with Research on the Prevention of Violence Against Workers.*

Wilkinson CW. *Violence Prevention At Work: A Business Perspective.*

Additional Information

Up-to-date information and statistics on workplace violence are available at the following websites:

Occupational Safety and Health Administration (OSHA)
Website: www.osha.gov (includes recommendations for prevention of workplace violence)

The Bureau of Labor Statistics
Website: http://stats.bls.gov

National Institute for Occupational Safety and Health
Website: www.cdc.gov/niosh

National Center for Injury Prevention and Control
Website: www.cdc.gov/ncipc

American Federation of State, County, and Municipal Employees
Website: www.afscme.org/health/faq-viol.htm

California OSHA Website on Workplace Security
Website: www.dir.ca.gov/DOSH/dosh_publications/index.html

Part Seven

Transportation Injuries and Safety

Chapter 48

Motor Vehicle Crashes, Injuries, and Fatalities

Motor vehicle travel is the primary means of transportation in the United States, providing an unprecedented degree of mobility. Yet for all its advantages, deaths and injuries resulting from motor vehicle crashes are the leading cause of death for persons of every age from 4 through 33 years old (based on 1998 data). Traffic fatalities account for more than 90 percent of transportation-related fatalities. The mission of the National Highway Traffic Safety Administration is to reduce deaths, injuries, and economic losses from motor vehicle crashes.

Fortunately, much progress has been made in reducing the number of deaths and serious injuries on our nation's highways. In 2000, the fatality rate per 100 million vehicle miles of travel fell to a new historic low of 1.5, down from 1.6, the rate from 1997 to 1999. The 1990 rate was 2.1 per 100 million vehicle miles traveled. A 71 percent safety belt use rate nationwide and a reduction in the rate of alcohol involvement in fatal crashes—to 40 percent in 2000 from 50 percent in 1990—were significant contributions to maintaining this consistently low fatality rate. However, much remains to be done. The economic cost alone of motor vehicle crashes in 1994 was more than $150.5 billion.

"Traffic Safety Facts 2000–Overview," National Center for Statistics and Analysis, National Highway Traffic Safety Administration (NHTSA), DOT HS 809 329, 2001; and "The Cost of Road Trauma: Single and Multiple Injury Cases," by Delia Hendrie, Greg Lyle, Diana Rosman, G. Anthony Ryan, Brian Fildes, Magda Les, excerpted from *Measuring the Burden of Injury—3rd International Conference*, U.S. Department of Transportation, 2001.

Table 48.1. Motor Vehicle Occupants and Nonoccupants Killed and Injured, 1990-2000

Year	Occupants							Nonoccupants				Total
	Passenger Cars	Light Trucks	Large Trucks	Motor-cycles	Buses	Other/ Unknown	Total	Pedes-trian	Pedal-cyclist	Other	Total	
Killed												
1990	24,092	8,601	705	3,244	32	460	37,134	6,482	859	124	7,465	44,599
1991	22,385	8,391	661	2,806	31	466	34,740	5,801	843	124	6,768	41,508
1992	21,387	8,098	585	2,395	28	387	32,880	5,549	723	98	6,370	39,250
1993	21,566	8,511	605	2,449	18	425	33,574	5,649	816	111	6,576	40,150
1994	21,997	8,904	670	2,320	18	409	34,318	5,489	802	107	6,398	40,716
1995	22,423	9,568	648	2,227	33	392	35,291	5,584	833	109	6,526	41,817
1996	22,505	9,932	621	2,161	21	455	35,695	5,449	765	154	6,368	42,065
1997	22,199	10,249	723	2,116	18	420	35,725	5,321	814	153	6,288	42,013
1998	21,194	10,705	742	2,294	38	409	35,382	5,228	760	131	6,119	41,501
1999	20,862	11,265	759	2,483	59	447	35,875	4,939	754	149	5,842	41,717
2000	20,492	11,418	741	2,862	22	714	36,249	4,739	690	143	5,572	41,821
Injured												
1990	2,376,000	505,000	42,000	84,000	33,000	4,000	3,044,000	105,000	75,000	7,000	187,000	3,231,000
1991	2,235,000	563,000	28,000	80,000	21,000	4,000	2,931,000	88,000	67,000	11,000	166,000	3,097,000
1992	2,232,000	545,000	34,000	65,000	20,000	12,000	2,908,000	89,000	63,000	10,000	162,000	3,070,000
1993	2,265,000	601,000	32,000	59,000	17,000	4,000	2,978,000	94,000	68,000	9,000	171,000	3,149,000
1994	2,364,000	631,000	30,000	57,000	16,000	4,000	3,102,000	92,000	62,000	9,000	164,000	3,266,000
1995	2,469,000	722,000	30,000	57,000	19,000	4,000	3,303,000	86,000	67,000	10,000	162,000	3,465,000
1996	2,458,000	761,000	33,000	55,000	20,000	4,000	3,332,000	82,000	58,000	11,000	151,000	3,483,000
1997	2,341,000	755,000	31,000	53,000	17,000	6,000	3,201,000	77,000	58,000	11,000	146,000	3,348,000
1998	2,201,000	763,000	29,000	49,000	16,000	4,000	3,061,000	69,000	53,000	8,000	131,000	3,192,000
1999	2,138,000	847,000	33,000	50,000	22,000	7,000	3,097,000	85,000	51,000	3,000	140,000	3,236,000
2000	2,052,000	887,000	31,000	58,000	18,000	10,000	3,055,000	78,000	51,000	5,000	134,000	3,189,000

In 2000, 41,821 people were killed in the estimated 6,394,000 police-reported motor vehicle traffic crashes, 3,189,000 people were injured, and 4,286,000 crashes involved property damage only.

This chapter contains statistics on motor vehicle fatalities based on data from the Fatality Analysis Reporting System (FARS). FARS is a census of fatal crashes within the 50 states, the District of Columbia, and Puerto Rico (although Puerto Rico is not included in U.S. totals). Crash and injury statistics are based on data from the General Estimates System (GES). GES is a probability-based sample of police-reported crashes, from 60 locations across the country, from which estimates of national totals for injury and property-damage-only crashes are derived.

"In 2000, there were an estimated 6,394,000 police-reported traffic crashes, in which 41,821 people were killed and 3,189,000 people were injured; 4,286,000 crashes involved property damage only." The 2000 fatality rate per 100 million vehicle miles of travel is 1.5

- In 2000, 41,821 people lost their lives in motor vehicle crashes—an increase of 0.2 percent from 1999.

- The fatality rate per 100 million vehicle miles of travel in 2000 was 1.5.

- The injury rate per 100 million vehicle miles of travel in 2000 was 116.

- The fatality rate per 100,000 population was 15.23 in 2000, slightly lower than the 1999 rate of 15.30.

- An average of 115 persons died each day in motor vehicle crashes in 2000—one every 13 minutes.

- Motor vehicle crashes are the leading cause of death for every age from 4 through 33 years old.

- Vehicle occupants accounted for 87 percent of traffic fatalities in 2000. The remaining 13 percent were pedestrians, pedalcyclists, and other nonoccupants.

Occupant Protection

In 2000, 49 states and the District of Columbia had safety belt use laws in effect. Use rates vary widely from state to state, reflecting factors such as differences in public attitudes, enforcement practices, legal provisions, and public information and education programs.

Table 48.2. Persons Killed and Injured and Fatality and Injury Rates, 1990-2000

Killed

Year	Killed	Resident Population (Thousands)	Fatality Rate per 100,000 Population	Licensed Drivers (Thousands)	Fatality Rate per 100,000 Licensed Drivers	Registered Motor Vehicles (Thousands)	Fatality Rate per 100,000 Registered Vehicles	Vehicle Miles Traveled (Billions)	Fatality Rate per 100 Million VMT
1990	44,599	249,464	17.88	167,015	26.70	184,275	24.20	2,144	2.1
1991	41,508	252,153	16.46	168,995	24.56	186,370	22.27	2,172	1.9
1992	39,250	255,030	15.39	173,125	22.67	184,938	21.22	2,247	1.7
1993	40,150	257,783	15.58	173,149	23.19	188,350	21.32	2,296	1.7
1994	40,716	260,327	15.64	175,403	23.21	192,497	21.15	2,358	1.7
1995	41,817	262,803	15.91	176,628	23.68	197,065	21.22	2,423	1.7
1996	42,065	265,229	15.86	179,539	23.43	201,631	20.86	2,486	1.7
1997	42,013	267,784	15.69	182,709	22.99	203,568	20.64	2,562	1.6
1998	41,501	270,248	15.36	184,980	22.44	208,076	19.95	2,632	1.6
1999	41,717	272,691	15.30	187,170	22.29	212,685	19.61	2,691	1.6
2000	41,821	274,634	15.23	190,625*	21.94*	217,028*	19.27*	2,750*	1.5*

Injured

Year	Killed	Resident Population (Thousands)	Injury Rate per 100,000 Population	Licensed Drivers (Thousands)	Injury Rate per 100,000 Licensed Drivers	Registered Motor Vehicles (Thousands)	Injury Rate per 100,000 Registered Vehicles	Vehicle Miles Traveled (Billions)	Injury Rate per 100 Million VMT
1990	3,231,000	249,464	1,295	167,015	1,934	184,275	1,753	2,144	151
1991	3,097,000	252,153	1,228	168,995	1,833	186,370	1,662	2,172	143
1992	3,070,000	255,030	1,204	173,125	1,773	184,938	1,660	2,247	137
1993	3,149,000	257,783	1,222	173,149	1,819	188,350	1,672	2,296	137
1994	3,266,000	260,327	1,255	175,403	1,862	192,497	1,697	2,358	139
1995	3,465,000	262,803	1,319	176,628	1,962	197,065	1,758	2,423	143
1996	3,483,000	265,229	1,313	179,539	1,940	201,631	1,728	2,486	140
1997	3,348,000	267,784	1,250	182,709	1,832	203,568	1,644	2,562	131
1998	3,192,000	270,248	1,181	184,980	1,726	208,076	1,534	2,632	121
1999	3,236,000	272,691	1,187	187,170	1,729	212,685	1,522	2,691	120
2000	3,189,000	274,634	1,161	190,625*	1,673*	217,028*	1,469*	2,750*	116*

*Revised 2000 data.

Sources: *Vehicle Miles of Travel and Licensed Drivers*, Federal Highway Administration; *Registered Vehicles*, R.L. Polk & Co. and Federal Highway Administration; *Population*, U.S. Bureau of the Census.

- From 1975 through 2000, it is estimated that safety belts saved 135,102 lives, including 11,889 lives saved in 2000. If all passenger vehicle occupants over age 4 wore safety belts, 21,127 lives (that is, an additional 9,238) could have been saved in 2000.

- In 2000, it is estimated that 316 children under age 5 were saved as a result of child restraint use. An estimated 4,816 lives were saved by child restraints from 1975 through 2000.

- Children in rear-facing child seats should not be placed in the front seat of cars equipped with passenger-side air bags. The impact of a deploying air bag striking a rear-facing child seat could result in injury to the child. NHTSA also recommends that children 12 and under sit in the rear seat away from the force of a deploying air bag.

- In 2000, 41 percent of passenger car occupants and 45 percent of light truck occupants involved in fatal crashes were unrestrained.

- In fatal crashes, 75 percent of passenger car occupants who were totally ejected from the vehicle were killed. Safety belts are effective in preventing total ejections: only 1 percent of the occupants reported to have been using restraints were totally ejected, compared with 22 percent of the unrestrained occupants.

Table 48.3. Restraint Use Rates for Passenger Car Occupants in Fatal Crashes, 1990 and 2000

Type of Occupant	Restraint Use Rate (Percent)	
	1990	2000
Drivers	45	62
Passengers		
Front Seat	42	62
Rear Seat	28	46
5 Years Old and Over	34	53
4 Years Old and Under	52	73
All Passengers	36	55
All Occupants	41	59

Speeding

Speeding—exceeding the posted speed limit, driving too fast for conditions, or racing—is one of the most prevalent factors contributing to traffic crashes. The economic cost to society of speeding-related crashes is estimated by NHTSA to be $27.4 billion per year. In 2000, speeding was a contributing factor in 29 percent of all fatal crashes, and 12,350 lives were lost in speeding-related crashes.

- In 2000, 593,000 people received minor injuries in speeding-related crashes. An additional 71,000 people received moderate injuries, and 39,000 received serious to critical injuries in speeding-related crashes (based on methodology from *The Economic Cost of Motor Vehicle Crashes1994*, NHTSA).

- In 2000, 85 percent of speeding-related fatalities occurred on roads that were not Interstate highways.

- For drivers involved in fatal crashes, young males are the most likely to be speeding. The proportion of all crashes that are speeding-related decreases with increasing driver age. In 2000, 34 percent of the male drivers 15 to 20 years old who were involved in fatal crashes were speeding at the time of the crash.

- Alcohol and speeding are clearly a deadly combination. Speeding involvement is prevalent for drivers involved in alcohol-related crashes. In 2000, 40 percent of the intoxicated drivers (BAC = 0.10 or higher) involved in fatal crashes were speeding, compared with only 13 percent of the sober drivers (BAC = 0.00) involved in fatal crashes.

Large Trucks

In 2000, 11 percent (4,719) of all the motor vehicle traffic fatalities reported involved heavy trucks (gross vehicle weight rating greater than 26,000 pounds), and 1 percent (562) involved medium trucks (gross vehicle weight rating 10,001 to 26,000 pounds).

- Of the fatalities that resulted from crashes involving large trucks (gross vehicle weight rating greater than 10,000 pounds), 78 percent were occupants of another vehicle, 8 percent were nonoccupants, and 14 percent were occupants of a large truck.

- Large trucks accounted for 9 percent of all vehicles involved in fatal crashes and 4 percent of all vehicles involved in injury and property-damage-only crashes in 2000.

- More than three-quarters (79 percent) of the large trucks involved in fatal crashes in 2000 collided with another motor vehicle in transport.

- Only 1 percent of the drivers of large trucks involved in fatal crashes in 2000 were intoxicated, compared with 19 percent for passenger cars, 20 percent for light trucks, and 27 percent for motorcycles.

- One out of nine traffic fatalities in 2000 resulted from a collision involving a large truck.

Table 48.4. Fatalities and Injuries in Crashes Involving Large Trucks, 2000

Type of Fatality	Number	Percentage of Total
Occupants of Large Trucks	741	14
Single-Vehicle Crashes	480	9
Multiple-Vehicle Crashes	261	5
Occupants of Other Vehicles in Crashes Involving Large Trucks	4,060	78
Nonoccupants (Pedestrians, Pedalcyclists, etc.)	410	8
Total	**5,211**	**100**

Type of Injury	Number	Percentage of Total
Occupants of Large Trucks	31,000	22
Single-Vehicle Crashes	16,000	12
Multiple-Vehicle Crashes	14,000	10
Occupants of Other Vehicles in Crashes Involving Large Trucks	106,000	76
Nonoccupants (Pedestrians, Pedalcyclists, etc.)	3,000	2
Total	**140,000**	**100**

Cars, Light Trucks, and Vans

In 2000, 31,910 occupants of passenger vehicles were killed in traffic crashes and an additional 2,938,000 were injured, accounting for 88 percent of all occupant fatalities (passenger cars 57 percent, light trucks and vans 31 percent) and 96 percent of all occupants injured (passenger cars 67 percent, light trucks and vans 29 percent).

- Occupant fatalities in single-vehicle crashes accounted for 42 percent of all motor vehicle fatalities in 2000. Occupant fatalities in multiple-vehicle crashes accounted for 45 percent of all fatalities, and the remaining 13 percent were nonoccupant fatalities (pedestrians, pedalcyclists, etc.).

- In 2000, 59 percent of passenger vehicle occupant fatalities occurred in vehicles that sustained frontal damage.

- Ejection from the vehicle accounted for 28 percent of all passenger vehicle occupant fatalities. The ejection rate for occupants of light trucks in fatal crashes was nearly twice the rate for passenger car occupants.

- Utility vehicles had the highest rollover involvement rate of any vehicle type in fatal crashes—36 percent, as compared with 24 percent for pickups, 19 percent for vans, and 15 percent for passenger cars.

- Utility vehicles also had the highest rollover rate for passenger vehicles in injury crashes—12 percent, compared with 7 percent for pickups, 4 percent for vans, and 3 percent for passenger cars.

- Nearly two-thirds (60 percent) of the passenger vehicle occupants killed in traffic crashes in 2000 were unrestrained.

- The intoxication rate for drivers of light trucks involved in fatal crashes (20 percent) is higher than that for passenger car drivers (19 percent).

Driver Age

There are more than 25 million people age 70 years and older in the United States. In 2000, this age group made up 9 percent of the total U.S. resident population, compared with 8 percent in 1990. From 1990 to 2000, this older segment of the population grew twice as fast as the total population.

- In 2000, 181,000 older individuals were injured in traffic crashes, accounting for 6 percent of all the people injured in traffic crashes during the year. These older individuals made up 13 percent of all traffic fatalities, 12 percent of all vehicle occupant fatalities, and 17 percent of all pedestrian fatalities.

- Older drivers involved in fatal crashes in 2000 had the lowest intoxication rate (4 percent) of all adult drivers.

- In two-vehicle fatal crashes involving an older driver and a younger driver, the vehicle driven by the older person was more than 3 times as likely to be the one that was struck (57 percent and 18 percent, respectively). In 44 percent of these crashes, both vehicles were proceeding straight at the time of the collision. In 27 percent, the older driver was turning left—6 times as often as the younger driver.

- When driver fatality rates are calculated on the basis of estimated annual travel, the highest rates are found among the youngest and oldest drivers. Compared with the fatality rate for drivers 25 through 69 years old, the rate for teenage drivers is about 4 times as high, and the rate for drivers in the oldest group is 9 times as high.

Table 48.5. Fatalities in Traffic Crashes, 1990 and 2000

	1990	2000
Nonoccupant Fatalities		
Pedestrians	6,482	4,739
Pedalcyclists	859	690
Other Nonoccupants	124	143
Occupant Fatalities		
Single-Vehicle Crashes		
Rollover	8,552	8,600
Nonrollover	9,607	8,830
Multiple-Vehicle Crashes		
Angle	8,312	8,376
Head-on	7,119	6,668
Rear-end	2,064	2,199
Sideswipe	720	683
Other/Unknown	760	893

- Young female drivers, under age 50, have a lower fatality rate than their male counterparts, on a per mile driven basis, while the rate is essentially the same for both male and female drivers over 50 years of age, with the exception of the oldest group (over 85 years).

Youth

In 2000, 16- to 24-year-olds represented 24 percent of all traffic fatalities, compared with 7 percent for ages 0 to 15, 45 percent for ages 25 to 54, and 24 percent for ages 55 and over.

- On a per population basis, drivers under the age of 25 had the highest rate of involvement in fatal crashes of any age group.

- The intoxication rate for 16- to 20-year-old drivers involved in fatal crashes in 2000 was 15 percent. The highest intoxication rates were for drivers 21 to 24 and 25 to 34 years old (27 percent and 24 percent, respectively).

- Almost one-fourth (23 percent) of all children between the ages of 5 and 9 years who were killed in motor vehicle traffic crashes were pedestrians. Nearly one-fifth (18 percent) of the traffic fatalities under age 16 were pedestrians.

- Passenger vehicle occupants 10 to 24 years old involved in fatal crashes had the lowest restraint use rate (49 percent), and those over age 65 had the highest rate (69 percent).

Male/Female Fatal Crash Involvement

In 2000, the fatal crash involvement rate per 100,000 population was almost 3 times as high for male drivers as for females. However, the population-based rates do not account for the actual on-road exposure, which is greater for males, or the percentage of the population that has driver licenses, also greater for males.

- Males accounted for 68 percent of all traffic fatalities, 68 percent of all pedestrian fatalities, and 89 percent of all pedalcyclist fatalities in 2000.

- The intoxication rate for male drivers involved in fatal crashes was 20 percent, compared with 11 percent for female drivers.

- Among female drivers of passenger vehicles involved in fatal crashes in 2000, 29 percent were unrestrained at the time of the collision, compared with 43 percent of male drivers in fatal crashes.

Pedestrians

In 2000, 78,000 pedestrians were injured and 4,739 were killed in traffic crashes in the United States, representing 2 percent of all the people injured in traffic crashes and 11 percent of all traffic fatalities.

- On average, a pedestrian is killed in a motor vehicle crash every 111 minutes, and one is injured every 7 minutes.

- Alcohol involvement—either for the driver or the pedestrian—was reported in 47 percent of the traffic crashes that resulted in pedestrian fatalities. Of the pedestrians involved, 31 percent were intoxicated. The intoxication rate for the drivers involved was only 13 percent. In 5 percent of the crashes, both the driver and the pedestrian were intoxicated.

Pedalcyclists

In 2000, 690 pedalcyclists were killed and an additional 51,000 were injured in traffic crashes. Pedalcyclists made up 2 percent of all

Table 48.6. Nonoccupant Traffic Fatalities, 1990-2000

Year	Pedestrian	Pedalcyclist	Other	Total
1990	6,482	859	124	7,465
1991	5,801	843	124	6,768
1992	5,549	723	98	6,370
1993	5,649	816	111	6,576
1994	5,489	802	107	6,398
1995	5,584	833	109	6,526
1996	5,449	765	154	6,368
1997	5,321	814	153	6,288
1998	5,228	760	131	6,119
1999	4,939	754	149	5,842
2000	4,739	690	143	5,572

traffic fatalities and 2 percent of all the people injured in traffic crashes during the year.

- Most of the pedalcyclists injured or killed in 2000 were males (78 percent and 89 percent, respectively), and most were between the ages of 5 and 44 years (87 percent and 65 percent, respectively).

- Almost one-third (27 percent) of the pedalcyclists killed in traffic crashes in 2000 were between 5 and 15 years old.

The Cost of Road Trauma: Single and Multiple Injury Cases

[Editor's note: The following data is based on road crashes in South Wales, Australia. It is included since the nature of injuries from road crashes do not vary greatly between developed countries.]

Casualties involved in road crashes often sustain multiple injuries, yet very little is known about the cost of single injury compared with multiple injury cases. The most common method of dealing with multiple injury cases in road safety research is to allocate a primary injury to casualties on the basis of the injury with the highest severity level. Subsequent analysis of the distribution and cost of road injury is then based on the classification of the primary injury.

The purpose of this study was to explore the cost of road trauma involving single and multiple injury cases. More specifically, the study was conducted to examine the marginal cost of each additional injury sustained by casualties in road crashes. The work is currently in progress, and this section presents some preliminary results. Information relating to the impact of second and subsequent injuries on the cost of a single injury is to be used in cost-effectiveness analyses of interventions such as vehicle design changes, which may prevent the occurrence of some, but not all, injuries sustained by motor vehicle occupants in a crash.

Road Injury Cost Database

The cost data used in this study was obtained from the Road Injury Cost Database. This database was constructed primarily from the unit records of personal injury claims paid to road crash casualties in New South Wales, Australia between July 1989 and June 1996. Finalized payments were available for 49,755 claimants. Personal injury insurance payments to individuals in the claims database were recorded for the following cost categories: legal and investigation, long term and home care, home and vehicle modifications, aids and appliances, economic loss, and general damages. Methods were developed to allocate the following person-based costs of road injury to claimant records: medical, hospital, rehabilitation, ambulance, future unpaid earnings, losses to non-victims, and personal injury insurance administration. Crash-based costs—namely property damage, travel delay, and motor vehicle insurance—are included in the Road Injury Cost Database but were not used for the analyses in this study.

Each claimant in the Road Injury Cost Database has up to five injuries coded on the basis of the 1985 revision of the Abbreviated Injury Scale (AIS), with lower extremity injuries divided into lower and upper leg injuries. A primary injury was allocated to claimants on the basis of the injury with the highest severity, and this classification was used for some comparisons of the cost of single and multiple injury cases. If a claimant sustained two or more injuries of the same maximum injury severity level, priority was assigned on the basis of the following ordering: head, spine, lower extremities, thorax, abdomen, upper extremities, neck, face, and external (MacKenzie, Shapiro and Siegel, 1988).

Incidence of Single and Multiple Injury Cases

Approximately one third of cases in the Road Injury Cost Database had a single injury (n = 16,603) and two thirds had multiple injuries (n = 33,152). The most commonly occurring single injuries were a minor injury (i.e. AIS 1)

- to the neck (n = 11,021),
- the spine (n = 8,151)
- and the external body regions (n = 3,683).

On the basis of the primary injury classification, the most frequently occurring multiple injuries were a minor injury

- to the spine (n = 7,283),
- the upper leg (n = 2,764) and
- the neck (n = 2,462).

A more detailed analysis of the multiple injury cases, based on all injuries sustained rather than the primary injury, indicated that the most commonly occurring injury combinations were as follows:

- neck AIS 1, spine AIS 1 (n = 5,497),
- neck AIS 1, upper extremity AIS 1 (n = 1,901);
- neck AIS 1, external AIS 1 (n = 1,709);
- neck AIS 1, spine AIS 1, upper extremity AIS 1 (n = 989);
- neck AIS 1, thorax AIS 1 (n = 834);
- external AIS 1, upper extremity AIS 1(n = 678);
- neck AIS 1, spine AIS 1, external AIS 1 (n = 622);
- external AIS 1; upper leg AIS 1 (n = 550);
- neck AIS 1, upper leg AIS 1 (n = 534); and
- upper extremity AIS 2, external AIS 1 (n = 480).

Comparison of the Predicted and Actual Costs of Multiple Injuries Using the Two Models

Table 48.7. compares costs for selected multiple injury combinations derived from the two models with the equivalent actual costs in the Road Injury Cost Database. For example, the actual average cost of cases with a minor head and minor neck injury was $18,920, while the costs predicted by the simple additive/non-additive model and the GLM model were $21,640 and $17,990 respectively. In general, the GLM costs were closer to the actual costs in the Road Injury Cost Database than those predicted by the simple additive/non-additive model, although this was not always the case (e.g. the simple model gave a closer fit for minor thorax/minor neck multiple injury cases).

Table 48.7. Actual Cost of Road Crash Casualties with Multiple Injuries

Multiple Injury Combinations	Actual Cost from Road Injury Cost Database
Minor head/minor neck	$18,920
Moderate head/minor neck	$33,860
Moderate head/minor external	$27,110
Minor spine/minor neck	$23,040
Moderate spine/minor neck	$60,470
Moderate spine/minor external	$70,610
Minor upper leg/minor external	$18,660
Minor thorax/minor neck	$17,580

References

MacKenzie, EJ, Shapiro, S and Siegel, JH. The economic impact of traumatic injuries. *JAMA*. 1988;260:3290-6.

Chapter 49

Alcohol-Related Impairment and Transportation Safety

The Extent of the Problem

In 2000 there were 16,653 fatalities in alcohol-related crashes. This is a 4 percent increase compared to 1999, and it represents an average of one alcohol-related fatality every 32 minutes.

- The 16,653 alcohol-related fatalities in 2000 (40 percent of total traffic fatalities for the year) represent a 25 percent reduction from the 22,084 alcohol-related fatalities reported in 1990 (50 percent of the total).

- NHTSA estimates that alcohol was involved in 40 percent of fatal crashes and in 8 percent of all crashes in 2000.

- In 2000, 31 percent of all traffic fatalities occurred in crashes in which at least one driver or nonoccupant had a blood alcohol concentration (BAC) of 0.10 grams per deciliter (g/dl) or greater.

- All states and the District of Columbia now have 21-year-old minimum drinking age laws. NHTSA estimates that these laws have reduced traffic fatalities involving drivers 18 to 20 years

This chapter includes "Impaired Driving Fact Sheet," National Center for Injury Prevention and Control, 1999; "Alcohol and Transportation Safety," *Alcohol Alert* No. 52, National Institute on Alcohol Abuse and Alcoholism (NIAAA), April 2001; and "Traffic Safety Facts 2000: Alcohol," U.S. Department of Transportation, DOT HS 809 320, 2001.

old by 13 percent and have saved an estimated 20,043 lives since 1975. In 2000, an estimated 922 lives were saved by minimum drinking age laws.

- Approximately 1.5 million drivers were arrested in 1999 for driving under the influence of alcohol or narcotics. This is an arrest rate of 1 for every 121 licensed drivers in the United States).

- About 3 in every 10 Americans will be involved in an alcohol-related crash at some time in their lives.

- From 1990 to 2000, intoxication rates (BAC of 0.10 g/dl or greater) decreased for drivers of all age groups involved in fatal crashes.

- Intoxication rates for drivers in fatal crashes in 2000 were 27 percent for motorcycles, 20 percent for light trucks, 19 percent for passenger cars, and 1 percent for large trucks.

Alcohol as a Factor in Traffic Fatalities Involving Young People

- In 1997, 14% of drivers aged 16-20 years and 26% of drivers aged 21-24 years who were involved in fatal crashes were legally drunk (BAC 0.10g/dL or greater).[1]

- Young men aged 18-20 years (too young to legally buy alcohol) report driving while impaired almost as frequently as men aged 21-34 years.[3]

- At all levels of blood alcohol concentration, the risk of being involved in a crash is greater for young people than it is for older people.[5]

Alcohol a Factor in Traffic Fatalities among Children

- In 1996, 21% of the 2,761 traffic fatalities among children aged 0-14 years involved alcohol.[6]

- Of the child passenger deaths that involve a driver with a BAC >0.10 g/dL, 60% of the time it is the driver of the child's car who is impaired.[6]

Other Subgroups That Are Most Likely to Be Involved in Fatal Alcohol-Related Crashes

- Male drivers who die in motor vehicle crashes are almost twice as likely as female drivers to be legally drunk (BAC of 0.10 g/dL or greater).[1]

- The highest intoxication rates among drivers in fatal crashes in 1997 were for those 21 to 24 years old (26.3%), followed by 25 to 34 years old (23.8%) and 35 to 44 years old (22.1%).[1]

- Drivers aged 21-34 years who have been arrested for driving while impaired are over four times as likely to eventually die in a crash involving alcohol than those who have not been arrested for driving while intoxicated.[7]

- Adult drivers aged 35 years or older who have been arrested for drunk driving are over 11 times more likely to eventually die in crashes involving alcohol than are those who have never been arrested.[7]

The Role of Drugs other Than Alcohol in Deaths Related to Motor Vehicle Crashes

- Drugs other than alcohol (e.g., marijuana and cocaine) have been identified as factors in 18% of deaths among motor vehicle drivers. Other drugs are generally used in combination with alcohol.[8]

- Most fatally injured drivers who have used drugs other than alcohol are male, or 25-54 years of age, or both.[8]

The Cost of Alcohol-Related Crashes

- In 1994, alcohol-related crashes cost the U.S. $45 billion in direct cost, loss of earnings, and household productivity.[9]

Do Most People Who Drink and Drive Have Serious Alcohol Problems?

- More than 70% of drivers convicted of driving while impaired are either heavy frequent drinkers (alcohol abuse) or alcoholics (alcohol dependent).[10]

Prevention

Effective measures include:[13]

- Promptly suspending the driver's licenses of people who drive while intoxicated.

- Lowering the permissible levels of blood alcohol concentration to 0.08 grams per deciliter (g/dL) for adults and zero tolerance for drivers younger than 21 years old in all states.

- Sobriety checkpoints.

- Continued public education, community awareness, and media campaigns about the dangers of alcohol-impaired driving.

- Reducing the legal limit for blood alcohol to 0.05 g/dL.[14,15]

- Raising state and federal alcohol excise taxes.[15]

- Implementing compulsory blood alcohol testing when traffic crashes result in injury.[15]

Table 49.1. Estimated Number and Percentage of Traffic Fatalities, by the Highest BAC (Blood Alcohol Concentration) of Any Person Involved in the Crash, United States, 1987-1997

Year	Total	BAC 0.00 g/dL No. (%)	BAC≥0.01 g/dL No. (%)	BAC ≥0.10 g/dL No. (%)
1987	46,390	22,749 (49.0)	23,641 (51.0)	18,529 (39.9)
1988	47,087	23,461 (49.8)	23,626 (50.2)	18,731 (39.8)
1989	45,582	23,178 (50.8)	22,404 (49.2)	17,862 (39.2)
1990	44,599	22,515 (50.5)	22,084 (49.5)	17,650 (39.6)
1991	41,508	21,621 (52.1)	19,887 (47.9)	15,928 (38.4)
1992	39,235	21,536 (54.9)	17,699 (45.1)	14,123 (36.0)
1993	40,115	22,653 (56.5)	17,461 (43.5)	13,982 (34.9)
1994	40,716	24,136 (59.3)	16,580 (40.7)	13,100 (32.2)
1995	41,798	24,524 (58.7)	17,274 (41.3)	13,564 (32.5)
1996	41,907	24,781 (59.1)	17,126 (40.9)	13,395 (32.0)
1997	41,967	25,778 (61.4)	16,189 (38.6)	12,704 (30.3)

Note: BAC distributions are estimates for drivers and nonoccupants of motor vehicles who were involved in fatal crashes.

Source: NHTSA Fatality Analysis Reporting System (FARS) 1998.

References

1. National Highway Traffic Safety Administration (NHTSA*)*. *Traffic Safety Facts 1997: Alcohol*. Washington, DC: NHTSA;1998.

2. National Center for Health Statistics. Health, United States, 1996-97. Hyattsville, MD: CDC; 1997. DHHS Publication No. (PHS) 97-1232.

3. Liu S, et al. *JAMA* 1997;277:122-5.

4. *Crime in the United States: 1996* Uniform Crime Reports. Washington, DC: FBI; 1997.

5. Mayhew DR, et al. *Accid Anal Prev* 1986;18:273-87.

6. CDC. *MMWR* 1997;46:1130-3.

7. Brewer RD, et al. *New Engl J Med* 1994;331:513-7.

8. National Highway Traffic Safety Administration (NHTSA). The incidence and role of drugs in fatally injured drivers. *Traffic Tech*. Washington, DC: NHTSA; 1993.

9. National Highway Traffic Safety Administration (NHTSA). *The Economic Cost of Motor Vehicle Crashes: 1994*. Washington, DC: NHTSA; 1996 July. DOT HS 808 425.

10. Miller BA, et.al. *Alcohol Clin Exp Res* 1986;10:651-6.

11. National Center for Health Statistics. *Healthy People 2000* Review, 1995-96. Washington, DC: PHS; 1990. DHHS Publication No. (PHS) 96-1256.

12. National Highway Traffic Safety Administration (NHTSA). *Partners in Progress: an Impaired Driving Guide for Action*. Washington, DC: NHTSA; 1997 Sept. DOT HS 808 365.

13. CDC. *MMWR* 1993;42:905-9.

14. Howat P, et al. Drug Alcohol Rev 1991;10(1):151-66. 15. National Committee on Injury Prevention and Control. *Am J Prev Med* 1989;5 (Suppl):123-27.

Alcohol and Transportation Safety

Research has shown that even low blood alcohol concentration (BAC) impairs driving skills and increases crash risk. (BAC is the proportion of alcohol to blood in the body. In the field of traffic safety, BAC is expressed as a percentage reflecting grams of alcohol per deciliter of blood—for example, 0.10 percent is equivalent to 0.10 grams per deciliter.) New information about BAC and impairment has led to policy changes, which have contributed to declines in alcohol-related crashes and fatalities. This section examines some aspects of alcohol-induced impairment and reviews selected strategies designed to reduce alcohol-related crashes and repeat drinking-and-driving offenses.

BAC and Impairment

A review of 112 studies concluded that certain skills required to operate essentially any type of motorized vehicle become impaired at even modest departures from zero BAC. At 0.05 percent BAC, most studies reported significant impairment. By 0.08 percent BAC, 94 percent of the studies reported impairment. Some skills are significantly impaired at 0.01 percent BAC, although other skills do not show impairment until 0.06 percent BAC.[1] At BACs of 0.02 percent or lower, the ability to divide attention between two or more sources of visual information can be impaired. Starting at BACs of 0.05 percent, drivers show other types of impairment, including eye movement, glare resistance, visual perception, and reaction time. Moskowitz and colleagues[2] reported that alcohol significantly impaired driving simulator performance at all BACs starting at 0.02 percent.

The risk of a fatal crash for drivers with positive BACs compared with other drivers (i.e., the relative risk) increases with increasing BAC, and the risks increase more steeply for drivers younger than age 21 than for older drivers.[3] Between 0.08 and 0.10 percent BACs, the relative risk of a fatal single-vehicle crash varies between 11 percent (for drivers age 35 and older) and 52 percent (for male drivers ages 16-20). Other forms of transportation also have been investigated. Studies using an automated device that simulates actual flight conditions have shown pilot performance to be impaired at BACs as low as 0.04 percent [4,5] and to remain impaired for as long as 14 hours after pilots reached BACs between 0.10 percent and 0.12 percent.[4,6] Another experiment using a simulated environment showed that experienced maritime academy students with BACs of 0.05 needed significantly more time than did other students to solve a problem related to power plant operation on board a merchant ship and were not aware of their impairment.[7]

474

Factors That Influence Alcohol-Induced Impairment

Alcohol Tolerance. Research suggests that the repeated performance of certain tasks while under the influence of alcohol can make a person less sensitive to impairment at a given BAC. However, although impairment from alcohol may not be evident during routine tasks, performance would worsen in novel or unexpected situations.[8]

Age. Based on miles driven, the highest driver fatality rates are found among the youngest and oldest drivers. Compared with the fatality rate for drivers ages 25-69, the rate for 16- to 19-year-old drivers is about four times as high, and the rate for drivers age 85 and older is nine times as high.[9,10] Among male drivers younger than age 21, a BAC increase of 0.02 percent more than doubles the relative risk for a single-vehicle fatal crash. Women in this age group, however, have lower relative risk than do men at every BAC.[3] Young drivers' greater crash risk is attributed, in part, to lack of driving experience [11] coupled with overconfidence.[12] The presence of other teenagers in the car may encourage risky driving and is associated with increased fatal crash risk among young drivers.[13]

Alcohol is less often a factor in crashes involving older drivers. In 1999 drivers age 65 and older killed in crashes were the least likely of any adult age group to have positive BACs.[14] Nevertheless, a person's crash risk per mile increases starting at age 55 and exceeds that of a young, beginning driver by age 80.[15] Factors associated with unsafe driving include problems with vision, attention, perception, and cognition.[16,17] Older drivers with alcoholism also are more vulnerable than are other elderly drivers to impairment and have greater crash risks.[15]

Sleep Deprivation. Drowsiness increases crash risk, and research shows that BACs as low as 0.01 percent increase susceptibility to sleepiness.[1] Alcohol consumption also increases the adverse effects of sleep deprivation. Subjects given low doses of alcohol following a night of reduced sleep perform poorly in a driving simulator, even with no detectable alcohol in the blood.[18,19]

Recent Declines in Drinking and Driving

Research shows that drinking and driving in the United States has decreased over the past decade, especially among young drivers. The proportion of all traffic fatalities that are alcohol related has decreased.

The overall percentage of drivers with positive BACs among all drivers surveyed on weekend nights also has decreased. In addition, crash statistics and driver surveys both show decreases in the proportion of drivers with BACs of 0.10 percent or higher, with the largest decreases among drivers younger than age 21.[20,21]

Prevention Strategies

Raising the Minimum Legal Drinking Age (MLDA). The National Highway Traffic Safety Administration (NHTSA) estimates that raising the MLDA to 21 has reduced traffic fatalities involving 18- to 20-year-old drivers by 13 percent and has saved an estimated 19,121 lives since 1975. Twenty of twenty-nine studies conducted between 1981 and 1992 reported significant decreases in traffic crashes and crash fatalities following an increase in MLDA. Three studies found no change in traffic crashes involving youth in various age groups, and six studies had mixed results.[22] Laws that prohibit selling or providing alcohol to minors generally are not well enforced, but community efforts to increase MLDA enforcement can be effective.[23,24]

Zero-Tolerance Laws. These laws, which set the legal BAC limit for drivers younger than age 21 at 0.00 or 0.02 percent, have been associated with 20 percent declines in the proportion of drinking drivers involved in fatal crashes who are younger than age 21 [25] and in the proportion of single-vehicle, nighttime fatal crashes among drivers younger than age 21.[26] Based on driver surveys, researchers have reported that young drivers may be more successful than are older drivers in separating drinking from driving, and these researchers have suggested that this difference could be attributable to zero-tolerance laws.[27]

BAC Laws That Lower Limits to 0.08 percent. The majority of States are now considering lowering the legal BAC limit for noncommercial drivers age 21 and older to 0.08 percent. In fact, according to NHTSA, 27 States have now approved legislation to lower BAC limits to 0.08 percent. Laws lowering the legal BAC limit for adult drivers to 0.08 percent are associated with declines in alcohol-related fatal crashes. One national study reported that States with 0.08 laws had smaller proportions of adult drivers in fatal crashes with BACs of 0.01-0.09 percent and with BACs of 0.10 percent and higher.[28]

Lower BAC Limits for DUI Offenders and Transportation Workers. In Maine, a law lowering the legal BAC limit to 0.05 percent for anyone convicted of driving under the influence (DUI) has been found to reduce significantly the number of fatal crashes among this population.[29] Because drinking and driving by transportation workers threatens public safety, the Federal Government prohibits commercial truck drivers, railroad and mass transit workers, maritime employees, and aircraft pilots from operating their vehicles with BACs of 0.04 percent or higher.

Community Prevention. Comprehensive community initiatives to reduce drinking and driving combine the efforts of public agencies and private citizens in implementing strategies, including media campaigns, police training, high school and college prevention programs, and increased liquor outlet surveillance. Such strategies have been found to reduce fatal crashes, alcohol-related fatal crashes, and traffic injuries.[30,31]

A community program in San Diego was implemented to reduce the binge drinking and impaired driving that result when young people cross the U.S.-Mexico border to drink in Tijuana, where the legal drinking age is 18 and beverage prices are lower. Researchers estimated that more than 250 drivers with BACs of 0.08 percent or higher on U.S. roads every Friday and Saturday night are border-crossers.[32] Targeted enforcement was found to reduce the number of late-night crossers by 26 percent.[33]

Alcohol Screening and Brief Intervention for Emergency Room Patients. Emergency room patients injured in alcohol-related crashes may have an increased motivation to change their drinking behavior.[34] Emergency room interventions have been shown to reduce future drinking and trauma re-admission[35] as well as drinking and driving, traffic violations, alcohol-related injuries, and alcohol-related problems among 18- and 19-year-olds.[36]

Reducing Repeated DUI Offenses

License Suspension. Laws that allow for administrative license suspension (ALS) at the time of arrest have been found to reduce both alcohol-related fatal crashes [28,37] and repeat DUI offenses.[38] A study of an Ohio ALS law found that first-time and repeat DUI offenders who had their licenses immediately confiscated had significantly lower rates of DUI offenses, moving violations, and crashes during the next

2 years compared with DUI offenders convicted before the ALS law went into effect.[38]

Although research shows that license suspension reduces repeat DUI offenses, there is also evidence that up to 75 percent of suspended drivers continue to drive. Evaluation of Oregon's "zebra sticker" law suggests that marking the license plates of vehicles driven by unlicensed drivers deters both driving while suspended (DWS) and DUI by suspended drivers. A similar law in Washington State was enforced differently and had no effect.[39]

Vehicle Impoundment/Immobilization. Two studies of an Ohio law that allowed for vehicle immobilization [40] or impoundment [41] for multiple DUI offenders both found that offenders whose vehicles were immobilized or impounded had lower recidivism rates compared with other offenders while their vehicles were not available and after they were returned.

Other Prevention Strategies. Alcohol ignition interlocks— breath-testing devices designed to prevent operation of a vehicle if the driver's BAC is above a predetermined low level—are used in some jurisdictions as an alternative to full license suspension. Research suggests that offenders who have interlocks installed have lower recidivism rates while the device is in use, but that recidivism rates rise after interlock removal.[42,43] Conversely, a few studies have reported that recidivism was significantly reduced both during interlock installation and after removal.[44,45]

At victim impact panels, drinking-and-driving offenders must listen to persons who were injured or who lost a loved one in an alcohol-related crash recount the event's impact on their lives. The effects of victim impact panels on recidivism have been mixed.[46-48]

Alcohol and Transportation Safety—A Commentary by NIAAA Director Enoch Gordis, M.D.

At what blood alcohol level (BAC) are individuals too impaired to drive a car safely? In the United States, the BAC limit for driving a car in many States is 0.10 percent. The United States, in fact, is the only industrialized nation to have a BAC limit this high. A large body of creditable research over many years has clearly shown that impairment of tasks necessary for safe driving begins at levels as low as 0.05 percent. At the 0.08 percent BAC level, currently under consideration in many States, individuals are significantly impaired and at risk for causing harm to themselves and others. To date, 27 States have lowered the legal BAC limit to 0.08 percent. In many of the States that still maintain the higher 0.10 percent BAC, debates about lowering it often have had little to do with scientific soundness—focusing, instead, on arguments that lower BAC limits infringe on the public's right to drink socially. This argument has no merit; a 160-pound man generally will have reached only a BAC of approximately 0.04 percent 1 hour after consuming two 12-ounce beers or two other standard drinks on an empty stomach. Until these debates consider the actual, rather than the perceived, results of lowered BACs, we all run the risk of being injured or killed in automobile crashes due to drivers who are significantly—but not legally—impaired.

References

1. Moskowitz, H., and Fiorentino, D. A Review of the Literature on the Effects of Low Doses of Alcohol on Driving-Related Skills. Washington, DC: National Highway Traffic Safety Administration (NHTSA), 2000.

2. Moskowitz, H.; Burns, M.; Fiorentino, D.; Smiley, A.; and Zador, P. *Driver Characteristics and Impairment at Various BACs*. Washington, DC: NHTSA, 2000.

3. Zador P.L.; Krawchuck S.A.; and Voas R.B. Alcohol-related relative risk of driver fatalities and driver involvement in fatal crashes in relation to driver age and gender: An update using 1996 data. *J Stud Alcohol* 61:387-395, 2000.

4. Morrow, D.; Leirer, V.; and Yesavage, J. The influence of alcohol and aging on radio communication during flight. *Aviat Space Environ Med* 61(1):12-20, 1990.

5. Ross, L.E.; Yeazel, L.M.; and Chau, A.W. Pilot performance with blood alcohol concentrations below 0.04%. *Aviat Space Environ Med* 63(11):951-956, 1992.

6. Yesavage, J.A., and Leirer, V.O. Hangover effects on aircraft pilots 14 hours after alcohol ingestion: A preliminary report. *Am J Psychiatry* 143(12):1546-1550, 1986.

7. Howland, J.; Rohsenow, D.J.; Cote, J.; Siegel, M.; and Mangione, T.W. Effects of low-dose alcohol exposure on simulated merchant ship handling power plant operation by maritime cadets. *Addict* 95(5):719-726, 2000.

8. Vogel-Sprott, M. *Alcohol Tolerance and Social Drinking: Learning the Consequences.* New York: Guilford Press, 1992.

9. *NHTSA. Traffic Safety Facts 1999: Older Population.* Washington, DC: NHTSA, 2000.

10. NHTSA. *Traffic Safety Facts 1999: Young Drivers.* Washington, DC: NHTSA, 2000.

11. Mayhew, D.R.; Donelson, A.C.; Beirness, D.J.; and Simpson, H.M. Youth, alcohol and relative risk of crash involvement. *Accid Anal Prev* 18(4):273-287, 1986.

12. Jonah, B.A. Accident risk and risk-taking behaviour among young drivers. *Accid Anal Prev* 18(4):255-271, 1986.

13. Preusser, D.F.; Ferguson, S.A.; and Williams, A.F. Effect of teenage passengers on the fatal crash risk of teenage drivers. *Accid Anal Prev* 30(2):217-222, 1998.

14. *NHTSA. Traffic Safety Facts 1999.* Washington, DC: NHTSA, 2000.

15. Waller, P.F. Alcohol, aging, and driving. In: Gomberg, E.S.L.; Hegedus, A.M.; and Zucker, R.A., ed. *Alcohol Problems and Aging.* NIAAA Research Monograph No. 33. NIH Pub. No. 98-4163. Bethesda, MD: NIAAA, 1998.

16. McGwin, G.; Chapman, V.; and Owsley, C. Visual risk factors for driving difficulty among older drivers. *Accid Anal Prev* 32:735-744, 2000.

17. McKnight, A.J., and Lange, J.E. *Automated screening techniques for drivers with age-related ability deficits.* In: 41st Annual Proceedings: Association for the Advancement of Automotive Medicine. Des Plaines, IL: Association for the Advancement of Automotive Medicine (AAAM), 1997.

18. Roehrs, T.; Beare, D.; Zorick, F.; and Roth, T. Sleepiness and ethanol effects on simulated driving. *Alcohol Clin Exp Res* 18(1):154-158, 1994.

19. Krull, K.R.; Smith, L.T.; Sinha, R.; and Parsons, O.A. Simple reaction time event-related potentials: Effects of alcohol and sleep deprivation. *Alcohol Clin Exp Res* 17(4):771-777, 1993.

20. *NHTSA. Traffic Safety Facts 1999: Alcohol.* National Center for Statistics and Analysis. Washington, DC: NHTSA, 2000.

21. Voas, R.B.; Wells, J.K.; Lestina, D.C.; Williams, A.F.; and Greene, M.A. *Drinking and Driving in the U.S.: The 1996 National Roadside Survey.* NHTSA Traffic Task No. 152. Arlington, VA: Insurance Institute for Highway Safety, 1997.

22. Toomey, T.L.; Rosenfeld, C.; and Wagenaar, A.C. The minimum legal drinking age: History, effectiveness, and ongoing debate. *Alcohol Health Res World* 20(4):213-218, 1996.

23. Wagenaar, A.C.; Murray, D.M.; Gehan, J.P.; et al. Communities mobilizing for change on alcohol: Outcomes from a randomized community trial. *J Stud Alcohol* 61(1):85-94, 2000.

24. Holder, H.D.; Saltz, R.F.; Grube, J.W.; et al. Summing up: Lessons from a comprehensive community prevention trial. *Addict* 92(Suppl. 2):S293-S301, 1997.

25. Voas, R.B.; Lange, J.E.; and Tippetts, A.S. Enforcement of the zero tolerance law in California: A missed opportunity? In: 42nd Annual Proceedings: Association for the Advancement of Automotive Medicine. Des Plaines, IL: *AAAM*, 1998.

26. Hingson, R.; Heeren, T.; and Winter, M. Lower legal blood alcohol limits for young drivers. *Public Health Rep* 109(6):738-744, 1994.

27. Roeper, P.J., and Voas, R.B. Underage drivers are separating drinking from driving. *Am J Public Health* 89(5):755-757, 1999.

28. Voas, R.B.; Tippets, A.S.; and Fell, J. The relationship of alcohol safety laws to drinking drivers in fatal crashes. *Accid Anal Prev* 32:483-492, 2000.

29. Hingson, R.; Heeren, T.; and Winter, M. Effects of Maine's 0.05% legal blood alcohol levels for drivers with DWI convictions. *Public Health Rep* 113(5):440-446, 1998.

30. Hingson, R.; McGovern, T.; Howland, J.; et al. Reducing alcohol impaired driving in Massachusetts: The Saving Lives Program. *Am J Public Health* 86(6):791-797, 1996.

31. Roeper, P.J.; Voas, R.B.; Padilla-Sanchez, L.; and Esteban, R. A long-term community-wide intervention to reduce alcohol related traffic injuries: Salinas, California. Drugs *Educ Prev Policy* 7(1)51-60, 2000.

32. Lange, J.E., and Voas, R.B. Youth escaping limits on drinking: Binging in Mexico. *Addict* 95(4):521-528, 2000.

33. Voas, R.B.; Lange, J.; Tippetts, A.S.; and Johnson, M. "Operation Safe Crossing: Using Science within a Community Intervention." Paper presented at the 15th International Conference on Alcohol, Drugs and Traffic Safety in Stockholm, Sweden, on May 22-26, 2000.

34. DiClemente, C.C.; Bellino, L.E.; and Neavins, T.M. Motivation for change and alcoholism treatment. *Alcohol Res Health* 23(2):86-92, 1999.

35. Gentilello, L.M.; Rivara, F.P.; Donovan, D.M.; et al. Alcohol interventions in a trauma center as a means of reducing the risk of injury recurrence. *Ann Surg* 230(4):473-483, 1999.

36. Monti, P.M.; Colby, S.M.; Barnett, N.P.; et al. Brief intervention for harm reduction with alcohol-positive older adolescents in a hospital emergency department. *J Consult Clin Psychol* 67(6):989-994, 1999.

37. Zador, P.L.; Lund, A.K.; Fields, M.; and Weinberg, K. *Fatal Crash Involvement and Laws against Alcohol-Impaired Driving*. Arlington, VA: Insurance Institute for Highway Safety, 1988.

38. Voas, R.B.; Tippetts, A.S.; and Taylor, E.P. *Impact of Ohio administrative license suspension*. In: 42nd Annual Proceedings: Association for the Advancement of Automotive Medicine. Des Plaines, IL: AAAM, 1998.

39. Voas, R.B.; Tippetts, A.; and Lange, J. Evaluation of a method for reducing unlicensed driving: The Washington and Oregon license plate sticker laws. *Accid Anal Prev* 29(5):627-634, 1997.

40. Voas, R.B.; Tippetts, A.S.; and Taylor, E. Temporary vehicle immobilization: Evaluation of a program in Ohio. *Accid Anal Prev* 29(5):635-642, 1997.

41. Voas, R.; Tippetts, A.; and Taylor, E. Temporary vehicle impoundment in Ohio: A replication and confirmation. *Accid Anal Prev* 30(5):651-656, 1998.

42. Voas, R.B.; Marques, P.R.; Tippetts, A.S.; and Beirness, D.J. Alberta Interlock Program: The evaluation of a province-wide program on DUI recidivism. *Addict* 94(12):1849-1859, 1999.

43. Tashima, H.N., and Helander, C.J. 1999 Annual Report of the California DUI Management Information System. Sacramento, CA: California Department of Motor Vehicles Research and Development Section, 1999.

44. Weinrath, M. Ignition interlock program for drunk drivers: A multivariate test. *Crime Delinquency* 43(1):42-59, 1997.

45. Beck, K.H.; Rauch, W.J.; Baker, E.A.; and Williams, A.F. Effects of ignition interlock license restrictions on drivers with multiple alcohol offenses: A randomized trial in Maryland. *Am J Public Health* 89(11):1696-1700, 1999.

46. Shinar, D., and Compton, R.P. Victim impact panels: Their impact on DWI recidivism. *Alcohol Drugs Driv* 11(1):73-87, 1995.

47. Fors, S.W., and Rojek, D.G. The effect of victim impact panels on DUI/DWI rearrest rates: A twelve-month follow-up. *J Stud Alcohol* 60(4):514-520, 1999.

48. C'de Baca, J.; Lapham, S.C.; Paine, S.; and Skipper, B.J. Victim impact panels: Who is sentenced to attend? Does attendance affect recidivism of first-time DWI offenders? *Alcohol Clin Exp Res* 24(9):1420-1426, 2000.

Additional Information

Insurance Institute for Highway Safety
1005 N. Glebe Road
Suite 800
Arlington, VA 22201
Tel: 703-247-1500
Fax: 703-247-1588
Website: www.highwaysafety.org

Mothers Against Drunk Driving
P.O. Box 541688
Dallas, TX 75354-1688
Toll-Free: 800-GET-MADD (438-6233)
Website: www.madd.org/madd/home

National Commission Against Drunk Driving
1900 L Street, N.W.
Suite 705
Washington, DC 20036
Tel: 202-452-6004
Fax: 202-223-7012
Website: www.ncadd.com

National Highway Traffic Safety Administration
400 7th St. S.W.
Washington, DC 20590
Toll-Free: 888-327-4236
Website: www.nhtsa.dot.gov
E-mail: custservice@nhtsa.dot.gov

Chapter 50

Motorcycle Risks and Safety Guidelines

The 2,862 motorcyclist fatalities in 2000 accounted for 7 percent of all traffic fatalities for the year. An additional 58,000 motorcycle occupants were injured.

- Per vehicle mile traveled in 1999, motorcyclists were 18 times as likely as passenger car occupants to die in a motor vehicle traffic crash and 3 times as likely to be injured.

- In 2000, 38 percent of all motorcycle drivers involved in fatal crashes were speeding. The percentage of speeding involvement in fatal crashes was approximately twice as high for motorcyclists as for drivers of passenger cars or light trucks, and the percentage of alcohol involvement was about 50 percent higher for motorcyclists.

- In 2000, 45 percent of fatally injured motorcycle operators and 52 percent of fatally injured passengers were not wearing helmets at the time of the crash.

- Nearly one out of seven motorcycle operators (15 percent) involved in fatal crashes in 2000 was operating the vehicle with an invalid license at the time of the collision.

"Motorcycles—Traffic Safety Facts 1997," National Highway Traffic Safety Administration; "Motorcycle Safety," DOT HS 807 709 Revised October, 1999; and "Traffic Safety Facts 2000: Motorcycle," U.S. Department of Transportation, DOT HS 809 329, 2001.

485

- Motorcycle operators involved in fatal crashes in 2000 had higher intoxication rates (BAC of 0.10 g/dl or greater) than any other type of motor vehicle driver. The intoxication rate for motorcycle operators involved in fatal crashes was 27 percent.

- NHTSA estimates that helmets saved the lives of 631 motorcyclists in 2000. If all motorcyclists had worn helmets, an additional 382 lives could have been saved.

- More than 100,000 motorcyclists have died in traffic crashes since the enactment of the Highway Safety and National Traffic and Motor Vehicle Safety Act of 1966.

- Per vehicle mile traveled in 1996, motorcyclists were about 15 times as likely as passenger car occupants to die in a motor vehicle traffic crash and about 3 times as likely to be injured.

- Per registered vehicle, the fatality rate for motorcyclists in 1996 was 3.1 times the fatality rate for passenger car occupants. The injury rate for passenger car occupants per registered vehicle was 1.4 times the injury rate for motorcyclists.

- In 1997, motorcyclists accounted for 5 percent of total traffic fatalities, 6 percent of all occupant fatalities, and 2 percent of all occupants injured.

- More than one-half (1,120) of all motorcycles involved in fatal crashes in 1997 collided with another motor vehicle in transport. In two-vehicle crashes, 78 percent of the motorcycles involved were impacted in the front. Only 5 percent were struck in the rear.

- Motorcycles are more likely to be involved in a fatal collision with a fixed object than are other vehicles. In 1997, 29 percent of the motorcycles involved in fatal crashes collided with a fixed object, compared to 23 percent for passenger cars, 18 percent for light trucks, and 8 percent for large trucks.

- Motorcycles are also more likely to be involved in an injury collision with a fixed object than are other vehicles. In 1997, 15 percent of the reported injury crashes involving motorcycles were fixed object crashes, compared to 8 percent for passenger cars, 9 percent for light trucks, and 6 percent for large trucks.

- In 1997, there were 999 two-vehicle fatal crashes involving a motorcycle and another vehicle. In 36 percent (363) of these crashes the other vehicle was turning left while the motorcycle was going straight, passing, or overtaking the vehicle. Both vehicles were going straight in 266 crashes (27 percent).

- Almost half (44 percent) of all motorcyclist fatalities in 1997 resulted from crashes in seven states: 235 in California, 184 in Florida, 117 in Texas, 114 in New York, 106 in Ohio, 84 in Pennsylvania, and 82 in Illinois.

- In 1997, 41 percent of all motorcyclists involved in fatal crashes were speeding, approximately twice the rate for drivers of passenger cars or light trucks. The percentage of alcohol involvement was more than 50 percent higher for motorcyclists than for drivers of passenger vehicles.

Licensing

- Nearly one out of five motorcycle operators (18 percent) involved in fatal crashes in 1997 were operating the vehicle with an invalid license at the time of the collision, while only 11 percent of drivers of passenger vehicles in fatal crashes did not have a valid license.

- Motorcycle operators involved in fatal traffic crashes were nearly twice as likely as passenger vehicle drivers to have a previous license suspension or revocation (20 percent and 12 percent, respectively).

- Almost 6 percent of the motorcycle operators involved in fatal crashes in 1997 had at least one previous conviction for driving while intoxicated on their driver records, compared to about 3 percent of passenger vehicle drivers.

Alcohol

- Motorcycle operators involved in fatal crashes in 1997 had higher intoxication rates, with blood alcohol concentrations (BAC) of 0.10 grams per deciliter (g/dl) or greater, than any other type of motor vehicle driver. Intoxication rates for vehicle operators involved in fatal crashes were 27.9 percent for motorcycles, 20.2 percent for light trucks, 18.2 percent for passenger cars, and 1.1 percent for large trucks.

- In 1997, 28.9 percent of all fatally injured motorcycle operators were intoxicated (BAC 0.10 g/dl or greater). An additional 11.2

percent had lower alcohol levels (BAC 0.01 to 0.09 g/dl). The intoxication rate was highest for fatally injured operators between 35 and 39 years old (43.7 percent), followed by ages 30 to 34 (39.7 percent), and ages 40 to 44 (37.0 percent).

- Almost half (42 percent) of the 876 motorcycle operators who died in single-vehicle crashes in 1997 were intoxicated. Three-fifths (57 percent) of those killed in single-vehicle crashes on weekend nights were intoxicated.

- Motorcycle operators killed in traffic crashes at night were 2.9 times as likely to be intoxicated as those killed during the day (41 percent and 14 percent, respectively).

- The reported helmet use rate for intoxicated motorcycle operators killed in traffic crashes was 50 percent, compared with 61 percent for those who were sober.

Helmets

- NHTSA estimates that helmets saved the lives of 486 motorcyclists in 1997. If all motorcyclists had worn helmets, an additional 266 lives could have been saved.

- Helmets are estimated to be 29 percent effective in preventing fatal injuries to motorcyclists.

- Helmets cannot protect the rider from most types of bodily injuries. However, a NHTSA study showed that motorcycle helmets are 67 percent effective in preventing brain injuries. (Source: 1996 Crash Outcome Data Evaluation System (CODES): Report to Congress on Benefits of Safety Belts and Motorcycle Helmets.)

- According to NHTSA's National Occupant Protection Use Survey, a nationally representative observational survey of motorcycle helmet, safety belt, and child safety seat use, helmet use was 64 percent in 1996. According to previous NHTSA surveys, helmet use was reported to be essentially 100 percent at sites with helmet use laws governing all motorcycle riders, as compared to 34 to 54 percent at sites with no helmet use laws or laws limited to minors.

- Reported helmet use rates for fatally injured motorcyclists in 1997 were 57 percent for operators and 49 percent for passengers, compared with 57 percent and 45 percent, respectively, in 1996.

- All motorcycle helmets sold in the United States are required to meet Federal Motor Vehicle Safety Standard 218, the performance standard which establishes the minimum level of protection helmets must afford each user.

- In 1997, 22 states, the District of Columbia, and Puerto Rico required helmet use by all motorcycle operators and passengers. In another 24 states, only persons under a specific age, usually 18, were required to wear helmets. Three states had no laws requiring helmet use.

- NHTSA estimates that $11.3 billion was saved from 1984 through 1997 because of the use of motorcycle helmets. An additional $9.8 billion would have been saved if all motorcyclists had worn helmets.

Motorcycle Safety

There are over 4 million motorcycles registered in the United States. The popularity of this mode of transportation is attributed to the low initial cost of a motorcycle, its use as a pleasure vehicle and, for some models, the good fuel efficiency. Motorcycle fatalities represent approximately five percent of all highway fatalities each year, yet motorcycles represent just two percent of all registered vehicles in the United States. One of the main reasons motorcyclists are killed in crashes is because the motorcycle itself provides virtually no protection in a crash. For example, approximately 80 percent of reported motorcycle crashes result in injury or death; a comparable figure for automobiles is about 20 percent. An automobile has more weight and bulk than a motorcycle. It has door beams and a roof to provide some measure of protection from impact or rollover. It has cushioning and airbags to soften impact and safety belts to hold passengers in their seats. It has windshield washers and wipers to assist visibility in the rain and snow. An automobile has more stability because it's on four wheels, and because of its size, it is easier to see. A motorcycle suffers in comparison when considering vehicle characteristics that directly contribute to occupant safety. What a motorcycle sacrifices in weight, bulk, and other crashworthiness characteristics is somewhat offset by its agility, maneuverability, ability to stop quickly, and ability to swerve quickly when necessary.

A motorcyclist should attend a motorcycle rider-training course to learn how to safely and skillfully operate a motorcycle. A motorcyclist has to be more careful and aware at intersections, where most motorcycle-vehicle collisions occur. Motorcyclists must remain visible to other motorists at all times. Don't ride in a car's "No Zone" (blind spot). Anticipate what may happen more than other vehicle drivers may. For example, anticipate that drivers backing their cars out of driveways may not see you; and place greater emphasis on defensive driving. Motorcyclists also must be more cautious when riding in inclement weather, on slippery surfaces, or when encountering obstacles on the roadway. They must place greater reliance on their helmet, eye protection, and clothing to increase riding comfort and to reduce the severity of injury should they become involved in a crash. Approximately half of all fatal single-vehicle motorcycle crashes involve alcohol. A motorcycle requires more skill and coordination to operate than a car. Riding a motorcycle while under the influence of any amount of alcohol significantly decreases an operator's ability to operate the motorcycle safely. An estimated 33 percent of motorcycle operators killed in traffic crashes are not licensed or are improperly licensed to operate a motorcycle. By not obtaining a motorcycle operator license, riders are bypassing the only method they and state licensing agencies have to ensure they have the knowledge and skill needed to safely and skillfully operate a motorcycle.

The causes of many motorcycle crashes can be attributed to:

- lack of basic riding skills
- failure to appreciate the inherent operating characteristics
- failure to appreciate the limitations of the motorcycle
- failure to use special precautions while riding
- failure to use defensive driving techniques
- lack of specific braking and cornering skills
- failure to follow speed limits

A motorcycle should be selected for a comfortable fit and functional requirements.

- Select a motorcycle that fits. A motorcyclist should be able to touch the ground with both feet when astride the vehicle.
- If you will be carrying a passenger, make sure the motorcycle you select has a passenger seat as well as footrests (footpegs) for the passenger.

- Check the location of the controls. Make sure you can reach and operate them easily and comfortably.

Functional Requirements

- Buy the power you need, but only as much as you can handle safely. Large motorcycles are heavy, and you must be strong enough to push it, or pick it up if it falls over. But smaller bikes (e.g., a 125cc machine) may not have the speed, performance, and ride you'll need if you plan to travel long distances.

- Consider the primary use of your bike. Don't buy a "trail" bike for highway use. Similarly, don't buy a "highway" bike if most of your riding will be off the road. Some motorcycles are built especially for trail use, with special tires and suspension. Other motorcycles have special characteristics for highway use, such as tires designed to grip pavement, and more powerful braking systems. If you have dual requirements, combination cycles are available that make a compromise between road and trail riding.

- The safe operation of a motorcycle requires different skill and knowledge than is needed for a passenger car.

- Never ride without a certified motorcycle helmet and eye protection.

- Insist on a helmet that has a U.S. Department of Transportation (DOT) label.

- Read your owner's manual thoroughly. Use it to get familiar with your motorcycle. Attend a motorcycle rider-training course. It is the best way to learn how to operate a motorcycle safely and skillfully. Rider-training classes provide unique knowledge and skills that you may not learn if a friend teaches you how to ride.

- Wear the right shoes, gloves, and clothing.

- Thick, protective garb not only provides comfort against the elements, but also may be all there is between you and the pavement in a crash.

After completing a motorcycle training course, practice before going out on the street. Depending on what type of bike you have, find an off-highway area or vacant parking lot and practice until use of all controls becomes automatic and you become thoroughly accustomed to requirements for balance, making turns, stopping, and shifting.

- Remember that a motorcyclist must abide by the same traffic rules and regulations as other motorists. Before taking your motorcycle on a public road, become familiar with traffic rules and regulations and any special requirements for motorcycles.

- Be aware that riding with a passenger requires even more skill than riding alone. Riding with a passenger should be delayed until you have considerable solo riding time and are ready to take on the responsibility of carrying a passenger.

- Obtain your learner's permit or motorcycle endorsement on your driver's license before you venture onto the streets. You will be required to display the knowledge and skill needed to operate a motorcycle safely before being issued a motorcycle operator's license. Never drink and ride. Alcohol slows reflexes and greatly limits your ability to operate a motorcycle. Even a very small amount of alcohol can reduce your ability to operate a motorcycle safely.

Protective Clothing and Equipment

Studies show that the head, arms, and legs are most often injured in a crash. Protective clothing and equipment serve a three-fold purpose for motorcyclists: comfort and protection from the elements; some measure of injury protection; and through use of color or reflective material, a means for other motorists to see the motorcyclist.

Helmet

This is the most important piece of equipment. Safety helmets save lives by reducing the extent of head injuries in the event of a crash. Many good helmets are available. Make sure it fits comfortably and snugly, and is fastened for the ride. In choosing a helmet, look for the DOT label on the helmet. The DOT label on helmets constitutes the manufacturer's certification that the helmet conforms to the federal standard. In many states, use of a helmet is required by law. Passengers should also wear a helmet.

A consumer information brochure on how to choose and care for a motorcycle helmet is available from the National Highway Traffic

Safety Administration, 400 Seventh Street, SW, NTS-22, Washington, DC 20590.

Eye Protection

Since many motorcycles don't have windshields, riders must protect their eyes against insects, dirt, rocks, or other airborne matter. Even the wind can cause the eyes to tear and blur vision, and good vision is imperative when riding. Choose good quality goggles, glasses with plastic or safety lenses, or a helmet equipped with a face shield. Goggles, glasses, and face shields should be scratch free, shatter proof, and well ventilated to prevent fog buildup. Only clear shields should be used at night since tinted shields reduce contrast and make it more difficult to see. Even if your motorcycle has a windshield, eye protection is recommended.

Jackets and Trousers

Clothing worn when riding a motorcycle should provide some measure of protection from abrasion in the event of a spill. These should be of durable material (e.g., special synthetic material or leather). Jackets should have long sleeves. Trousers (not shorts) should not be baggy or flared at the bottom to prevent entanglement with the chain, kick starter, footpegs, or other protrusions on the sides of a motorcycle.

Gloves

Durable gloves are recommended. They should be of the non-slip type to permit a firm grip on the controls. Leather gloves are excellent, as are special fabric gloves with leather palms and grip strips on the fingers. Gauntlet-type gloves keep air out of the rider's sleeves. Appropriate gloves are available for all types of weather.

Footwear

Proper footwear affords protection for the feet, ankles, and lower parts of the legs. Leather boots are best. Durable athletic shoes that cover the ankles are a good second choice. Sandals, sneakers, and similar footwear should not be used since they provide little protection from abrasion or a crushing impact. Avoid dangling laces that can get in the way.

Note: Upper body clothing should be brightly colored. Some riders wear lightweight reflective orange or yellow vests over their jackets.

Retro-reflective material used on clothing, helmet, and the motorcycle helps to make the rider visible to other motorists, especially at night. A high percentage of car-vehicle crashes occur because the driver of the other vehicle "failed to see the rider in time to avoid the crash."

Follow These Rules

- Treat other motorists with courtesy and respect.

- Avoid tailgating.

- Avoid riding between lanes of slow moving or stopped traffic.

- Know and obey traffic laws, including ordinances in your community.

- Avoid excessive noise by leaving the stock muffler in place or using a muffler of equivalent noise reduction.

- Use signals when appropriate.

Be Courteous

The practices of some riders are offensive to other motorists (e.g., weaving in and out of stalled traffic, riding on shoulders). Being inconsiderate of other motorists creates a negative image for all riders, and can cause crashes.

Drive Defensively

- Be especially alert at intersections because approximately 70 percent of motorcycle-vehicle collisions occur there! Watch for vehicles that may unexpectedly turn in front of you or pull out from a side street or driveway. At intersections where vision is limited by shrubbery, parked vehicles, or buildings, slow down, make doubly sure of traffic, and be prepared to react quickly.

- Check the rearview mirrors before changing lanes or stopping. A quick stop without checking rear traffic may result in a rear-end crash. When changing lanes, use signals and make a visual check to assure that you can change lanes safely.

- Watch the road surface and traffic ahead to anticipate problems and road hazards. Road hazards that are minor irritations for an automobile can be a major hazard for a rider. Hazards include potholes, oil slicks, puddles, debris or other objects on the roadway, ruts, uneven pavement, and railroad tracks. Painted roadway markings and manhole covers can be extremely slippery when wet. Go around most hazards. To do so safely, you must be able to spot such hazards from a distance. Slow down before reaching the obstacle and make sure you have enough room before changing direction. Railroad tracks should be crossed at an angle as close to 90 degrees as possible.

- Experienced motorcyclists often have this advice for new riders: "Assume that you are invisible to other motorists and operate your motorcycle accordingly." Position yourself to be seen. Ride in the portion of the lane where it is most likely that you will be seen by other motorists. Avoid the car's "No Zone" (i.e., blind spot). Use your headlights, day and night. All motor vehicles have blind spots where other vehicles cannot be seen with mirrors.

  These blind spots are to the left and right rear of the vehicle. Do not linger in motorists' blind spot. Wear brightly colored, preferably fluorescent, clothing. Use retro-reflective materials on clothing and motorcycle, especially at night.

- Maintain a safe speed consistent with driving conditions and your capabilities. Gravel on the road and slippery road surfaces can be hazardous. Avoid sudden braking or turning.

When riding in the rain, riders find they get better traction by driving in the tracks of vehicles in front of them. But avoid following too closely, and riding on painted lines and metal surfaces such as manhole covers because they offer less traction. If caught in a sudden shower while riding, pull off the highway under some shelter (e.g., overpass) and wait for the rain to stop. If you must ride in the rain, remember that conditions are most dangerous during the first few minutes of rainfall because of oil and other automobile droppings on the roadway. If possible, sit out the beginning of a rain shower.

Don't tailgate, and don't let other drivers tailgate you. Following too closely behind another vehicle may make it difficult for you to brake suddenly. Further, you won't have time to avoid road hazards and traffic situations ahead. If another vehicle is following too closely, wave it off with a hand signal or tap your brake pedal. If they continue to follow too closely, change lanes or pull off the road, and let them pass.

Pass only when it is safe to do so. Do not pass or ride on the shoulder. Pull over to the left third of the lane before passing and make sure that you are at a safe following distance. Use turn signals, and avoid crowding the other vehicle as you pass. Remember to make a head check before changing lanes.

Use brakes wisely. Use both brakes together. Brake firmly and progressively and bring the motorcycle upright before stopping. Remember that driving through water can adversely affect the brakes. After passing through water, look for following traffic, and when safe to do so check your brakes by applying light pressure.

Dogs can be a problem for riders. Don't become distracted and don't kick at a dog. As you approach a dog, downshift, when you reach the dog, accelerate quickly away.

The Owner's Manual

Read the owner's manual from cover to cover. It tells you how to operate your motorcycle, maintain it, and diagnose problems.

Carry the owner's manual and recommended tools and spare parts on your motorcycle. Adhere closely to the manufacturer's recommended maintenance schedule. Before each day's riding, perform a visual and operational check of the motorcycle and its operating systems. Check lights, turn signals, tires, brakes, fuel and oil levels, mirrors, and control cables. Replace broken, worn or frayed cables at once. Lubricate and adjust your chain as prescribed in your owner's manual.

Riders must ride aware, know their limits and ride within them. They must also be aware of and understand their motorcycle's limitations and the environment in which they ride.

Additional Information

Motorcycle Safety Foundation
2 Jenner Street, Suite 150
Irvine, CA 92618
Tel: 949-727-3227
Website: www.msf-usa.org

For location of a RiderCourse nearest you call toll-free: 800-446-9227

Chapter 51

ATV-Related Death and Injury

There was a statistically significant increase in the estimated number of injuries for 2000, up about 12 percent over the number for 1999. The increase occurred across all age categories and is not explained by an increase in ATVs in use.

ATV-related deaths and injuries showed a general decline from the late 1980s through the early 1990s. Since then, however, there has been a gradual increase in both. Statistically significant increases in the estimated number of injuries were found for the last three years.

Characteristics of ATVs and Fatalities

A review of the fatalities indicated that 1,409 victims (35% of the 4,082 total) were under 16 years of age and 602 victims (15% of the total) were under 12 years of age.

The percent of fatalities reported that involved four-wheel ATVs has increased from 7 percent or less prior to 1985 to about 90 percent for 2000. This percent increase is expected since production of the three-wheel vehicle ceased in the mid-1980s.

Estimated Hospital Emergency Room-Treated Injuries

Table 51.2. shows estimates of ATV-related injuries treated in hospital emergency rooms nationwide between 1996 and December 31,

"Annual Report: All-Terrain Vehicle (ATV)-Related Deaths and Injuries," United States Consumer Product Safety Commission, May 2001.

2000. Children under age 16 years accounted for about 40 percent of the total of estimated injuries from January 1, 1985 through December 31, 2000.

The age group 25-34 had the greatest percentage increase, which was about 17 percent more that the group's estimate for 1999. The age group 15 and under showed an increase of about 15 percent. The 35-44 age group increased by approximately 9 percent, while both the 16-24 and 45-54 age groups increased by about 8 percent. The 55 and older age group had the smallest relative increase, 4 percent.

Summary

Estimated numbers of deaths and injuries for all ATVs generally declined from the late 1980s through the early 1990s, thereafter, there is a gradual increase in the number of deaths. Injuries were relatively stable from 1993 through 1997, but showed statistically significant increases for the years 1997-98; 1998-99; and 1999-2000.

Table 51.1. Reported ATV[1]-Related Deaths by Year 1996-December 31, 2000

Year	Number of Deaths
2000[2]	218
1999[2]	296
1998	251
1997	241
1996	247

Source: U.S. Consumer Product Safety Commission, Directorate for Epidemiology, Division of Hazard Analysis.

[1]Unknown number of wheels

[2]Reporting is incomplete

Table 51.2. Annual Estimates of ATV[1]-Related Hospital Emergency Room-Treated Injuries1, January 1, 1996-December 31, 2000.

Year	All Ages	Age <16 Years
2000*	95,300	33,000
1999*	85,000	28,700
1998*	70,200	26,000
1997*	54,600	21,300
1996*	53,600	20,200

[1]Unknown number of wheels

* Estimates adjusted by factors to account for out of scope (non-ATV) cases based on injury surveys in 1997. The adjustment factors were 0.95 for 1990-1996 and 0.935 (amended from 0.984) for 1997 onward.

Table 51.3. Annual ATV-Related Injury Estimates by Calendar Years 1996-2000 by Age Groups

Age Group	1996	1997	1998	1999	2000
Under 16	20,200	21,300	26,000	28,700	33,000
16-24	13,400	14,300	20,000	25,100	27,100
25-34	10,500	9,600	12,200	15,100	17,700
35-44	5,800	5,400	7,700	9,800	10,700
45-54	2,300	2,300	2,800	3,800	4,100
55 and over	1,300	1,700	1,400	2,500	2,500

Source: U.S. Consumer Product Safety Commission (CPSC). Directorate for Epidemiology, Division of Hazard Analysis (EPHA).

Chapter 52

Bicycles, Head Injuries, and Helmet Recommendations

In 2000, 690 pedalcyclists were killed and an additional 51,000 were injured in traffic crashes. Pedalcyclists made up 2 percent of all traffic fatalities and 2 percent of all the people injured in traffic crashes during the year.

- Most of the pedalcyclists injured or killed in 2000 were males (78 percent and 89 percent, respectively), and most were between the ages of 5 and 44 years (87 percent and 65 percent, respectively).

- Almost one-third (27 percent) of the pedalcyclists killed in traffic crashes in 2000 were between 5 and 15 years old.

The Problem

Bicycle-related head injuries account for about:

- 900 deaths per year
- 17,000 hospitalizations

"Traffic Safety Facts 2000: Pedalcyclist," U.S. Department of Transportation, DOT HS 809 329, 2001; "The Problem," National Bike Safety Network Sources: Centers for Disease Control and Prevention (CDC), 1998; "National Bike Helmet Use Survey," Released by McDonald's and the U.S. Consumer Product Safety Commission, April 1999; and "Preventing Bicycle-Related Head Injuries," National Center for Injury Prevention and Control (NCIPC), January 2000.

- 567,000 emergency department visits
- Two-thirds of bicycle-related deaths
- One-third of non-fatal bicycle injuries

There is:

- One head injury death every 15 hours
- One emergency department visit due to head injury every 3 minutes

Cost of bicycle-related head injuries:

- Cost society more than $3 billion in 1991
- 32% of bicycle-related head injury deaths in 1992 were children aged 5-14 years

Age is a factor for bicycle-related injuries and deaths:

- Rate of injury is highest for children aged 5-15 years
- Rate of death is highest for children aged 10-14 years

Gender is a factor for bicycle-related injuries and deaths:

- Males are 2.4 times more likely to be killed per bicycle trip.

Helmet use is a factor. Universal helmet use could:

- Save one life each day
- Prevent one head injury every 4 minutes

Table 52.1. Pedalcyclist Traffic Fatalities, 1990-2000.

Year	Fatalities	Year	Fatalities
1990	859	1996	765
1991	843	1997	814
1992	723	1998	760
1993	816	1999	754
1994	802	2000	690
1995	833		

Helmet Use Survey

- About 50% of all bicycle riders in the U.S. regularly wear bike helmets while riding a bike, according to the first national survey of bike helmet usage patterns since 1991.

- Of the 50% of bikers who regularly wear a bike helmet, 43% said they always wear a helmet and 7% said they wear a helmet more than half the time.

- The percentage of bikers who reported regularly wearing a helmet rose from 18% in 1991 to about 50% of all bike riders in the new survey.

- About 38% of adult bike riders regularly wear a bike helmet; about 69% of children under 16, as reported by their parents, regularly wear a bike helmet while riding a bike.

- Bike helmet ownership among bike riders rose from 27% in 1991 to 60% in the new survey.

- Bike ridership rose 20% from an estimated 66.9 million riders in 1991 to 80.6 million riders in the new survey, or about three times the U.S. population increase over that time period.

- Half of all bike riders, however, do not regularly wear a helmet, which is the single most effective protection against head injury.

The McDonald's Corporation and the U.S. Consumer Product Safety Commission (CPSC) have been working together on a national education campaign to encourage bike riders, especially youngsters, to wear bike helmets. As part of this effort, Yankelovich Partners conducted a national survey of bike helmet usage patterns. This is the first such survey since 1991.

In 1991, CPSC conducted the first national survey of bike helmet usage patterns. The survey reported that 18% of all bike riders wore bike helmets all or more than half of the time. Since then, there has been a heightened awareness of the importance of wearing bike helmets. CPSC's bike helmet safety standard, state helmet laws, public education campaigns, and better-fitting and better-looking bike helmets have all contributed to a climate that encourages helmet use.

To ascertain whether these efforts resulted in more bike riders wearing helmets, Yankelovich Partners conducted this new survey. It is similar in scope and questions to the 1991 CPSC survey.

Bike Helmet Ownership and Use

In the new survey, about 60% of bicyclists reported owning a bicycle helmet (Table 52.2). About 45% of adults reported that they owned a helmet. About 84% of children under 16, as reported by their parents, owned a helmet.

About 50% of all bike riders reported that they regularly wore a bike helmet while riding a bike. This included 43% who said they always wore a helmet and another 7% who said they wore a helmet more than half the time. "Regular" helmet usage is defined as wearing a bike helmet "all or almost all the time" or "more than half the time."

About 38% of adult bike riders reported regularly wearing a bike helmet. About 69% of children under 16, as reported by their parents, regularly wore a bike helmet while riding a bike. In contrast, 43% of all bicyclists reported never or almost never wearing a helmet. Another 7% said they wore a helmet less than half the time.

Reasons for Choosing and Wearing a Bike Helmet

Of those who owned a helmet, 95% said that comfort or fit was an important factor in choosing a bike helmet for themselves or a child (Table 52.4). Safety certification was an important factor for 93%. Ease of strap adjustment also ranked high among bike helmet owners, with 88% citing this as a factor in choosing a helmet. In addition, 70% mentioned cost as an important factor; 64% cited helmet appearance.

Of those bikers who wore a helmet all or some of the time, 98% said they wore a helmet for safety reasons (Table 52.5). In addition, bikers reported that they wore a helmet because a parent or spouse insisted on it (70%), and/or they lived where a law required bike helmet use (44%).

Table 52.2. Riders Who Own a Bicycle Helmet

Response	Percent
Yes	60%
No	40%
Total	100%

Table 52.3. Time Spent Wearing a Helmet

Response	Percent
Always or almost always	43%
More than half the time	7%
Less than half the time	7%
Never or almost never	43%

Reasons for Not Wearing a Bike Helmet

Bikers reported several reasons for not wearing a bike helmet. For those who only sometimes wore a helmet, the major reasons included: riding only a short distance (26%), forgetting to wear a helmet (25%), and feeling that the helmet was uncomfortable (20%) (Table 52.6).

For those who did not own a helmet, the major reasons for not wearing a bike helmet included: they had not gotten around to it (20%), and the helmet was not comfortable (18%) (Table 52.7).

Table 52.4. Reasons for Choosing the Helmet Purchased

Importance of Factors	Very (%)	Somewhat (%)	Not (%)	Unknown (%)
Comfort or Fit	82%	13%	3%	2%
Safety Certification	81%	12%	5%	2%
Ease of Strap Adjustment	54%	34%	10%	2%
Appearance	29%	35%	33%	3%
Cost	26%	44%	28%	2%

Table 52.5. Reasons for Wearing a Helmet All or Some of the Time*

Response	Percent
Safety	98%
Parent or spouse insists	70%
Local legal requirements	44%

*Includes multiple responses

Table 52.6. Reasons for Not Wearing a Helmet All of the Time*

Response	Percent
When riding a short distance	26%
Forgetting to wear it	25%
Helmet uncomfortable	20%

*Includes multiple responses

Table 52.7. Reasons for Not Owning a Helmet*

Response	Percent
Haven't gotten around to it	20%
Helmets are not comfortable	18%
Helmets are unnecessary	11%
Helmets are not attractive	9%
Do not ride very often	7%

*Includes multiple responses

Bike Helmet Use for Other Sports

The bikers surveyed also reported wearing a bike helmet for other sports. Nationally, 20% reported wearing a helmet for other activities. Of this group, most (67%) reported wearing the helmet while in-line skating. Skate boarding was mentioned by 10% of this group.

Bike Riding Patterns

Those interviewed for this survey said they rode bicycles, on average, between six and seven months of the year.

- Most bike riders (61%) said they frequently rode their bikes on neighborhood streets with little traffic.

- Thirty-one percent said they frequently rode on sidewalks or playgrounds.

- Only 10% said they frequently rode on major thoroughfares, highways, or streets with significant traffic.

- Twenty percent said they frequently or sometimes rode bikes at night. However, 80% said they rarely or never rode at night.

Views about Bicycle Deaths and Injuries

Each year, bicycle crashes kill about 900 people; about 200 of those killed are children under age 15. Each year, about 567,000 people go to hospital emergency departments with bicycle-related injuries; about 350,000 of those injured are children under 15. Of those children, about 130,000 suffer head injuries.

In the survey, however, most bikers underestimated the annual number of bicycle-related deaths and emergency department injuries. For example, 72% of those who responded believed there were 500 or fewer bicycle-related deaths every year. Similarly, 96% believed there were fewer than 50,000 bicycle-related injuries treated in hospital emergency departments every year.

Comparisons with 1991 Survey on Bike Helmet Usage

The new survey showed that national bike helmet use rose to about 50% from the 18% reported in the 1991 CPSC survey. Bike helmet ownership rose to 60% from 27% in 1991 (Table 52.8).

Bike ridership also rose. In the new survey, there were an estimated 80.6 million bike riders. This increased from an estimated 66.9

million riders in 1991 (Table 52.8). Over this time period, bike rider-ship increased about 20%, or about three times the 7% population increase of the U.S.

In the new survey, more than 80% of the bike riders with helmets indicated that comfort or fit and safety certification were very important factors in choosing a bike helmet. In 1991, 77% listed comfort and 75% listed safety certification as very important factors.

In the new survey, 98% cited safety as a reason for wearing a helmet when riding a bike, and 70% mentioned having family members, such as a parent or spouse, insist upon use of a bike helmet (Table 52.9). In the 1991 survey, more than 90% mentioned safety and family members' insistence upon using a helmet as an important reason for wearing a helmet.

In the new survey, 44% cited living where a law required bike helmet use. In 1991, only 12% cited a legal requirement as a reason for wearing a bike helmet (Table 52.9).

For those who did not have a helmet, 11% said that helmets were not necessary in the new survey (Table 52.10). In 1991, 21% said that helmets were unnecessary. In the new survey, only 3% said that helmets were too expensive or that they could not afford one. In 1991, 8% felt that helmets were too expensive.

Table 52.8. Comparisons with 1991 Survey

Response	1991	1998
Helmet use	18%	50%
Helmet ownership	27%	60%
Number of bike riders	66.9 million	80.6 million

Table 52.9. Reasons for Wearing a Helmet All or Some of the Time, 1991 and 1998*

Response	1991	1998
Safety	94%	98%
Parent or spouse insists	93%	70%
Local legal requirement	12%	44%

*Includes multiple responses

Table 52.10. Reasons for Not Owning a Helmet, 1991 and 1998

Response	1991	1998
Helmets are unnecessary	21%	11%
Helmets are too expensive	8%	3%
Never thought about it	21%	10%

Description of Bike Riders Surveyed

- According to the new survey, 80.6 million people rode a bicycle during the preceding year.

- Approximately one-half (49%) of those interviewed lived in suburban neighborhoods. The other half was split between urban (27%) and rural (24%) areas. Twenty-three percent lived in the West, 27% lived in the Midwest, 30% lived in the South, and 20% lived in the Northeast.

- Helmet usage and helmet ownership were highest among those who lived in the Northeast and West and lowest in the Midwest.

- Fifty-two percent of those interviewed had a college bachelor's degree or higher. Of those who regularly wore helmets, 57% had a bachelor's degree or higher.

- Of those who responded to the question about annual household income, 57% made more than $45,000 per year and 35% made more than $60,000 per year. Household incomes were not much higher for those who regularly wore helmets: 60% of these households made more than $45,000 and 36% made more than $60,000.

- Of the bike riders surveyed, 51% were male. Sixty-two percent were 16 years or older. About three-quarters identified themselves as Caucasian. Ten percent identified themselves as African-American, 6% as Hispanic, and 1% as Asian. Seven percent were from another ethnic background or did not respond to the question.

Description of New Bike Helmet Survey

The new survey was based on telephone interviews completed with a nationally representative sample of 1,020 bicycle riders in the United

States. The survey employed a single stage list-assisted random-digit-dialing sample design and was conducted by Yankelovich Partners, an experienced and well-known marketing research firm headquartered in Connecticut.

The survey focused on the current helmet usage patterns of bicycle riders in the United States: how many riders own helmets, the frequency of use, and the reasons riders do or do not use helmets. The survey also collected information about the characteristics of riders (e.g., age, gender, and experience) and their riding patterns (e.g., how much they ride, where they ride).

Yankelovich Partners developed the questionnaire during the summer of 1998. In order to evaluate helmet usage patterns over time, the survey's helmet questions were designed to be similar to those asked in the 1991 CPSC bicycle survey.

The survey was conducted during August 1998. When households were reached, respondents were asked how many household members had ridden a bicycle during the last year. Each of the riders was a potential respondent. If there was more than one rider, one was selected to be interviewed. This was done by selecting the rider with (alternately) the most recent or the next birthday. If the selected rider was under 16, a parent or guardian was asked to respond on the child's behalf.

Attempts were made to contact about 11,000 U.S. households. Of the 3,347 households contacted, 1,069 had at least one bicycle rider in the household. Interviews were completed with a total of 1,020 respondents. The sample was weighted to make population projections of bicycle riders in the continental United States.

Preventing Bicycle-Related Head Injuries

What Can Be Done?

- Riders should wear bicycle helmets **every time they ride**.

- In the event of a crash, wearing a bicycle helmet reduces the risk of serious head injury by as much as 85% and the risk for brain injury by as much as 88%.[6] Helmets have also been shown to reduce the risk of injury to the upper and mid-face by 65%.[7] In fact, if each rider wore a helmet, an estimated 500 bicycle-related fatalities and 151,000 nonfatal head injuries would be prevented each year—that's one death per day and one injury every four minutes.[8]

- Unfortunately, estimates on helmet usage suggest that only 25% of children ages 5-14 years wear a helmet when riding.[9] The percentage is close to zero when looking at teen riders. Children and adolescents' most common complaints are that helmets are not fashionable, or "cool," their friends don't wear them, and/or they are uncomfortable (usually too hot). Riders also convey that they do not think about the importance of bike helmets, nor about the need to protect themselves from injury, particularly if they are not riding in traffic.

- Accordingly, the national health goal for 2010 is for 50% of teenage bicyclists in 9th-12th grade to wear wear helmets.[10]

Strategies Available to Get Bicyclists to Wear Helmets

- The primary strategies to increase bike helmet use include education, legislation, and helmet distribution programs. Educational programs have been conducted in different communities and schools around the nation, with generally positive results. The most successful programs are multifaceted and often multi-site campaigns that combine education with helmet giveaways or discount programs and state or local legislation requiring helmet use.

- Some evidence suggests that legislative efforts are more cost-effective than school- or community-based programs.[11]

How Many States Have Bicycle Helmet Laws?

By early 1999, 15 states and more than 65 local governments had enacted some form of bicycle helmet legislation. Most of these laws pertain to children and adolescents.[13]

What Standards Exist to Ensure That Helmets Are Truly Protective?

The U.S. Consumer Product Safety Commission issued a new safety standard for bike helmets in 1999. The new standard ensures that bike helmets will adequately protect the head and that chin straps will be strong enough to prevent the helmet from coming off in a crash, collision, or fall. In addition, helmets intended for children up to age five must cover a larger surface of the head than before. All bike helmets made or imported into the United States must meet the CPSC standard.[14]

How Can You Help Prevent Injuries While Bicycling?

- Wear a bicycle helmet every time you ride. A bicycle helmet is a necessity, not an accessory.

- Wear your bicycle helmet correctly. A bicycle helmet should fit comfortably and snugly, but not too tightly. It should sit on top of your head in a level position, and it should not rock forward and back or from side to side. Always keep the helmet straps buckled.

- Only buy a bicycle helmet if it meets or exceeds the safety standards developed by the U.S. Consumer Product Safety Commission.

- Learn the rules of the road and obey all traffic laws. Ride with the traffic, on the right side of the road. Use appropriate hand signals. Respect traffic signals, which are meant for riders as well as drivers. Stop at all intersections, not just those intersections with pedestrian markings. Stop and look both ways before entering a street.

- Children should not ride in the street until they are 10 years old, demonstrate good riding skills, and are able to observe the basic rules of the road. And, of course, children should always wear helmets when they ride.

References

1. *NHTSA Traffic Safety Facts, 1997: Bicyclists*. Washington, D.C.: National Highway Traffic Safety Administration

2. Insurance Institute for Highway Safety (IIHS). *1997 Fatality Facts: Bicycles*. Arlington (VA): IIHS, 1997.

3. U.S. Consumer Product Safety Commission. *National Electronic Injury Surveillance System (NEISS)*. Washington, DC: Consumer Product Safety Commission; 1997.

4. Sosin DM, Sacks JJ, Webb KW. Pediatric head injuries and deaths from bicycling in the United States. *Pediatrics* 1996;98(5):868-70.

5. U.S. Consumer Products Safety Commission (CPSC). *Bicycle-related head injury or death*. Washington (DC): CPSC, 1994.

6. Thompson RS, Rivara FP, Thompson DC. A case-control study of the effectiveness of bicycle safety helmets. *N Engl J Med.* 1989; 320:1361-7.

7. Thompson DC, Nunn ME, Thompson RS, Rivara FP. Effectiveness of bicycle safety helmets in preventing serious facial injury. *JAMA* 1996; 276:1974-1975.

8. Sacks JJ, Holmgreen P, Smith S, Sosin D. Bicycle-associated head injuries and deaths in the United States from 1984-1988. *JAMA* 1991;266:3016-8.

9. Sacks JJ, Kresnow M, Houston B, Russell J. Bicycle helmet use among American children, 1994. *Injury Prevention* 1996;2:258-62.

10. Public Health Service (PHS). *Healthy People 2010 Objectives: Draft for Public Comment*. Washington (DC): US Department of Health and Human Services, PHS; 1999.

11. Hatziandreu EJ, Sacks JJ, Brown R, Taylor WR, Rosenberg ML, Graham JD. The cost effectiveness of three programs to increase use of bicycle helmets among children. *Public Health Reports* 1995 May-Jun;110(3):251-9.

12. CDC. Injury Control Recommendations: Bicycle Helmets. *MMWR* 44(RR-1)1995.

13. Bicycle Helmet Safety Institute (BHSI). *Mandatory helmet laws: summary*. Arlington (VA): BHSI, 1997.

14. Federal Register. U. S. Consumer Product Safety Commission. *Safety standard for bicycle helmets; Final rule*. FR Doc. 98-4214, February 13, 1998.

Chapter 53

Pedestrian Safety

The Extent of the Problem

In 2000, 78,000 pedestrians were injured and 4,739 were killed in traffic crashes in the United States, representing 2 percent of all the people injured in traffic crashes and 11 percent of all traffic fatalities.

- On average, a pedestrian is killed in a motor vehicle crash every 111 minutes, and one is injured every 7 minutes.

- Alcohol involvement—either for the driver or the pedestrian—was reported in 47 percent of the traffic crashes that resulted in pedestrian fatalities. Of the pedestrians involved, 31 percent were intoxicated. The intoxication rate for the drivers involved was only 13 percent. In 5 percent of the crashes, both the driver and the pedestrian were intoxicated.

- Pedestrian fatalities are the second-leading cause of motor vehicle-related deaths, following occupant fatalities. Pedestrian-related fatalities account for about 13% of all motor vehicle-related deaths.[2]

- Hit-and-run pedestrian crashes account for one out of every six pedestrian deaths.[2]

"Traffic Safety Facts 2000: Pedestrians," U.S. Department of Transportation, DOT HS 809 329, 2001; "Walking Safety," SafeUSA, 1998; and "Pedestrian Injury Prevention," National Center for Injury Prevention & Control (NCIPC), 2000.

513

Is the Pedestrian Injury Problem Getting Any Better?

The situation is improving. Pedestrian deaths, expressed as a rate per 100,000 people, have decreased 43% from 1975 to 1998.[2] Factors contributing to this decrease may include more and better sidewalks, pedestrian paths, playgrounds away from streets, one-way traffic flow, and restricted on-street parking.[3] Some of the reduction is likely due to the decreasing amount of time Americans spend walking.

What Is the Role of Alcohol in Pedestrian Injuries?

- Alcohol is a major factor in adult pedestrian deaths. In 1998, about one-third of pedestrians 16 years of age or older who were killed by a motor vehicle were legally intoxicated with blood alcohol concentrations (BAC) of 0.10 % or more.[1] Looking only at nighttime crashes, the percentage of pedestrians who were legally intoxicated jumps to 52%.[2]

- In 46% of traffic crashes that resulted in a pedestrian fatality during 1998, either the driver or the pedestrian had a measurable blood alcohol level.[1]

What Age Groups Are at Greatest Risk for Pedestrian Injury?

Children

Children are at risk for pedestrian injuries and fatalities. In 1998, children 15 years and younger represented 23% of the total population and accounted for 30% of all nonfatal pedestrian injuries, 11% of all pedestrian fatalities, and 18% of non-traffic related fatalities (this includes incidents in driveways and other non-public roads).[1,4] Among children between the ages of 5 and 9 who were killed in traffic crashes, 25% were pedestrians.[1]

Older Adults

In 1998, adults 70 years and older comprised 9% of the population and accounted for 18% of all pedestrian fatalities. The death rate for this group, 4.57 per 100,000 people, is the highest of any age group.[1]

Males

In 1998, the pedestrian fatality rate for males was more than twice that for females. Non-fatal injury rates for male pedestrians were also higher; the pedestrian injury rate, per 100,000 people, was 31 for males and 21 for females.[1]

People of Color

In 1997, the pedestrian fatality rate for blacks was nearly twice that for whites; for American Indian and Native Alaskan populations, the fatality rate was close to three times the rate for whites.[4] Researchers believe that these rate differences are due, in part, to differences in walking patterns. The Nationwide Personal Transportation Survey in 1995 found that blacks walk 82% more than whites.[5] Environmental and socioeconomic factors are also likely contributors to these rate differences.

When Are Pedestrian Injuries Most Likely to Occur?

- In 1998, more pedestrian fatalities occurred on Fridays and Saturdays than on any other day of the week.[1]

- In 1998, 46% of pedestrian deaths occurred between 6:00 p.m. and midnight.[2] Among children under 16 years old, 44% of the pedestrian fatalities in 1998 occurred between 4:00 and 8:00 p.m.[1]

Where Do Most Pedestrian Deaths Occur?

Urban areas

In 1998, 69% of pedestrian deaths occurred in urban areas.[1] Case fatality rates, however, are higher in rural areas—for nearly all age groups. Researchers have suggested that these higher fatality rates may be due to higher driving speeds (greater impact during a crash), and less immediate access to emergency medical care.[6,7]

Intersections

In 1998, 38% of pedestrian deaths among people 65 years and older and 14% of pedestrian deaths among children 4 years old and younger took place at an intersection.[2]

What Are the National Objectives with Regard to Injuries among Pedestrians?

According to *Healthy People 2010*, written by the U.S. Department of Health and Human Services in cooperation with many other federal agencies:

- The objective is to "reduce pedestrian deaths on public roads" to no more than 1 per 100,000 people.[8] In 1998, the rate was 1.93 per 100,000 population (for all pedestrian deaths).[1]

- A second pedestrian-related objective is to "reduce nonfatal pedestrian injuries on public roads" to 21 per 100,000 people.[8] In 1998, the rate was 26 per 100,000 population (for all pedestrian nonfatal injuries).[1]

What Are Some Appropriate Public Health and Environmental Strategies to Reduce Pedestrian Deaths?

- Physically separate pedestrians from motor vehicle traffic by putting up physical barriers, using pedestrian bridges, overpasses, underpasses, traffic islands, and other similar measures.

- Design communities that favor pedestrian access (e.g., more sidewalks and pedestrian malls) and combine residential, work, and shopping areas into close geographic units. Such proximity would decrease residents' reliance on motor vehicles for daily errands and activities.

- Adopt traffic calming measures, such as narrow streets and street corners that have shorter radii, making motor vehicle traffic slower and more orderly. Time intersection crossing signals to allow longer periods of time for pedestrians to cross the intersection.

- Lower posted speed limits on streets with heavy pedestrian traffic, and enhance enforcement. Pass laws restricting the legal blood alcohol concentration of pedestrians and continue to enforce existing DUI laws for drivers.

- Improve pedestrian visibility for drivers (e.g., better reflective clothing, personal lights, and street lighting).

- Encourage people of all ages to walk rather than drive—for their physical health, to protect the environment, and to reduce the number of cars on the street.

- Improve or maintain careful adult supervision of young children crossing the street.

- Incorporate pedestrian skills training into school health education curriculum.

- Relocate bus stops to areas with less traffic, and hire crossing guards and escorts to assist young children.[9]

Walking Safety

Adults should supervise children as they cross the street and teach them to look left-right-left again before crossing a street and to keep looking as they cross. You greatly reduce the chances of getting injured as a pedestrian if you follow these simple safety tips:

- Supervise young children and do not leave them alone to play, especially near a street or the driveway.

- Make sure that the children's play area is at least 200 feet from any dangerous area (such as a street, driveway, a vacant lot, or water). If it is within 200 feet, the play area should be fenced.

- Obey the school safety patrol, crossing guard, or police officer when walking near a school.

- Teach children to cross streets at a corner, use crosswalks (whenever possible), and obey the traffic signals. Teach them to check for approaching vehicles before crossing even with the green light or "walk" sign on.

- Make sure children under age 10 are supervised when crossing the street. You may also need to supervise older children, especially when they cross streets with heavy traffic or more than two lanes.

- Teach children to look left-right-left again before crossing a street and to keep looking as they cross. Practice this behavior with them until they master it.

- Teach children to walk facing on-coming traffic if no sidewalks are available.

- Wear light-colored clothing if walking at dawn, at dusk, or after dark. Even better, wear reflective tape (placed diagonally across the back) and carry a flashlight.

- Make sure that doors leading to the outside of the house, including garage doors, cannot be opened by young children. This is to prevent children from getting out of the house unnoticed by their parents and being injured in traffic.

- Do not drink alcohol and walk near traffic.

- As a driver, take extra care to look out for children who might enter the road unexpectedly.

Who Is Affected?

Walking is a great way to get exercise and simply to get around. Unfortunately, walking is not always safe. In 1997, more than 5,000 pedestrians were killed in traffic-related incidents in the United States. Most were young children, the elderly, and persons who were intoxicated. These deaths among children are highest in the five- to nine-year-old age group and are higher among boys than girls. In fact, in 1996 pedestrian injury deaths were the fourth leading cause of death overall for children aged.[5-9]

In 1997, at least 77,000 pedestrians were injured but did not die. Of these, roughly 26,000 were children under the age of 16. Child pedestrians tend to sustain more serious injuries to the head and neck than adults, in part because of children's smaller size.

How children are injured as pedestrians varies by age. For example:

- Toddlers' pedestrian injuries are mainly from being run over by a driver backing a vehicle in the driveway. Toddlers' small size makes them difficult for drivers to see, especially if they are playing behind the vehicle.

- Preschoolers' injuries are typically from darting out between two parked cars on a residential street. Children this small are easily hidden from the view of drivers by parked cars, trucks, or bushes. Preschool children often are not able to judge distances and vehicle speeds accurately.

- Pedestrian injuries among children ages 6-12 mainly occur from collisions with a car in the middle of the block and on busy streets. Many parents overestimate their children's street-crossing ability. The truth is that many elementary-school-aged children still don't understand traffic signals and patterns and can confuse left and right when crossing a street. Also, adult drivers often incorrectly assume that a child always will yield the right-of-way.

Among adults, alcohol use is a major reason for pedestrian deaths. One-third of all fatally injured pedestrians aged 16 and older have blood alcohol concentrations (BACs) above the legal limit. The situation worsens at night. More than half of all adult pedestrians killed at night have BACs above the legal limit.

References

1. *NHTSA Traffic Safety Facts, 1998: Pedestrians.* Washington, DC: National Highway Traffic Safety Administration, 1999. DOT HS 808 958. Available: www.nhtsa.dot.gov/people/ncsa/pdf/Ped98.pdf, January 7, 2000.

2. Insurance Institute for Highway Safety (IIHS). *Safety Facts: Pedestrians.* Arlington (VA): IIHS, 1999. Available: www.iihs.org/safety_facts/fatality_facts/peds.htm, January 7, 2000.

3. National Highway Traffic Safety Administration. *Traffic safety facts, 1997.* Washington, DC: Department of Transportation, National Highway Traffic Safety Administration, 1998.

4. National Center for Health Statistics (NCHS). National Mortality Data, 1997. Hyattsville (MD): NCHS 1998.

5. US Department of Transportation, Federal Highway Administration, Office of Highway Policy Information. *Our nation's travel: 1995 NPTS Early Results Report,* 1997. Washington, DC: US Department of Transportation, Federal Highway Administration, 1997; report no. FHWA-PL-97-028. Available at www-cta.ornl.gov/npts, April 1999.

6. Mueller BA; Rivara FP; Bergman AB. Urban-rural location and the risk of dying in a pedestrian-vehicle collision. *Journal of Trauma-Injury Infection & Critical Care* 1988;28(1):91-4.

7. Baker, S.P.; O'Neill, B.; Ginsberg, M.; and Li, G. 1991. *The injury fact book* (2nd edition). New York, NY: Oxford University Press.

8. U.S. Department of Health and Human Services. *Healthy People 2010*. Washington (DC): January 2000.

9. Stevenson MR, Sleet DA. Which prevention strategies for child pedestrian injuries? A review of the literature. *Community Health Education* 1996-97;16(3):207-17.

Part Eight

Recreation-Related Injuries and Prevention

Chapter 54

Water Accidents and Safety Guidelines

Drowning

How Large Is the Problem of Unintentional Drowning in the United States?

- In 1998, 4,406 people drowned, including 1,003 children younger than 15 years old.[1]

- In 1992, the U.S. Coast Guard received reports of 6,000 crashes involving recreational boats that resulted in 3,700 injuries and 816 deaths.[2]

Which Groups of People Are More Likely to Drown?

Children: Drowning is the second leading cause of injury-related death for children (aged 1 through 14 years), accounting for 940 deaths in 1998.[1]

Males: In 1998, males comprised 81% of people who drowned in the United States.[1]

This chapter includes "Drowning Prevention," National Center for Injury Prevention and Control (NCIPC), October 2000; "CPSC Warns Backyard Pools Can Be a Fatal Attraction to Toddlers," U.S. Consumer Product Safety Commission (CPSC), June 11, 2001; and "Boating Under the Influence," Office of Boating Safety, U.S. Coast Guard, 2001.

Blacks: In 1998, the overall age-adjusted drowning rate for blacks was 1.6 times higher than for whites. Black children ages 5 through 19 years drowned at 2.5 times the rate of whites.[1] Black children ages 1 through 4 years had a lower drowning rate than white children, largely because drowning in that age group typically occurs in residential swimming pools, which are not as accessible to minority children in the United States.[1,3,4]

Where Do Childhood Drownings Occur Most Often?

Most children drown in swimming pools. According to the U.S. Consumer Product Safety Commission (CPSC), emergency departments reported that among children younger than 5 years old, about 320 fatal drownings in 1991 and nearly 2,300 non-fatal near-drownings in 1993 occurred in residential swimming pools. Between 60%-90% of drownings among children aged 0-4 years occur in residential pools; more than half of these occur at the child's own home. Compared with in-ground pools without four-sided fencing, 60% fewer drownings occur in in-ground pools with four-sided isolation fencing.[5]

Drowning Is a Leading Cause of Death to Children Under 5

About 350 children under 5-years-old drown in pools each year nationwide, and over half of these incidents occur in June, July, and August. Among unintentional injuries, drowning is the second leading cause of death to this age group after motor vehicle incidents. Another 2,600 children are treated in hospital emergency rooms each year for near-drowning incidents. Most of these cases involve residential pools. The U.S. Consumer Product Safety Commission (CPSC) wants to reduce the number of children drowning.

Many people assume that, at a residence with a pool, the danger of drowning occurs only when the family is outside or using the pool. But, a common scenario takes place when young children leave the house without a parent or caregiver realizing it. Children are drawn to water, not knowing the terrible danger pools can pose.

"Drowning happens quickly and silently, often without any splashing or screaming," said CPCS Chairman Ann Brown. "It can occur in just the couple of minutes it takes to answer the telephone."

The key to preventing these tragedies is to have layers of protections. This includes placing barriers around your pool to prevent access, using pool alarms, closely supervising your child, and being prepared in case of an emergency. CPSC offers these tips to prevent drowning:

- Fences and walls should be at least 4 feet high and installed completely around the pool. Fence gates should be self-closing and self-latching. The latch should be out of a small child's reach.

- If your house forms one side of the barrier to the pool, then doors leading from the house to the pool should be protected with alarms that produce a sound when a door is unexpectedly opened.

- A power safety cover—a motor-powered barrier that can be placed over the water area—can be used when the pool is not in use.

- Keep rescue equipment by the pool and be sure a phone is poolside with emergency numbers posted. Knowing cardiopulmonary resuscitation (CPR) can be a lifesaver.

- For above-ground pools, steps and ladders to the pool should be secured and locked, or removed when the pool is not in use.

- If a child is missing, always look in the pool first. Seconds count in preventing death or disability.

- Pool alarms can be used as an added precaution. Underwater pool alarms generally perform better and can be used in conjunction with pool covers. CPSC advises that consumers use remote alarm receivers so the alarm can be heard inside the house or in other places away from the pool area.

How Often Is Alcohol Use Involved in Drowning?

Alcohol use is involved in about 25%-50% of adolescent and adult deaths associated with water recreation. It is a major contributing factor in up to 50% of drownings among adolescent boys.[6,7]

What Can Government Agencies Do to Prevent Drowning?

- Mandate and enforce legal limits for blood alcohol levels during water recreation activities.

- Provide public service announcements about the danger of combining alcohol with water recreation.

- Eliminate advertisements that encourage alcohol use during boating.

- Restrict the sale of alcohol at water recreation facilities.

How Can People Guard Against Drowning?

You can greatly reduce the chances of you or your children becoming drowning or near-drowning victims by following a few simple safety tips:

- Whenever young children are swimming, playing, or bathing in water, make sure an adult is *constantly* watching them. By definition this means that the supervising adult should not read, play cards, talk on the phone, mow the lawn, or do any other distracting activity while watching children.

- Never swim alone or in unsupervised places. Teach children to always swim with a buddy.

- Keep small children away from buckets containing liquid: 5-gallon industrial containers are a particular danger. Be sure to empty buckets when household chores are done.

- Never drink alcohol during or just before swimming, boating, or water skiing. Never drink alcohol while supervising children.

Table 54.1. States with the Highest Rates of Unintentional Drowning per 100,000 population* (1998)[1]

State	Number of people drowned	Rate per 100,000 persons (1996)
Alaska	47	7.41
Mississippi	95	3.47
Louisiana	129	3.03
Idaho	34	2.90
Florida	396	2.64
Alabama	112	2.60
Arkansas	59	2.53
Hawaii	33	2.53
South Carolina	92	2.49
Oregon	76	2.38
United States	4,406	1.65

*Ranking based on age-adjusted rate.

Source: NCHS 2000 Vital Statistics System

Teach teenagers about the danger of drinking alcohol and swimming, boating, or water skiing.

- To prevent choking, never chew gum or eat while swimming, diving, or playing in water.

- Learn to swim. Enroll yourself and/or your children aged 4 and older in swimming classes. Swimming classes are not recommended for children under age 4.

- Learn CPR (cardio-pulmonary resuscitation). This is particularly important for pool owners and individuals that regularly participate in water recreation.

- *Do not use* air-filled swimming aids (such as "water wings") in place of life jackets or life preservers with children. These can give parents and children a false sense of security and increase the risk of drowning.

- Check the water depth before entering. The American Red Cross recommends 9 feet as a minimum depth for diving or jumping.

If you have a swimming pool at your home:

- Install a four-sided, isolation pool-fence with self-closing and self-latching gates around the pool. The fence should be at least 4 feet tall and completely separate the pool from the house and play area of the yard.

- Prevent children from having direct access to a swimming pool.

- Install a telephone near the pool. Know how to contact local emergency medical services. Post the emergency number, 911, in an easy to see place.

- Learn CPR.

Additional Tips for Open Water

- Know the local weather conditions and forecast before swimming or boating. Thunderstorms and strong winds can be extremely dangerous to swimmers and boaters.

- Restrict activities to designated swimming areas, which are usually marked by buoys.

- Be cautious, even with lifeguards present.

- Use U.S. Coast Guard-approved personal flotation devices (life jackets) when boating, regardless of distance to be traveled, size of boat, or swimming ability of boaters.

- Remember that open water usually has limited visibility, and conditions can sometimes change from hour to hour. Currents are often unpredictable—they can move rapidly and quickly change direction. A strong water current can carry even expert swimmers far from shore.

- Watch for dangerous waves and signs of rip currents—water that is discolored, unusually choppy, foamy, or filled with debris.

- If you are caught in a rip current, swim parallel to the shore. Once you are out of the current, swim toward the shore.

References

1. National Center for Health Statistics (NCHS). National Mortality Data, 1998. Hyattsville (MD): NCHS 2000.

2. US Coast Guard Boating Statistics, 1992. Washington, DC: US Department of Transportation (COMDTPUB P16754.8).

3. Branche CM. What is happening with drowning rates in the United States? In: JR Fletemeyer and SJ Freas (eds). *Drowning: New perspectives on intervention and prevention.* Boca Raton, Florida: CRC Press LLC, 1999.

4. Branche-Dorsey CM, Russell JC, Greenspan AI, Chorba TC. Unintentional injuries: the problems and some preventive strategies. In: IL Livingston (ed). *Handbook of Black American Health: The mosaic of conditions, issues, policies and prospects.* Westport, CT: Greenwood Publishing Group, 1994.

5. US Consumer Product Safety Commission Clearinghouse, Washington DC, (301) 504-0424.

6. National Safety Council, 1993. *Accident Facts, 1993* Ed. Itasca, Illinois: Author.

7. Howland J, Hingson R. Alcohol as a risk factor for drowning: a review of the literature (1950-1985). *Accident Analysis and Prevention* 1988;20:19-25.

Boating Under the Influence of Alcohol

Boating under the influence (BUI) of alcohol is illegal. That said, while 76 million people enjoy boating on America's waterways each year, many are not aware of the very real, life threatening dangers associated with consuming alcohol and boating. To help reduce the incidents of BUI, the United States Coast Guard (USCG) has initiated a major, nationwide campaign to warn Americans about the dangers of alcohol consumption and boating.

Liquor Is Quicker on the Water

Alcohol, with its well-known ability to impair performance, creates an even more hazardous situation when added to the stress of the marine environment. This is because the marine environment—the fluid base, motion, vibration, engine noise, and elements of sun, wind, and spray—accelerates impairment. The operator's coordination, judgment, and reaction time are reduced by fatigue caused by these stressors. A boat operator with a blood alcohol concentration above 10 percent is estimated to be more than 10 times as likely to be killed in a boating accident than boat operators with zero blood alcohol concentration. Further, alcohol can be more treacherous for boaters since they are less experienced and less confident on the water than on the highway. Recreational boaters do not have the advantage of experiencing daily operation of a boat. In fact, boaters average only about 110 hours of boating in a whole year. And in areas with seasonal boating, there can be months between boating outings or fishing trips.

Effects of Alcohol Consumption

Add boating stressors to those usual factors resulting from drinking alcohol, and a truly perilous condition is present. Drinking alcohol produces certain physiological responses that directly affect safety and well being.

- Judgment and skills deteriorate, affecting peripheral vision, balance, and ability to process information.

- Physical performance and reaction time are reduced.

- Alcohol reduces depth perception, night vision, focus, and the ability to distinguish colors, especially red and green.

- Alcohol consumption can result in inner ear disturbance, which can make it impossible for a person suddenly immersed in water to distinguish up from down.

- Alcohol creates a sense of warmth and may prevent a person in cold water from getting out before hypothermia sets in.

Boating Under the Influence (BUI) Is Illegal Nationwide

It is unlawful in every State to operate a boat while under the influence of alcohol or drugs. In addition to State BUI laws, there is also a Federal law, enforced by the Coast Guard, prohibiting BUI. This law applies to all boats, including foreign vessels in U.S. waters and U.S. vessels on the high seas.

Penalties for BUI Are Severe

The Coast Guard and every State have stringent penalties for violation of BUI laws, including the possibility of not only a large fine, suspension or revocation of operator privileges, but perhaps a jail term. The Coast Guard and the States, in a mutual effort to remove impaired boat operators from the water, cooperate fully. In sole State waters, States have authority to enforce their own BWI statutes. Within State waters that are also subject to the jurisdiction of the U.S., there is concurrent jurisdiction. If, in these waters, a boater is apprehended under Federal law, the Coast Guard will, unless precluded by State law, request that State enforcement officers assume custody of an intoxicated boater.

What Will Happen to the Impaired Operator?

When the Coast Guard determines that an operator is impaired, the voyage will be terminated. The vessel will be brought to mooring either by Coast Guard tow, a member of the Coast Guard crew, or a competent, sober person on board of the recreational vessel. Depending on the circumstances, the operator may then be arrested, detained until sober, or turned over to State or local authorities.

Threefold Approach

Because operating a boat under the influence is so dangerous, the Coast Guard is using a threefold approach to reducing alcohol-related accidents:

- Improved law enforcement in cooperation with the States.

- An improved accident reporting system to identify alcohol-related accidents.

- Widespread education and public awareness of the dangers of alcohol. Every boater, whether an operator or passenger, should cooperate in spreading this word.

Boating Safety Education

Throughout the country each year, over 2,000 safe boating courses are offered by groups such as the U.S. Coast Guard Auxiliary, the U.S. Power Squadrons, the American Red Cross, and individual States. Courses cover many aspects of boating safety—from boat handling to reading the weather. All courses include knowledge and warning about alcohol and boating. For more information on finding a course near you that will fit your schedule—call the toll-free U.S. Coast Guard Infoline at 1-800-368-5647 or view Boating Safety Courses at www.uscg.mil.

Suggested Ways to Avoid the Hazards of Alcohol

Boating doesn't need any stimulus to make it fun. Fishing doesn't need any liquid bait to improve the catch. Consider these alternatives to alcohol and boating:

- Take along a variety of sodas, a jug of water, ice tea, or lemonade, or take along non-alcoholic beer

- Take along plenty of food

- Wear clothes that will keep you cool

- Plan to limit your trip to the number of hours you can spend on the water without becoming tired

- Enjoy your outing more by having the party ashore after you dock—in the picnic area, in the Yacht Club, in your backyard—where you'll have time between the fun and getting back into a boat or your car

- If you dock somewhere for lunch or dinner and drink alcohol, wait a reasonable time before heading back home

- If necessary, be sure to have a sober designated driver as the boat operator. Or better yet, in case of emergency, have two designated non-drinking operators

- No alcohol aboard is the safe way to go—remember, intoxicated passengers can fall overboard too

Additional Information

U.S. Consumer Product Safety Commission
Washington, DC 20207
Toll-Free Hotline: 800-638-2772
Fax: 800-809-0924
Website: www.cpsc.gov
E-mail: info@cpsc.gov

U.S. Coast Guard
2100 Second Street, SW,
Washington, DC 20593
Telephone: 202-267-2229
Website: www.uscg.mil

United States Lifesaving Association (USLA)
P.O. Box 366
Huntington Beach, California 92648
Toll-Free: 866-FOR-USLA (367-8752)
Website www.usla.org

Chapter 55

Amusement Ride Injuries and Deaths

This chapter describes U.S. Consumer Product Safety Commission (CPSC) data on amusement ride-related fatalities and hospital emergency room-treated injuries. Fatality data are presented for calendar years 1987 through 1999. Injury data are presented for calendar years 1993 through 1999. Hazard scenario data derived from in-depth investigations and incident reports are presented for the period from January 1, 1990 through April 30, 2000.

- An estimated 10,400 hospital emergency room-treated injuries occurred in 1999, with about 7,000 involving fixed rides and 3,000 involving mobile rides. An estimated 23.5 injuries per million attendance occurred at fixed-site parks in 1999. Attendance data are not currently available for mobile rides.

- There was a marginally significant upward trend in fixed-site and total amusement ride-related injuries from 1993 through 1999 due to a sharp increase in fixed-site injuries beginning in 1997.

- The estimated annual average number of non-occupational amusement ride-related fatalities from 1987 through 1998 was 4.3 fatalities each year, and there was a marginally significant upward trend in fatalities from 1993 through 1999.

"Amusement Ride-Related Injuries and Deaths in the United States: 1987-1999," by C. Craig Morris, Ph.D., U.S. Consumer Product Safety Commission (CPSC), July 2000.

- A hazard sketch summarizing CPSC investigations of amusement ride incidents revealed hazard patterns associated with mechanical failure, operator behavior, consumer behavior, other factors, and combinations of these factors.

Definition of Amusement Rides

Section 3(a)(1) of the Consumer Product Safety Act describes an amusement ride as: "any mechanical device which carries or conveys passengers along, around, or over a fixed or restricted route within a defined area for the purpose of giving its passengers amusement, which is customarily controlled or directed by an individual who is employed for that purpose and who is not a consumer with respect to that device, and which is not permanently fixed to a site."

Although fixed-site amusement rides are excluded from CPSC jurisdiction by Section 3 (a)(1), CPSC data collection systems receive data on amusement rides that do not, at the outset, distinguish between fixed-site and mobile rides. Additional analysis must be undertaken in order to determine which incidents involve mobile rides and whether a fixed-site ride that was the subject of an incident is also a mobile ride. Data regarding fixed-site ride incidents are included in this report, along with data on mobile ride incidents, since those data are immediately available to CPSC through the process described above and are useful for comparison purposes. Only non-occupational incidents, which involve non-employee victims injured while on, in, or around an amusement ride, are included in this report.

Amusement Ride-Related Injuries

Method

Data on non-occupational amusement ride-related injuries were obtained from CPSC's National Electronic Injury Surveillance System (NEISS). The NEISS is a stratified probability sample of hospitals with emergency rooms and 6 or more beds in the United States. There are currently 100 participating hospitals in the NEISS. NEISS hospital coders identify injury incidents associated with amusement rides by using the NEISS product code for amusement rides (1293). In this analysis, all NEISS records for calendar years 1993 through 1999 containing product code 1293 were reviewed. Based on information in narrative comments in the records, a single experienced coder (the author) classified each case into 1 of 5 mutually exclusive and exhaustive categories: not a ride (out of scope), fixed-site ride, mobile-site ride, unknown-site ride, or unknown if ride. Cases involving coin-operated rides or free-play attractions often found at restaurants or shopping centers, alpine and water slide amusements, wave machines, "moon walks," inflatable slides, mechanical bulls, playground equipment, etc., are examples of cases coded not a ride. Cases involving roller coasters or "whirling" rides are examples of cases coded fixed-site, mobile-site, or unknown-site ride: if the comment stated the name of an amusement park or that the incident occurred at a park or involved an amusement park ride, then the case was coded fixed-site; if the comment stated that the incident occurred at a carnival, fair, or festival, then the case was coded mobile-site; if the comment gave no site information, then the case was coded unknown-site. Cases involving a "merry go round," with no indication of whether it was playground equipment or an amusement ride as defined by the Consumer Product Safety Act, are examples of cases coded unknown if ride.

Estimate Adjustments

Adjustments of amusement ride-related injury estimates for prior years appear in this report. First, all NEISS cases from 1993 to 1999 were reviewed by an experienced coder to verify consistency in the coding of cases. A few codings were adjusted to improve consistency. Second, the NEISS sample of hospitals was updated in 1997 to reflect changes in the distribution and size of emergency room hospitals in the U.S. since the previous sample update in 1990. Periodic updates are required for the sample of NEISS hospitals to accurately represent the universe of hospitals with emergency rooms in the U.S. Data were collected concurrently from both the old and updated NEISS samples for 9 months in 1997 to provide a statistical basis for adjustments of prior estimates. Third, unknown-site estimates were allocated to fixed-site and mobile-site estimates in the proportions observed in known-site estimates each year. The adjusted estimates in this report differ from estimates given in previous CPSC publications.

Results

Table 55.1 gives the unallocated NEISS estimates for calendar years 1993 through 1999. Note that the fixed-site and mobile-site injury estimates in Table 55.1 underestimate actual totals due to the exclusion of unknown-site cases, all of which involve fixed-site or mobile amusement rides. The adjusted estimates in Table 55.2 correct for the underestimation of fixed-site and mobile injuries in Table 55.1 by allocating the unknown-site estimates to the known fixed-site and mobile estimates in the same proportions observed in the known-site estimates.

Table 55.2 gives the allocated NEISS estimates for calendar years 1993 through 1999. As previously explained, the adjusted estimates in Table 55.2 correct for the underestimation of fixed-site and mobile injuries in Table 55.1 by allocating the unknown-site estimates to the

Table 55.1. Unallocated Estimated Non-Occupational Amusement Ride Injuries by Year and Site of Ride

Year	Fixed	Mobile	Unknown-Site	Total	ME (Total)
1999	5,980	2,580	1,820	10,380	5,560
1998	4,760	2,110	2,500	9,370	3,950
1997	4,590	2,170	1,280	8,050	4,600
1996	3,220	2,530	900	6,650	4,010
1995	3,530	2,680	1,330	7,540	4,340
1994	3,080	2,420	1,260	6,760	3,930
1993	3,750	2,240	1,710	7,700	3,980

Note: Details may not sum to totals due to rounding. Margin of error (ME) for 95% confidence level.

Source: U.S. Consumer Product Safety Commission.

Table 55.2. Allocated Estimated Non-Occupational Amusement Ride Injuries by Year and Site of Ride

Year	Fixed	Mobile	Total	ME (Total)
1999	7,260	3,120	10,380	5,560
1998	6,500	2,870	9,370	3,950
1997	5,460	2,580	8,050	4,600
1996	3,720	2,930	6,650	4,010
1995	4,290	3,260	7,540	4,340
1994	3,790	2,970	6,760	3,930
1993	4,830	2,880	7,700	3,980

Note: Details may not sum to totals due to rounding. Margin of error (ME) for 95% confidence level.

Source: U.S. Consumer Product Safety Commission.

known fixed-site and mobile estimates in the same proportions observed in the known-site estimates.

Table 55.3 gives estimated fixed-site injuries divided by estimated attendance at amusement parks[7] each year. The upward trend in risk is marginally significant, p < .07, 1-tail exact Kendall Tau test. Unknown-site estimates were allocated to fixed-site and mobile estimates as described above. Attendance data for mobile rides are not available.

Because an increasing trend in amusement ride-related injuries began in 1997, the same year the NEISS sample of hospitals was updated, it is important to determine whether the increase might be attributable to revision of the NEISS sample, i.e., replacement of about 30 hospitals in the sample of about 100 hospitals. Hospitals continuously present in NEISS from 1995 through 1999 were identified to determine the trend in amusement ride-related injuries at those hospitals. Table 55.4 gives sample counts, not estimates, from these hospitals. Although the total count dropped from 121 in 1995 to 95 in 1996, it steadily increased to 117 in 1997, 124 in 1998, and 167 in 1999. The increasing trend from 1996 to 1999 was statistically significant by an exact Kendall Tau 1-tailed test, p = .04. Thus, the trend in fixed-site and total amusement ride-related injuries does not appear to be an artifact of the updated NEISS sample in 1997.

Analysis of individual NEISS hospital data for calendar years 1995 through 1999 revealed one hospital (#58) that both records more amusement ride-related cases each year and exhibits a larger increasing trend over the period than all other NEISS hospitals. However,

Table 55.3. Risk of Non-Occupational Fixed-Site Amusement Ride Injury by Year

Year	Attendance (millions)	Risk
1999	309	23.5
1998	300	21.6
1997	300	18.2
1996	290	12.8
1995	280	15.3
1994	267	14.2
1993	275	17.5

Note: Risk is number of injuries per million attendance.

Source: U.S. Consumer Product Safety Commission and International Association of Amusement Parks and Attractions.

as discussed in Appendix A, reporting amusement ride-related injury estimates with hospital 58 excluded is inappropriate because the NEISS sample with hospital 58 removed is not statistically representative of all emergency room hospitals in the U.S.

In conclusion, current NEISS data indicate a total in 1999 of about 10,400±5,600 emergency room-treated, amusement ride-related injuries, with about 7,000 involving fixed-site rides and about 3,000 involving mobile rides. From 1993 through 1999, there was a marginally significant upward trend in fixed-site and total amusement ride-related injuries and in the risk of fixed-site injury defined as the estimated number of injuries per million attendance at amusement parks. It should be noted that, although there are fewer mobile as compared to fixed-site ride injuries, the amount of exposure is probably different for mobile versus fixed-site rides, so the relative risk of injury attributable to one versus the other cannot be determined without comparable exposure information for both types of rides.

Amusement Ride-Related Fatalities

CPSC's files were searched for records of fatalities involving amusement rides during calendar years 1987 through 1999. These files were the death certificate file (DTHS), the injury or potential injury incident file (IPII), and the National Electronic Injury Surveillance System file (NEISS). Information in the narrative field of the records was used to classify cases using the criteria defined above in the Method section for the NEISS injury analyses.

DTHS and IPII files recorded 49 non-occupational fatalities from 1987 through 1999; NEISS files recorded no amusement ride-related fatalities during this period. Due to the logistical difficulty of captur-

Table 55.4. Non-Occupational Amusement Ride-Related Injury Counts for Hospitals in NEISS from 1995 through 1999 by Year and Site of Ride

Year	Fixed	Mobile	Unknown	Total
1999	87	44	36	167
1998	62	29	33	124
1997	63	29	25	117
1996	49	33	13	95
1995	60	43	18	121

Source: U.S. Consumer Product Safety Commission.

ing all fatalities related to any product or event, these counts do not account for all amusement ride-related fatalities. Methods for estimating true totals given 2 or more independent data sources are known as "capture-recapture" or "multiple record systems" methods.[8,9] Capture-recapture analyses were conducted on 43 documented cases during 1987 through 1998 to estimate the total and annual average number of non-occupational amusement ride-related fatalities during that period. Lags in fatality reporting preclude estimation of fatalities for the last full calendar year. The capture-recapture analyses treated the DTHS and IPII files as independent samples of all non-occupational amusement ride-related deaths during the study period. The estimated number of non-occupational amusement ride-related fatalities from 1987 through 1998 was 52 (95% confidence interval = 43 to 62), for an estimated annual average of 4.3 fatalities each year during that period.

Documented non-occupational fatalities from 1987 through 1999 were classified by ride type, location (state), and ride site. Site refers to fixed-site rides as in amusement parks, mobile rides as in carnivals

Table 55.5. Non-Occupational Amusement Ride-Related Fatalities by Year and Ride Site

Year	Fixed	Mobile	Unknown	Total
1999	6	0	0	6*
1998	3	2	2	7*
1997	1	0	3	4
1996	2	1	0	3
1995	3	1	0	4
1994	2	0	0	2
1993	1	1	2	4
1992	0	2	0	2
1991	3	0	0	3
1990	0	0	0	0
1989	3	0	0	3
1988	2	1	4	7
1987	4	0	0	4
Total	30	8	11	49

* Data for 1998-1999 are incomplete; counts will increase if additional reports are received.

Source: U.S. Consumer Product Safety Commission.

Table 55.6. Non-Occupational Amusement Ride-Related Fatalities from 1987 through 1999 by Ride Type and Mobility

Type of Ride	Fixed	Mobile	Unknown	Total
Roller Coaster	12	0	3	15
Whirling	2	4	4	10
Water	5	0	0	5
Train	2	1	0	3
Ferris Wheel	2	0	0	2
Sleigh	1	0	0	1
Unknown	6	3	4	13
Total	30	8	11	49

Table 55.7. Non-Occupational Amusement Ride-Related Fatalities from 1987 through 1999 by State and Ride Mobility

State	Fixed	Mobile	Unknown	Total
CA	3	1	2	6
CT	1	0	0	1
FL	1	1	2	4
GA	0	0	1	1
IL	1	2	0	3
IN	1	0	0	1
MA	1	0	0	1
MD	0	0	1	1
MN	2	0	0	2
NE	1	0	0	1
NJ	5	0	1	6
NM	0	1	0	1
NV	0	0	1	1
NY	4	1	0	5
OH	2	0	1	3
OK	0	0	1	1
PA	1	0	0	1
SC	2	0	0	2
TN	0	0	1	1
TX	2	2	0	4
UT	2	0	0	2
VA	1	0	0	1
Total	30	8	11	49

Note: Data for 1998-1999 are incomplete; counts will increase if additional reports are received.

Source: U.S. Consumer Product Safety Commission.

or fairs, or rides of unknown site. From 1987 through 1999, there were 49 documented fatalities, including 30 fixed ride-related fatalities, 8 mobile ride-related fatalities, and 11 fatalities involving unknown ride mobility status. The following tables give documented fatalities by year and ride mobility (Table 55.5), ride type and mobility (Table 55.6), and state and ride mobility (Table 55.7).

Table 55.5 gives fatalities by year and site. The fatalities observed in 1998[7] and 1999[6] were the most since 1988. From 1993 through 1999, there was a marginally significant upward trend in both fixed-site and total fatalities, both p = .08, exact Kendall Tau 1-tailed tests.

Table 55.6 gives documented non-occupational amusement ride fatalities by type and mobility. The majority of deaths were associated with roller coasters and "whirling" rides.

Table 55.7 gives the number of documented non-occupational amusement ride fatalities by state and mobility. States with the largest number of documented fatalities included California,[6] New Jersey,[6] and New York.[5]

Hazard Patterns Associated with Amusement Ride-Related Incidents

A review of in-depth investigation (INDP) reports by CPSC staff from Jan 1, 1990 through April 30, 2000 revealed several hazard patterns associated with amusement ride-related incidents. The investigated cases were neither a probability sample nor complete account of all such incidents, so estimates of the proportions or numbers of incidents involving the scenarios observed in these investigations are not provided. Review of the 85 cases revealed hazard patterns involving mechanical failure, operator behavior, consumer behavior, other factors, and combinations of these factors.

Mechanical failures associated with amusement ride-related incidents included missing safety pins, broken welds or structural components, exposed electrical wires, broken drive chains, malfunctioning lap bars or other safety restraints, failure to shutoff, improper detachment of cars, and improper detachment of structural components.

Operator behaviors associated with amusement ride-related incidents included abruptly stopping the ride (e.g., following an apparent mechanical failure), improperly assembling or maintaining the ride, and defeating safety equipment such as brakes and automatic overheat cutoff switches.

Consumer behaviors associated with amusement ride-related incidents included intentionally rocking cars, standing up, defeating safety restraints, sitting improperly (e.g., sideways or with feet above lap bar), holding a child above the safety restraint, and in one instance, a disembarking passenger intentionally restarting the ride by pressing the start button as other passengers were disembarking.

The **other hazard** pattern applies to rides that can injure people while apparently functioning normally, without any unusual or inappropriate behavior on the part of consumers or operators. An example is a hand-powered ride called the "Spaceball" in which the occupant is spun extremely rapidly. Five reports of eye hemorrhage, and one report of retinal tear and possible cerebral edema, were associated with this ride. CPSC files document reported cases of amusement ride-related cerebral and retinal hemorrhage, subdural hematoma, loss of consciousness, headache, and dizziness. Fatalities with little or no overt trauma have occurred during or after rides that induce abrupt changes in speed and direction.

Several incidents involved combinations of the above hazard patterns. In one incident, for example, an operator abruptly stopped a ride upon hearing an unusual "thumping" sound due to a bent rail. In another case, the victim reported that the operator spun him longer and more vigorously than usual in a ride called the "Spaceball."

References

1. Cassidy S. *Deaths and Injuries Associated with Amusement Rides*, 21 May 1996, US Consumer Product Safety Commission, Washington, DC.

2. Morris CC. *Amusement Ride-Related Injuries and Deaths*, 10 Oct 1997, US Consumer Product Safety Commission, Washington, DC.

3. Morris CC. *Amusement Ride-Related Injuries and Deaths*, 16 June 1998, US Consumer Product Safety Commission, Washington, DC.

4. Morris CC. *Amusement Ride-Related Injuries and Deaths in the United States*, 15 July 1999, US Consumer Product Safety Commission, Washington, DC.

5. Kessler E, Schroeder T. *National Electronic Injury Surveillance System (NEISS) Estimated Generalized Relative Sampling*

Errors, Sep 1998, US Consumer Product Safety Commission, Washington, DC.

6. Gibbons JD. *Nonparametric Measures of Association*, 1993, Sage Publications, Newbury Park, CA.

7. Personal communication from the International Association of Amusement Parks and Attractions, Alexandria, VA to James DeMarco, US Consumer Product Safety Commission, Washington DC.

8. Hook EB, Regal RR. Capture-recapture methods in epidemiology: methods and limitations, 1995, *Epidemiologic Reviews*, 17(2);243-264.

9. Fienberg SE. The multiple recapture census for closed populations and incomplete 2K contingency tables, 1972, *Biometrika*, 59(3);591-603.

Chapter 56

Unpowered Scooter-Related Injuries

Injuries associated with unpowered scooters have increased dramatically since May 2000.[1] These scooters are a new version of the foot-propelled scooters first popular during the 1950s. Most scooters are made of lightweight aluminum with small, low-friction wheels similar to those on in-line skates. They weigh under 10 pounds and fold for easy portability and storage. Up to 5 million scooters are expected to be sold in 2000, an increase from virtually zero last year (Consumer Product Safety Commission [CPSC], unpublished data, 2000). This report summarizes the results of a descriptive analysis of scooter-related injuries during the past 34 months and provides recommendations to reduce these injuries.

CPSC and CDC analyzed preliminary data from CPSC's National Electronic Injury Surveillance System (NEISS) from January 1998 through October 2000 and the Injury and Potential Injury Incident File (IPII) during January-October 2000. NEISS is a probability sample of 100 U.S. hospitals with 24-hour emergency departments (EDs) and more than six beds. NEISS collects data from these hospitals on all persons seeking treatment for consumer product-related injury in the hospitals' EDs. Estimates of injuries in the United States associated with specific consumer products or activities can be made from NEISS data. Data were weighted according to the probability

---

"Unpowered Scooter-Related Injuries–United States, 1998–2000," *MMWR Weekly*, December 15, 2000/49(49);1108-1110, and "Popularity of Scooters Leads to Dramatic Rise in Injuries This Year," Press Release, National SAFE KIDS Campaign.

of hospital selection in the NEISS sample to provide estimates for the U.S. population.[2] IPII consists of anecdotal information reported to CPSC from many sources (e.g., coroners and medical examiners; newspaper reports; consumer complaints through the CPSC hotline or CPSC's website; and referrals from federal, state, and local officials). NEISS was used to estimate scooter-related injuries, and IPII was used to identify scooter-related deaths. Because the new scooters were introduced in large numbers into the United States market in 2000, the 1998 and 1999 data relate to the older versions of scooters.

During January-October 2000, an estimated 27,600* (95% confidence limits [CL]=22,190–33,010) persons sought ED care for scooter-related injuries. In August, September, and October 2000, the estimated number of injuries requiring ED care was 6,529 (95% CL=4,610–8,450), 8,628 (95% CL=6,090–11,170), and 7,359 (95% CL=5,200–9,520), respectively (Figure 56.1); October data are incomplete and may change slightly as additional injury reports are filed. The estimated number of injuries during August-October represents 80% of the estimated total number of injuries for all of 2000. Each of the preceding 3 months also exceeded the 12-month total for either 1998 or 1999. The estimated number of injuries seen in EDs in September 2000 was nearly 18 times higher than in May 2000.

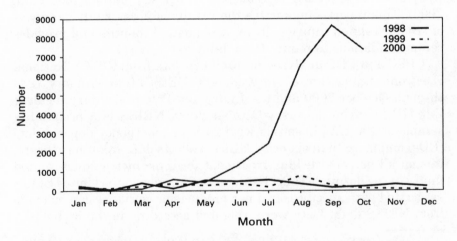

Figure 56.1. *Estimated Number of Emergency Department Visits for Unpowered Scooter-Related Injuries, by Month—United States, January 1998-October 2000.*

Approximately 85% of persons treated in EDs were children aged under 15 years, and 23% were aged under 8 years; two-thirds were male. The most common type of injury was a fracture or dislocation (29%), of which 70% were to the arm or hand. Other injuries included lacerations (24%), contusions/abrasions (22%), and strains/sprains (14%). Forty-two percent of all injuries occurred to the arm and hand, 27% to the head and face, and 24% to the leg and foot.

Two persons have died while using a scooter. An adult fell and struck his head while showing his daughter how to ride the scooter. A 6-year-old boy rode into traffic and was struck by a car.

Reported by: GW Rutherford, Jr, MS, R Ingle, MA, Consumer Product Safety Commission. Div of Unintentional Injury Prevention, National Center for Injury Prevention and Control, CDC.

Editorial Note

The findings in this report demonstrate the rapid increase in injuries associated with riding the new lightweight, folding, unpowered scooters, which are a fast-growing activity in the United States. Because these scooters are a recent phenomenon, scientific data about the efficacy of safety equipment to protect against scooter-related injuries are not available. However, lessons learned from similar recreational activities (e.g., in-line skating) can guide users in adopting reasonable safety precautions, such as wearing protective gear.

On the basis of data from in-line skating and bicycling, many of these injuries might have been prevented or reduced in severity had protective equipment been worn. Helmets can prevent 85% of head injuries,[3] elbow pads can prevent 82% of elbow injuries, and knee pads can prevent 32% of knee injuries.[4] Although wrist guards are effective in preventing injuries among in-line skaters, the protection they provide against injury for scooter riders is unknown because wrist guards may make it difficult to grip the scooter handle and steer it.

The public health community can be proactive and support efforts to decrease scooter-related injury in children by increasing awareness among parents and health care providers of the injury potential and the need for safety measures when using scooters. Many children may not be prepared developmentally to handle the multitask challenges they may experience while riding a scooter. Changes in the product and rider behavior also may make riding scooters safer. The mechanisms and circumstances of scooter-related injury require further research.

Give the Gift of Safety When Purchasing Scooters

The National SAFE KIDS Campaign wants every parent and child to understand the potential for serious injury that exists when children ride these scooters without the proper protective gear. In addition, parents should make sure their child's scooter hasn't been recalled by the U.S. Consumer Product Safety Commission. You can check on the Internet at http://www.safekids.org/recalls.html.

"Parents may have a false sense of security when it comes to their kids and scooters," said Heather Paul, Ph.D., executive director of the National SAFE KIDS Campaign. "Because these scooters have handlebars, brakes and are low to the ground, adults might feel their children can easily control them. Without the appropriate safety gear, children can sustain severe injury, including hear trauma."

According to the Toy Manufacturers of America, scooters topped the list of best-selling toys reaching between 2 and 5 million in 2001. Safety gear is relatively affordable and can be purchased for as little as $35.00—less than half the cost of an average scooter. In addition, SAFE KIDS recommends the following guidelines:

- Children should always wear appropriate safety gear, including a helmet, and elbow and knee pads when riding a scooter.

- Be sure protective gear fits properly and does not interfere with the rider's movement vision or hearing.

- Children ages 8 and under should not use scooters without close adult supervision.

- Before using a scooter, the rider or parent should check it thoroughly for hazards such as loose, broken, or cracked parts, sharp edges on metal boards; slippery top surfaces; and wheels with nicks and cracks. Ride scooters on smooth, paved surfaces free from traffic. Avoid riding on streets or surfaces with water, sand, gravel, or dirt.

- Don't ride scooters at night.

- Never hitch a ride from a car, bus, truck, bicycle, etc., and limit usage of the scooter to one person at a time.

- Exercise caution when riding a scooter downhill. If a steep hill is encountered, step off the scooter and walk to the bottom of the hill.

"These are common sense guidelines, but when you look at the overwhelming number of scooter-related injuries this year, it appears the safety message is getting lost. Parents and caregivers must do better. We also encourage the manufacturers of these scooters to stress safety in their brochures and advertising materials," Paul said.

References

1. Consumer Product Safety Commission. National Electronic Injury Surveillance System [computer file]. Washington, DC: Consumer Product Safety Commission, November, 2000.

2. Kessler E, Schroeder T. The NEISS sample (design and implementation). Washington, DC: Consumer Product Safety Commission, October 1998.

3. Thompson RS, Rivara FP, Thompson DC. A case-control study of the effectiveness of bicycle safety helmets. *N Engl J Med* 1989;320:1361-7.

4. Schieber RA, Branche-Dorsey CM, Ryan GW, Rutherford GW, Stevens JA, O'Neil J. Risk factors for injuries from in-line skating and the effectiveness of safety gear. *N Engl J Med* 1996;335:1630-5.

*Estimates are based on the approximate range at the 95% confidence level of relative sampling error. For this analysis, the corresponding relative sampling error for the estimated number of injuries during January-October is 0.1.

Chapter 57

Fireworks-Related Injuries, Deaths, and Fires

Fireworks-Related Injuries

- In 1999, 16 persons died and an estimated 8,500 were injured from fireworks in the United States. Estimated emergency department-treated injuries decreased 32% from 1994, when an estimated 12,500 fireworks injuries were sustained.[1]

- Seven of every 100 people injured from fireworks require hospitalization.[1]

Who Is Most Likely to Be Injured?

- Over 40% of those injured from fireworks are children 14 years of age and younger.[1]

- Males are injured three times as frequently as females.[1]

- Boys between 5 and 14 years of age have the highest fireworks-related injury rate.[1]

- Those who are actively participating in fireworks-related activities are more frequently injured, and sustain more severe injuries, than bystanders.[2]

Reprinted from www.nfpa.org with permission, "Fireworks-Related Injuries, Deaths, and Fires in the U.S. March 2001," © 2001, National Fire Protection Association, Quincy, MA 02269; and "Fireworks-Related Injuries," National Center for Injury Prevention and Control, reviewed June, 2001.

When and Where Do These Injuries Happen?

- Injuries occur on and around holidays associated with fireworks celebrations, especially Independence Day and New Year's Eve. Two-thirds of all fireworks injuries occur during the month of July.[3]

- Homes are where most of these injuries occur, followed by recreational settings, streets or highways, and parking lots or occupational settings.[4]

What Kinds of Injuries Occur?

- Fireworks-related injuries most frequently involve hands and fingers (40%), the head and face (20%), and eyes (18%). More than half of the injuries are burns (55%); contusions and lacerations were second most frequent (25%).[1]

- Fireworks can also cause life-threatening residential fires.[1]

What Types of Fireworks Are Associated with the Most Injuries?

- Nearly two-thirds of fireworks-related injuries are caused by backyard, "class C" fireworks such as firecrackers, bottle rockets, Roman candles, fountains, and sparklers, that are legal in many states. Specifically, fireworks-related injuries are most commonly associated with firecrackers (51%), bottle rockets (12%), and sparklers (7%).[5]

- The most severe injuries are typically caused by "class B" fireworks, such as rockets, cherry bombs, and M-80s, which are federally banned from public sale.[2]

- Illegal firecrackers represent 29% of all firecracker injuries.[5]

How and Why Do These Injuries Occur?

- **Availability:** In spite of federal regulations and varying state prohibitions, "class C" and "class B" fireworks are often accessible by the public. It is not uncommon to find fireworks distributors near state borders, where residents of states with strict fireworks regulations can take advantage of more lenient state laws.

- **Fireworks type:** Among "class C" fireworks, bottle rockets can fly into one's face and cause eye injuries; sparklers can ignite one's clothing (sparklers burn at more than 1,000°F); and firecrackers can injure one's hands or face if they explode at close range.[6]

- **Being too close:** Injuries may result from being too close to fireworks when they explode; for example, when someone bends over to look more closely at a firework that has been ignited, or when a misguided bottle rocket hits a nearby person.[6]

- **Unsupervised use:** One study estimates that children are 11 times more likely to be injured by fireworks if they are unsupervised.[6]

- **Lack of physical coordination:** Younger children often lack the physical coordination to handle fireworks safely.

- **Curiosity:** Children are often excited and curious around fireworks which can increase their chances of being injured (e.g., when they re-examine a firecracker "dud" that fails to ignite).[6]

- **Experimentation:** "Homemade" fireworks (e.g., ones made of the powder from several firecrackers) can lead to dangerous explosions.[6]

How Much Do These Injuries Cost Each Year?

- Firework-related injuries are estimated to cost approximately $100 million per year.[7]

- According to the National Fire Protection Association, fireworks resulted in $15.6 million in direct property damage in 1998.[8]

What Effect Do Laws Have on Fireworks Injuries?

- Studies suggest that state laws regulating the sale and use of fireworks affect the number of injuries incurred. For example, in one state, the number of injuries seen in emergency departments more than doubled following the legalization of fireworks.[3]

- Under the Federal Hazardous Substances Act, the federal government prohibits the sale of the most dangerous types of fireworks to consumers. These banned fireworks include large reloadable shells, cherry bombs, aerial bombs, M-80 salutes, and larger firecrackers that contain more than two grains of powder. Mail-order kits to build these fireworks are also prohibitied.[9]

What Is the Safest Way to Prevent Fireworks Injuries?

- The safest way to prevent fireworks-related injuries is to leave fireworks displays to trained professionals.

References

1. U.S. Consumer Product Safety Commission. (June 11, 2001) *1999 Fireworks Annual Report: Fireworks-related deaths, emergency department treated injuries, and enforcement activities during 1999.* [Online]. Available: www.cpsc.gov/library/1999fwreport6.PDF

2. Smith GA, Knapp JF, Barnett, TM, Shields BJ. The rockets' red glare, the bombs bursting in air: fireworks-related injuries to children. *Pediatrics.* 1996; 98(1):1-9.

3. McFarland LV, Harris JR, Kobayashi JM, Dicker RC. Risk factors for fireworks-related injury in Washington State. *JAMA* 1984;251:3251-3254.

4. U.S. Consumer Product Safety Commission. (28 June 1993). *Safety commission holds seventh annual fireworks safety news conference. 1993.* [Online]. Available: www.cpsc.gov/gophroot/

5. U.S. Consumer Product Safety Commission. *Fireworks*—Publication #12.

6. Consumer Product Safety Commission. (5 May 1996). *CPSC stops hazardous products at the docks: Preventing fireworks injuries and deaths.* [Online]. Available: www.cpsc.gov/cpscpub/pubs/success/firework.html

7. CDC. Fireworks-related injuries, Marion County, Indiana, 1986-1991. *MMWR Morbidity and Mortality Weekly Report.* 1992;41:451-453.

8. National Fire Protection Association. *Fireworks-related injuries, deaths, and fires in the U.S., 2001.*

9. California Department of Forestry and Fire Protection; State Fire Marshal. (No date). *California 4th of July fireworks safety: Fireworks injuries by type of device.* [Online].

The Problem with Fireworks in the U.S.

Every year, thousands of people are injured by fireworks, both legal and illegal. Fireworks-related injuries treated in U.S. hospital emergency rooms did not change in 1998 and stayed at roughly the average level of 1974-1983.[1] The recent level is substantially lower than the levels of 1984-1995, but it is still too high.

Since at least 1910, the National Fire Protection Association, (NFPA) has crusaded to stop the dangerous private use of fireworks, which accounts for nearly all of the toll from fireworks.[2] Many states still permit untrained citizens to purchase and use fireworks—objects designed to explode, throw off showers of hot sparks, and reach surface temperatures as high as 1,200°F. The thousands of serious injuries and extensive property loss nearly all arise from this misguided activity, rather than the only acceptably safe way to enjoy fireworks, which is in public fireworks displays conducted in accordance with NFPA 1123, Code for Fireworks Display. Anything else is a violation of IFMA's (International Fire Marshals Association) Model Fireworks Law, which reflects NFPA's zero-tolerance policy for consumer use of fireworks.

School-age children suffer most from the widespread private use of fireworks, whether as spectators or, too often, as active participants. On the July 4 Independence Day holiday in a typical year, fireworks cause more fires in the United States than all other causes of fire on that day combined. But because most people encounter the risk of fireworks only once a year, many Americans do not realize how great that risk is.

Fires and Losses Caused by Fireworks

Table 57.1 summarizes estimated fire losses due to fireworks for the period from 1980 through 1998. In 1998, an estimated 21,700 fires involving fireworks were reported to U.S. fire departments. These fires were estimated to have killed no civilians, injured 44 civilians, and caused $15.6 million in direct property damage.

Table 57.1 shows that fireworks-related fires have typically caused at least $20 million in property loss (not adjusted for inflation) each year in recent years. Each year, a substantial share of the structure fire property loss due to fireworks typically involves bottle rockets or other fireworks rockets, based on details of large-loss incidents reported individually to NFPA.

Table 57.1. Fires and Losses Associated with Fireworks, 1980–1998 Fires Reported to U.S. Fire Departments

A. Fires

Year	Residential Structures	Nonresidential Structures	Vehicles	Outdoors and Other	Total
1980	2,900	1,100	500	21,800	26,400
1981	2,900	1,300	500	27,100	31,800
1982	1,700	1,000	500	24,600	27,800
1983	1,400	800	500	25,300	28,000
1984	2,500	1,200	1,000	34,700	39,400
1985	2,700	1,500	900	46,600	51,600
1986	2,400	1,200	1,000	30,500	35,100
1987	2,000	1,100	800	33,200	37,100
1988	2,400	1,400	900	47,400	52,100
1989	1,800	900	800	29,800	33,400
1990	1,700	800	800	30,000	33,300
1991	1,600	900	800	24,700	28,000
1992	1,400	900	700	22,500	25,500
1993	1,300	800	800	27,300	30,200
1994	1,400	900	700	35,100	38,000
1995	1,200	700	700	24,800	27,400
1996	1,100	600	600	22,500	24,800
1997	1,000	700	500	17,900	20,100
1998	800	500	500	19,800	21,700

Note: The year 1998 is the latest for which national fire estimates are possible. These are fires reported to U.S. municipal fire departments and so exclude fires reported only to Federal or state agencies or industrial fire brigades. Fires are estimated to the nearest hundred. Row sums may not equal row totals because of rounding error.

Source: National estimates based on NFIRS and NFPA survey.

B. Civilian Deaths

Year	Residential Structures	Nonresidential Structures	Vehicles	Outdoors and Other	Total
1980	0	0	0	0	0
1981	0	0	0	0	0
1982	0	0	0	0	0
1983	0	0	0	0	0
1984	3	0	0	0	3
1985	8	0	3	4	15
1986	4	0	0	0	4
1987	4	3	0	0	7

Table 57.1. Fires and Losses Associated with Fireworks, 1980–1998 Fires Reported to U.S. Fire Departments (continued)

B. Civilian Deaths (continued)

Year	Residential Structures	Nonresidential Structures	Vehicles	Outdoors and Other	Total
1988	20	0	0	0	20
1989	4	0	0	0	4
1990	3	0	0	0	3
1991	0	0	0	0	0
1992	0	0	0	1	1
1993	0	0	0	0	0
1994	12	0	0	0	12
1995	0	0	0	1	1
1996	9	18	0	0	27
1997	0	0	0	3	3
1998	0	0	0	0	0

Note: The year 1998 is the latest for which national fire estimates are possible. These are fires reported to U.S. Municipal fire departments and so exclude fires reported only to Federal or state agencies or industrial fire brigades. Civilian deaths are estimated to the nearest one. Row sums may not equal row totals because of rounding errors.

Source: National estimates based on NFIRS and NFPA survey.

C. Civilian Injuries

Year	Residential Structures	Nonresidential Structures	Vehicles	Outdoors and Other	Total
1980	31	3	0	16	50
1981	29	16	4	17	66
1982	10	23	2	63	99
1983	45	3	0	28	76
1984	38	10	8	31	87
1985	73	10	29	32	144
1986	55	46	2	22	126
1987	55	10	0	28	93
1988	39	16	16	28	99
1989	49	4	19	34	107
1990	46	6	3	57	112
1991	54	13	10	30	107
1992	42	11	8	42	103
1993	23	18	2	23	66
1994	96	6	5	46	153
1995	53	0	3	37	93
1996	20	21	2	23	67

Table 57.1. Fires and Losses Associated with Fireworks, 1980–1998 Fires Reported to U.S. Fire Departments (continued)

C. Civilian Injuries (continued)

Year	Residential Structures	Nonresidential Structures	Vehicles	Outdoors and Other	Total
1997	21	7	17	23	68
1998	6	0	7	31	44

Note: The year 1998 is the latest for which national fire estimates are possible. These are fires reported to U.S. municipal fire departments and so exclude fires reported only to Federal or state agencies or industrial fire brigades. Civilian injuries are estimated to the nearest one. Row sums may not equal row totals because of rounding error.

Source: National estimates based on NFIRS and NFPA survey.

D. Direct Property Damage (in Millions)

Year	Residential Structures	Nonresidential Structures	Vehicles	Outdoors and Other	Total
1980	$11.7	$3.2	$0.4	$0.3	$15.5
1981	$12.0	$5.8	$0.3	$0.5	$18.6
1982	$9.0	$1.6	$0.4	$0.4	$11.4
1983	$6.5	$5.2	$0.5	$0.4	$12.6
1984	$18.9	$5.6	$1.9	$0.5	$26.9
1985	$22.5	$7.4	$1.2	$5.5	$36.5
1986	$24.2	$29.1	$1.6	$0.7	$55.7
1987	$17.1	$7.1	$0.8	$0.3	$25.3
1988	$22.4	$14.4	$1.3	$0.9	$38.9
1989	$56.5	$2.7	$1.1	$1.7	$62.1
1990	$22.1	$3.8	$1.5	$0.6	$28.1
1991	$14.1	$3.3	$1.5	$0.2	$19.1
1992	$13.6	$15.9	$1.4	$2.6	$33.4
1993	$12.5	$6.2	$1.2	$1.4	$21.3
1994	$10.1	$7.5	$2.0	$2.3	$21.9
1995	$21.6	$8.6	$1.7	$0.6	$32.5
1996	$12.3	$7.0	$1.3	$6.2	$26.8
1997	$12.9	$8.4	$1.0	$0.3	$22.7
1998	$9.1	$3.1	$1.4	$2.0	$15.6

Note: The year 1998 is the latest for which national fire estimates are possible. These are fires reported to U.S. municipal fire departments and so exclude fires reported only to Federal or state agencies or industrial fire brigades. Direct property damage is estimated to the nearest hundred thousand dollars. Row sums may not equal row totals because of rounding error.

Source: National estimates based on NFIRS and NFPA survey.

Table 57.2 shows that deaths due to fireworks-related fires and deaths that were directly caused by fireworks are not the same. Fireworks may start fires that subsequently cause deaths, and fireworks may kill directly without producing a fire that requires a fire department response. Table 57.2 shows statistics on both types of fireworks-related deaths for 1980 through 1997. The year 1997 is the latest for which death certificate data are available. Most fireworks-related injuries do not involve fires that are reported to fire departments. In 1998, for example, an estimated 44 civilians were injured in reported fires caused by fireworks, but fireworks-related injuries reported to hospital emergency rooms alone totaled 8,500 the same year. Other fireworks-related injuries, such as those treated in doctors' offices or at home, are not documented in any national database, but they would surely push the total even higher.

Table 57.2. Deaths Associated with Fireworks Accidents, 1980–1997

Year	Estimated Civilian Deaths in Fires Reported to U.S. Fire Departments	Recorded on U.S. Death Certificates
1980	0	10
1981	0	4
1982	0	5
1983	0	13
1984	3	7
1985	15	11
1986	4	8
1987	7	5
1988	20	4
1989	4	5
1990	3	5
1991	0	4
1992	1	2
1993	0	10
1994	12	4
1995	1	2
1996	27	9
1997	3	8

Note: In any year, the figures in these two columns may partially overlap.
Sources: For death certificate tallies, Injury Facts, Chicago (1985-1992) and Itasca, IL (1993-2000): National Safety Council, 1985-2000; for national estimates of fire deaths, NFPA analysis based on NFIRS and NFPA survey.

In 1999, an estimated 8,500 people suffered fireworks-related injuries severe enough to require treatment in hospital emergency rooms, according to the National Electronic Injury Surveillance System (NEISS) of the U.S. Consumer Product Safety Commission (CPSC). Figure 57.1 shows the trend in fireworks-related injuries reported to emergency rooms since 1974, with statistics for 1985-96 shown both as they were reported and as they have been revised to fit with two adjustments in the sample, in 1990 and 1996.

Note: From 1985 to 1989 and from 1991 to 1996, ranges of estimates are given reflecting the transitions between sampling plans.

Source: CPSC National Electronic Injury Surveillance System (NEISS).

The age breakdowns for 1999 fireworks injury victims treated in hospital emergency rooms are shown in Figure 57.2. The relative risks by age group, as may be seen in Figure 57.3, do not clearly show what past studies have shown, which is that children age 10-14 have the highest risk, with older children age 15-19 close behind. In Figure 57.3, these two age groups are indistinguishable from children age 5-9 and adults age 20-24, respectively.

Males accounted for roughly three-fourths of fireworks injuries. Among adults age 45 to 64, however, females accounted for roughly as many fireworks injuries as males.

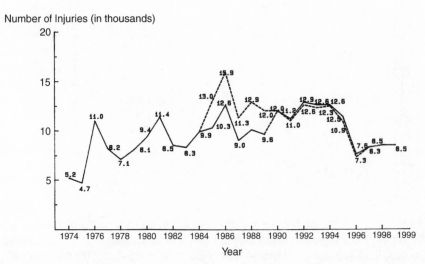

Figure 57.1. *Fireworks Injuries Reported to Hospital Emergency Rooms*

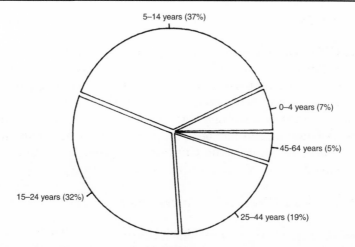

Figure 57.2. *1999 Fireworks Injuries by Age of Victim from June 23-July 23 Only. Source: CPSC National Electronic Injury Surveillance System (NEISS).*

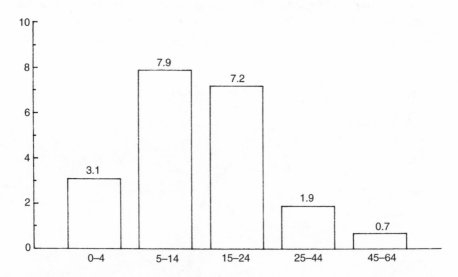

Figure 57.3. *Risk of 1999 Fireworks Injury* by Age of Victim. Source CPSC NEISS, US Census Bureau.*

*Number of 1999 fireworks injuries per 100,000 persons in 1999. Adjusted by fixed factor to reflect total injuries for year vs. injuries in one-month study period.

Other Patterns

The CPSC conducted a detailed analysis of fireworks-related injuries in 1999 in the one-month period around July 4. In a typical year, two-thirds to three-fourths of all fireworks injuries occur during that period. In 1999, only 67 percent took place then. The remaining injuries that occur at other times of the year reflect, in part, certain local traditions, such as the use of fireworks during Christmas and New Year holidays nationally, the Chinese New Year in some areas, and Mardi Gras in parts of the South.

What Kinds of Fireworks Cause the Injuries?

Figure 57.4 shows the percentage of injuries caused by each type of fireworks device. If unknown-type fireworks are allocated over known and unknown-type firecrackers are allocated over known, then 31 percent of injuries involved fireworks illegal under Federal law, either homemade or altered devices (none in 1999) or illegally large firecrackers. Using the same allocations, 67 percent of injuries involved fireworks that were permitted under Federal law, but would not be allowed under the long-standing Model Fireworks Law of the International Fire Marshals Association. Public displays of fireworks accounted for 2 percent of the injuries, under the same allocation rules.

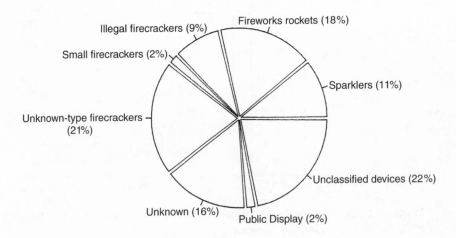

Figure 57.4. *1999 Fireworks Injuries by Type of Fireworks from June 23 to July 23 Only. Source: CPSC National Electronic Injury Surveillance System (NEISS).*

These figures clearly show that subsequential progress in reducing the high annual toll of fireworks injuries will require effective action to reduce those injuries caused by fireworks that are not covered by current Federal law. Simply enforcing the existing law will not affect the fireworks that cause most of the problem.

It is possible that limited laws, such as the current Federal law, are actually more difficult to enforce than a broader law would be, because the existence of some legal fireworks for the public encourages a climate of acceptance and creates a distribution network, both of which make it easier for amateurs to obtain illegal fireworks.

What Else Do We Know?

The largest share of 1999 emergency-room fireworks injuries involved the hand or finger (41 percent), followed by the head or face other than the eye (21 percent), the eye (18 percent), the arm (9 percent), the leg (5 percent), the trunk (4 percent), and the foot or toe (2 percent). (See Figure 57.5.)

The majority of 1999 emergency-room fireworks injuries (56 percent) were burns, followed by contusions, abrasions, or lacerations (23 percent); fractures or sprains (5 percent); and other (16 percent). (See Figure 57.6.)

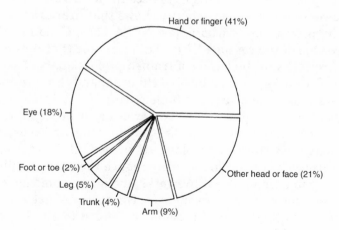

Figure 57.5. *1999 Fireworks Injuries by Part of Body Injured for June 23 to July 23 Only. Source: CPSC National Electronic Injury Surveillance System (NEISS).*

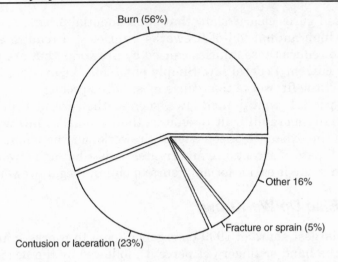

Burn (56%)

Other 16%

Fracture or sprain (5%)

Contusion or laceration (23%)

Figure 57.6. *1999 Fireworks Injuries by Type of Injury for June 23 to July 23 Only. Source: CPSC National Electronic Injury Surveillance System (NEISS).*

What's It All Mean?

Fireworks have been one of the leading causes of injuries serious enough to require hospital emergency room treatment. However, the fact that public fireworks displays account for a very small share of the fireworks problem consistently shows that fireworks can be used safely by professionals who follow NFPA 1123, Code for Fireworks Display. One of the reasons NFPA 1123 works is that it puts the control of fireworks in the hands of trained professionals.

Most fireworks injuries involve children, and those in the school-age years consistently face the highest risk.

Most fireworks injuries involve devices that are legal under current Federal law, demonstrating that tougher enforcement alone would leave most of the problem untouched. Universal use of the Model Fireworks Law could sharply reduce their tragic toll.

At the same time, illegal fireworks, including homemade devices, also account for many serious injuries. Efforts to enforce existing laws must be maintained and, if possible, extended to address the problem of homemade devices.

We must find a way to convince the average person that safe use of fireworks means no use at all by untrained people. "Safe and sane" fireworks are neither. When things go wrong with fireworks, they go very wrong very fast, far faster than any fire protection provisions can reliably respond. And fireworks are a classic attractive nuisance for children. If children are present to watch, they will be tempted to touch. Children can move too fast and be badly hurt too quickly if they are close to fireworks, as they inevitably are at home fireworks displays. Why would anyone, especially a parent, who knows the facts about fireworks want to take that chance when he or she can enjoy a festive—and safe—Independence Day at readily available public displays?

The fire protection community must spread the word in order to reduce the awful tolls of injury, death, and damage caused by the use of fireworks by amateurs.

References

1. All fireworks-related injury statistics from hospital emergency rooms come from reports by CPSC and private communications from Linda E. Smith of the CPSC. Linda Smith also provided the rules for setting the range of fireworks injury estimates during the period from 1985 to 1989, reflecting the change in the sample, and in 1991 to 1996, reflecting the latest change in the sample. Reports referenced include Michael A. Greene and Patrick M. Race, *1999 Fireworks Annual Report*; Michael A. Greene, *1998 Fireworks-Related Injuries*; Ron Monticone and Linda Smith, *1997 Fireworks-Related Injuries*; Sheila L. Kelly, *Fireworks Injuries, 1994*; Dr. Terry L. Kissinger, *Fireworks Injuries-Results of a 1992 NEISS Study*; Linda Smith and Sheila Kelly, *Fireworks Injuries, 1990*; Deborah Kale and Beatrice Harwood, *Fireworks Injuries-1981*; and the May/June 1974 issue of *NEISS News*. All were published by the U.S. Consumer Product Safety Commission.

2. Federal law permits public use of what are now referred to as "consumer fireworks" (formerly known as "common" or Class C fireworks), which are defined as "any small fireworks device designed primarily to produce visible effects by combustion" that comply with specific construction, chemical composition, and labeling regulations. These include a 50-mg maximum limit of explosive composition for ground devices and a 130-mg maximum limit of explosive composition for aerial devices.

"Safe and sane" fireworks include devices such as sparklers, fountains, snakes, party poppers, and ground spinners. Laws based on this approach allow considerable private use of fireworks, but exclude any explosive type devices that lift off the ground that are allowed under Federal law.

Chapter 58

BB Gun Injuries

Each year in the United States, approximately 30,000 persons with BB and pellet gun*-related injuries are treated in hospital emergency departments (EDs).[1] Most (95%) injuries are BB or pellet gunshot wounds (GSWs); 5% are other types of injuries (e.g., lacerations sustained inadvertently while cleaning or shooting a gun or contusions resulting from being struck with the butt of a gun).[1] Most (81%) persons treated for BB and pellet GSWs are children and teenagers (aged less than or equal to 19 years). To assist in developing strategies for preventing these injuries, CDC analyzed data from an ongoing special study of nonfatal gun-related injuries conducted using the National Electronic Injury Surveillance System (NEISS) of the U.S. Consumer Product Safety Commission; this study has characterized the epidemiology of BB and pellet GSWs among children and teenagers in the United States during June 1992-May 1994.[2] This report summarizes the circumstances of six cases of BB and pellet gun-related injuries identified through NEISS and presents the findings of the analysis of NEISS data.

NEISS includes a probability sample of 91 hospitals selected from all hospitals with at least six beds and that provide 24-hour emergency service.[2] Data were weighted to provide national estimates of injuries treated in hospital EDs in the United States and its territories.[1]

"BB and Pellet Gun-Related Injuries–United States, June 1992-May 1994," *MMWR Weekly*, December 15, 1995/ 44(49); 909-13, reviewed May 2001.

Case Reports

- A 9-year-old boy was struck by a BB beneath his lower left eye-lid after he stepped from behind a board at which other children were shooting. The children had been left unsupervised following a youth club target practice session.

- A 16-year-old boy sustained a severe midbrain injury from a self-inflicted combination BB/pellet gun GSW through the roof of his mouth.

- A 9-year-old girl incurred a pellet injury to the back of her right ankle after four boys fired a pellet gun at her from a passing car while she was walking on a sidewalk.

- A 10-year-old boy sustained injuries to his neck and trachea after being struck by a BB from a gun that had been fired unintentionally by an unspecified person.

- A 13-year-old boy was shot in the neck with a BB gun while he and a friend were playing in a house. The friend, who believed the gun was unloaded, had aimed the gun at the 13-year-old and pulled the trigger.

- A 16-year-old boy sustained a penetrating injury to his right eye after being struck by a BB that ricocheted from a gun fired by a friend.

Summary of NEISS Data

During June 1992-May 1994, a total of 959 BB and pellet GSWs among children and teenagers were reported through NEISS. Based on these reports, an estimated 47,137 (95% confidence interval {CI} = 39,746-54,528) children and teenagers were treated for BB or pellet GSWs in hospital EDs during this period (an average of 23,600 per year or 65 per day) (Table 58.1). The incidence of BB or pellet gun-related injuries was highest for males (53.5 per 100,000 population) and children aged 10-14 years (66.6 per 100,000 population) (Table 58.1), and the sex- and age group-specific rate was highest for males aged 10-14 years (114.3 per 100,000 population {95% CI=94.1-134.5}).

Although most (64%) persons with GSWs were transported to EDs by private vehicles, 8% of those treated were taken to EDs by emergency medical services (Table 58.2). Injuries to the eye, face, and head and neck accounted for 31% of all injuries. Hospitalization was required for 5% of cases; of these, 37% were associated with severe injury to the eye.

Data on victim-shooter relationship were complete for 71% of cases (Table 58.2). Based on these data, 31% of injuries were self-inflicted, and 33% were caused by friends, acquaintances, or relatives. Data on 76% of the incidents indicated the type of injury: although most (66%) resulted from unintentional shootings, approximately 10% were assaults; suicide attempts were rare (0.1%). Locale of the injury incident was known for approximately 55% of cases; approximately 45% of injuries occurred in and around a home, apartment, or condominium.

Reported by: Office of Statistics and Programming, Div of Violence Prevention and Div of Unintentional Injury Prevention, National Center for Injury Prevention and Control, CDC.

Table 58.1. Characteristics of Children and Teenagers Aged <=19 Years Treated in Hospital Emergency Departments for BB and Pellet Gun-Related Injuries–United States, June 1992-May 1994

Characteristic	No. *	(%)	Rate +	(95% CI &)
Sex				
Male	40,605	(86.1)	53.5	(45.1-61.9)
Female	6,532	(13.9)	9.0	(6.7-11.3)
Age (yrs)				
0-4 @	1,040	(2.2)		
5-9	8,033	(17.0)	21.6	(16.5-26.7)
10-14	24,400	(51.8)	66.6	(54.9-78.3)
15-19	13,664	(29.0)	39.6	(31.8-47.4)
Total	47,137	(100.0)	31.8	(26.8-36.8)

*Based on weighted data from 959 BB and pellet gunshot injuries reported through the National Electronic Injury Surveillance System.

+ Annualized rate per 100,000 population.

& Confidence interval.

@ Rate was not calculated because of the small number (21) of cases in this age group; interpret estimate with caution.

An estimated 3.2 million nonpowder guns are sold in the United States each year; 80% of these have muzzle velocities greater than 350 feet per second (fps) and 50% have velocities from 500 fps to 930 fps (AC Homan, US Consumer Product Safety Commission, unpublished data, 1994). Most of these guns are intended for use by persons aged 8-18 years. At close range, projectiles from many BB and pellet guns, especially those with velocities greater than 350 fps, can cause tissue damage similar to that inflicted by powder-charged bullets fired from low-velocity conventional firearms.[3] Injuries associated with use of these guns can result in permanent disability or death;[4] injuries from BBs or pellets projected from air guns involving the eye particularly are severe.[5] For example, based on data from the National

Table 58.2. BB and Pellet Gun-Related Injuries Treated in Hospital Emergency Departments (EDs) for Children and Teenagers Aged <=19 Years, by Selected Characteristics–United States, June 1992-May 1994

Characteristic	No.*	(%)
Mode of transport to ED		
Private vehicle	30,298	(64.3)
Walked in	7,788	(16.5)
Emergency medical service/		
Fire rescue/Ambulance	3,742	(8.0)
Police vehicle	468	(1.0)
Other/Not stated	4,841	(10.2)
Primary body part injured		
Extremity	25,453	(54.0)
Trunk	7,276	(15.4)
Face	6,788	(14.4)
Head/Neck	4,747	(10.1)
Eye	2,839	(6.0)
Other	34	(0.1)
ED Discharge Disposition		
Not hospitalized	44,759	(95.0)
Hospitalized	2,378	(5.0)
Victim-Shooter relationship		
Self	14,636	(31.0)
Friend/Acquaintance	9,280	(19.7)

Eye Trauma System and the United States Eye Injury Registry—a system of voluntary reporting by ophthalmologists—projectiles from air guns account for 63% of reported perforating eye injuries that occur in recreational settings.[6]

Despite the large number of BB and pellet gun-related injuries treated in hospital EDs each year,[1] there are no nationally specified safety standards for nonpowder guns. Although voluntary industry standards were established in 1978 and revised in 1992,[7] the effectiveness of these standards for preventing injuries has not been determined. These voluntary standards specify two types of warning labels, including one on the gun itself ("WARNING: Before using read Owner's Manual available free from {company name}"), and one on

Table 58.2. BB and Pellet Gun-Related Injuries Treated in Hospital Emergency Departments (EDs) for Children and Teenagers Aged <=19 Years, by Selected Characteristics–United States, June 1992-May 1994 (continued)

Characteristic	No.*	(%)
Victim-Shooter relationship, continued		
Relative	6,445	(13.7)
Stranger	1,260	(2.7)
Other/Shooter not seen	1,821	(3.9)
Not Stated	13,695	(29.1)
Type of Injury		
Unintentional	30,960	(65.7)
Assault	4,903	(10.4)
Suicide attempt	34	(0.1)
Not stated	11,240	(23.8)
Locale of injury incident		
Home/Apartment/Condominium	21,413	(45.4)
Street/Highway	1,821	(3.9)
Other property	1,389	(2.9)
School/Recreation area	1,104	(2.3)
Farm	90	(0.2)
Not stated	21,320	(45.2)
Total	47,137	(100.0)

*Based on weighted data from 959 BB and pellet gunshot injuries reported through the National Electronic Injury Surveillance System.

the packaging ("WARNING: Not a toy. Adult supervision required. Misuse or careless use may cause serious injury or death. May be dangerous up to {specific distance} ** yards ({specific distance} meters).").[7] The voluntary standards also specify that the owner's manual should provide instructions about handling and operating the gun safely, selecting safe and proper targets, caring for and maintaining the gun properly, storing of the gun in an unloaded state and in a safe and proper manner, and always confirming that the gun is unloaded when removed from storage or received from another person.[7] However, these standards do not include specifications regarding other important injury-prevention measures pertinent to minors (e.g., limits on maximum velocity and impact force of BBs and pellets or design modifications to clearly indicate when a gun is loaded).[8]

In the United States, 14 states have enacted laws to regulate the sale or possession of nonpowder guns. Although most of these states restrict the purchase, possession, or use of these guns by minors aged less than 16 years or aged less than 18 years, such age restrictions on the purchase of these guns are void in most of these states when a minor has obtained permission from a parent or guardian.

Analysis of the NEISS data indicate that BB and pellet GSWs treated in hospital EDs typically result from an unintentional shooting of a young or adolescent male who either shot himself or was shot by a friend, acquaintance, or relative. Many of these shootings occur when using or playing with a gun in or around the home. These findings suggest that ready access to a BB or pellet gun and ammunition stored in the home and/or the lack of supervision during use of the gun may contribute substantially to the risk for injury among children and adolescents, especially for boys aged 10-14 years. Although most BB and pellet gun injuries are unintentional, the findings from this analysis and from a statewide ED-based surveillance system in Massachusetts[9] also indicate that BB and pellet guns sometimes have been used to purposefully inflict harm.

Unintentional BB and pellet gun-related injuries that occur during unsupervised activities are preventable. Parents considering the purchase of a BB or pellet gun for their children should be aware of the potential hazards of these guns, and should help to ensure the safety of their children in the presence of a BB or pellet gun. Children and teenage users should recognize that these guns are not toys but are designed and intended specifically for recreational and competitive sport use. Parents or other adults should provide direct supervision at all times for each child who is using or observing the use of these guns. Each user should be educated about the potential danger of these guns, the importance of gun-safety practices, and how to safely handle and fire the gun. The use of protective eyewear should be enforced during shooting activities. When not in use, all guns in the home should be kept locked up and unloaded. Subsequent efforts to reduce the severity and frequency of injuries associated with BB and pellet guns should include determination of the effectiveness of a variety of interventions (e.g., technological, regulatory, environmental, and behavioral).

References

1. McNeill AM, Annest JL. The ongoing hazard of BB and pellet gun-related injuries in the United States. *Ann Emerg Med* 1995;26:187-94.

2. Annest JL, Mercy JA, Gibson DR, Ryan GW. National estimates of nonfatal firearm-related injuries: beyond the tip of the iceberg. *JAMA* 1995;273:1749-54.

3. Harris W, Luterman A, Curreri PW. BB and pellet guns: toys or deadly weapons? *J Trauma* 1983;23:566-9.

4. Wascher RA, Gwinn BC. Air rifle injury to the heart with retrograde caval migration. *J Trauma* 1995;38:379-81.

5. Schein OD, Enger C, Tielsch JM. The context and consequences of ocular injuries from air guns. *Am J Ophthalmol* 1994;117: 501-6.

6. Parver LM. The National Eye Trauma System. *Int Ophthalmol Clin* 1988;28:203.

7. Committee on Standards, American Society for Testing and Materials. Standard consumer safety specification for non-powder guns. Conshohocken, Pennsylvania: American Society for Testing and Materials, 1992.

8. Greensher J, Aronow R, Bass JL, et al. Injuries related to "toy" firearms: Committee on Accident and Poison Prevention. *Pediatrics* 1987;79:473-4.

9. CDC. Emergency department surveillance for weapon-related injuries — Massachusetts, November 1993-April 1994. *MMWR* 1995;44:160-3,169.

*In this report, the terms BB gun and pellet gun refer to nonpowder guns that use compressed air or gas to propel lead pellets or steel BBs.

**Distance is dependent on the type of gun and muzzle velocity.

Chapter 59

In-Line Skates and Skateboard Injuries

Each year, more than 100,000 people are treated in hospital emergency departments for injuries related to in-line skating, and nearly 40,000 seek emergency treatment for skateboarding injuries. The majority of these patients are under age 25. Many injuries can be prevented if skaters wear proper safety gear and avoid risky skating behavior.

Prevention Tips for In-Line Skaters and Skateboarders

To help your child avoid injuries while in-line skating and skateboarding, follow these safety tips from the American Academy of Pediatrics, the Centers for Disease Control and Prevention (CDC), the U.S. Consumer Product Safety Commission, and other sports and health organizations. (Note: Adult skaters should heed this advice, too.)

- Make sure your child wears all the required safety gear every time he or she skates. All skaters should wear a helmet, knee and elbow pads, and wrist guards. If your child does tricks or plays roller hockey, make sure he or she wears heavy duty gear.

- Check your child's helmet for proper fit. The helmet should be worn flat on the head, with the bottom edge parallel to the ground. It should fit snugly and should not move around in any direction when your child shakes his or her head.

"Skates and Skateboards Safety," SafeUSA, 2000.

- Choose in-line skates or a skateboard that best suits your child's ability and skating style. If your child is a novice, choose in-line skates with three or four wheels. Skates with five wheels are only for experienced skaters and people who skate long distances. Choose a skateboard designed for your child's type of riding—slalom, freestyle, or speed. Some boards are rated for the weight of the rider.

- Find a smooth skating surface for your child; good choices are skating trails and driveways without much slope (but be careful about children skating into traffic). Check for holes, bumps, and debris that could make your child fall. Novice in-line skaters should start out in a skating rink where the surface is smooth and flat and where speed is controlled.

- Don't let your child skate in areas with high pedestrian or vehicle traffic. Children should not skate in the street or on vehicle parking ramps.

- Tell your child never to skitch. Skitching is the practice of holding on to a moving vehicle in order to skate very fast. People have died while skitching.

- If your child is new to in-line skating, lessons from an instructor certified by the International In-line Skating Association may be helpful. These lessons show proper form and teach how to stop. Check with your local parks and recreation department to find a qualified instructor.

- If your child gets injured while skating, see your doctor. Follow all the doctor's instructions for your child's recovery, and get the doctor's permission before your child starts skating again.

Who Is Affected?

Millions of people in the U.S.—the majority of them under age 25—take part in in-line skating and skateboarding as a form of recreation and exercise. But these sports can be dangerous, especially when safety precautions are ignored. Each year, more than 100,000 skaters are injured seriously enough to need medical care in hospital emergency departments, doctors' offices, clinics, and outpatient centers. Most of these injuries occur when skaters lose control, skate over an obstacle, skate too fast, or perform a trick.

While most skating injuries are minor or require only outpatient care, 36 fatalities have been reported since 1992. Thirty-one of those skating deaths were from collisions with motor vehicles. Among all age groups, 63 percent of skating injuries are fractures, dislocations, sprains, strains, and avulsions (tears). More than one-third of skating injuries are to the wrist area, with two-thirds of these injuries being fractures and dislocations. Approximately 5 percent are head injuries. Safety gear has been shown to be highly effective in preventing injuries among skaters. Pads can reduce wrist and elbow injuries by about 85 percent and knee injuries by 32 percent. Although studies have not determined the degree to which helmets reduce head injuries among skaters, helmets have been shown to be highly protective among bicyclists.

Despite the proven safety benefits and relative low cost of helmets and pads, many skaters don't wear them. Nearly two-thirds of injured in-line skaters and skateboarders were not wearing safety gear when they crashed. One study found that one-third of skaters wear no safety gear, and another one-third use only some of the recommended safety equipment. Teens are least likely to wear all the safety gear. Nine out of ten beginning skaters wear all the safety gear, but studies have shown that many skaters shed the helmet and pads as they gain experience.

References

American Academy of Orthopaedic Surgeons. *Injuries from in-line skating. Position statement.* Available at www.aaos.org/wordhtml/papers/position/inline.htm. Accessed July 8, 1999.

American Academy of Pediatrics. In-line skating injuries in children and adolescents. *Pediatrics* 1998;101(4):720-721.

CDC. Toy safety–United States, 1984. *Morbidity and Mortality Weekly Report* 1985;34(5):755-6, 761-2.

National Pediatric Trauma Registry. *Falls while skating or skateboarding.* NPTR fact sheet #9. April 1999. Available at www.nemc.org/rehab/factshee.htm. Accessed July 7, 1999.

Schieber R, Branche-Dorsey C, Ryan G. Comparison of in-line skating injuries with rollerskating and skateboarding injuries. *JAMA* 1994;271(23):1856-1858.

Schieber R, Branche C. In-line skating injuries: Epidemiology and recommendations for prevention. *Sports Medicine* 1995;19(6):427-432.

U.S. Consumer Product Safety Commission. *CPSC projects sharp rise in in-line skating injuries.* News release, June 21, 1995. Available at www.cpsc.gov/cpscpub/prerel/prhtml95/95135.html. Accessed July 12, 1999.

U.S. Consumer Product Safety Commission. *Safety commission warns about hazards with in-line roller skates: Safety alert.* CPSC document #5050. Available at www.cpsc.gov/cpscpub/pubs/5050.html. Accessed July 12, 1999.

U.S. Consumer Product Safety Commission. *Holiday skateboard and roller skates safety.* Available at www.cpsc.gov/kids/skate.html. Accessed July 12, 1999.

Safety Resources

American Academy of Pediatrics
141 Northwest Point Blvd
Elk Grove Village, IL 60007-1098
Toll-Free: 847-434-4000
Fax: 847-434-8000
Website: www.aap.org/policy/re9739.html

In 1998, AAP issued a statement on in-line skating injuries in children and adolescents.

American Academy of Orthopaedic Surgeons
6300 North River Road
Rosemont, IL 60018-4262
Toll-Free: 800-346-2267
Tel: 847-823-7186
Fax: 847-823-8125
Fax on Demand: 800-999-2939
Website: www.aaos.org

Through the public information link on the AAOS home page (www.aaos.org), you can access fact sheets on a variety of popular sports, including in-line skating.

Brain Injury Association
105 North Alfred Street
Alexandria, VA 22314
Toll-Free: 800-444-6443
Tel: 703-236-6000
Fax: 703-236-6001
Website: www.biausa.org/sportsfs.htm
E-mail: familyhelpline@biausa.org

BIA's fact sheet on sports and concussion safety provides data on brain injuries for several sports, including in-line skating.

U.S. Consumer Product Safety Commission
Washington, DC 20207
Toll-Free: 800-638-2772
Fax: 800-638-2772
Website: www.cpsc.gov/kids/skate.html
E-mail: info@cpsc.gov

CPSC offers kids advice on skateboard and in-line skating safety.

National SAFE KIDS Campaign
1301 Pennsylvania Ave., N.W.
Suite 1000
Washington, DC 20004
Tel: 202-662-0600
Fax: 202-393-2072
Website: www.safekids.org
E-mail: info@safekids.org

Visit the SAFE KIDS home page to access fact sheets on sports and recreation injuries.

National Youth Sports Safety Foundation
333 Longwood Avenue, Suite 202
Boston, Massachusetts 02115
Tel: 617-277-1171
Fax: 617-277-2278
Website: www.nyssf.org
E-mail: NYSSF@aol.com

NYSSF has a variety of fact sheets on sports safety available for purchase.

Chapter 60

Winter Sports Injury Prevention

For many children, winter is not the end of outdoor fun. From sledding to skiing, snowmobiling to ice skating, children find lots to do when the snow starts to fall. Unfortunately, the cold season can also lead to tragedy.

For 10-year-old Joshua of Minnesota, it was a deadly snowmobile incident. Five-year-old Jonathan from Massachusetts nearly drowned. Frostbite affected 3-year-old Nicole of Colorado. Winter does not need to be a tragic time for children. When properly prepared, they can enjoy a safe and fun-filled winter wonderland.

"The inviting snow draws children to ice-covered lakes and ski slopes each winter, regardless of the frigid temperatures and the risks," says Heather Paul, Ph.D., executive director of the National SAFE KIDS Campaign. "Parents should watch their children closely, limit their outdoor playtime, and make sure that they are dressed appropriately for the weather." The National SAFE KIDS Campaign recommends the following tips to help keep your children safe.

Winter Drowning

Most parents associate drowning with summer months, but the increased use of hot tubs and whirlpools as well as the danger of hidden bodies of water or weak ice make winter drowning a risk as well. To minimize drowning dangers, parents and caregivers should:

"Stay Safe in Your Winter Wonderland," National SAFE KIDS Campaign, 2000; and "Winter Sports Injury Prevention," SafeUSA, 2000.

- Supervise children in or near a pool, hot tub, or any open body of water.

- Make sure pools and spas are secure. If you have a pool or spa, install four-sided isolation fencing that is at least 5 feet high. The fence should have a self-closing and self-latching gate. Do not use the exterior of the house as one side of the fence.

- Allow children to skate only on ponds or lakes that have been approved for skating.

Frostbite

Exposure to cold without adequate protection can result in frostbite. Parents can protect their children by following these precautions:

- Dress children warmly. Several thin layers will help keep children dry as well as warm. Clothing should consist of thermal long johns, turtlenecks, one or two shirts, pants, sweater, coat, warm socks, boots, gloves or mittens, and a hat.

- Set reasonable time limits on outdoor play. Call children in periodically to warm up with drinks such as hot chocolate.

- When possible, avoid taking infants outdoors when it is colder than 40 degrees Fahrenheit. Infants lose body heat quickly.

If a child complains of numbness or pain in the fingers, toes, nose, cheeks, or ears while playing in the snow, or if his skin is blistered, hard to the touch or glossy, be alerted to the possibility of frostbite and take the following steps:

- Take the child indoors.

- Call a doctor.

- Tell the child to wiggle the affected body part(s) to increase blood supply to that area.

- Warm the frozen part(s) against the body. Hold fingers to the chest, for example.

- Immerse frozen part(s) in warm, not hot, water. Frozen tissue is fragile and can be damaged easily. Avoid warming with high heat from radiators, fireplaces, or stoves, and avoid rubbing or breaking blisters.

Pedestrian Safety

Slippery driveways and sidewalks can be particularly hazardous in the winter. Keep them well shoveled, and apply materials such as rock salt or sand to improve traction.

- Make sure that children under age 10 do not cross streets alone, and make sure children wear appropriate shoes and brightly colored (not white) clothing while walking in snowy conditions.

- Use retroreflective clothing or stickers for maximum protection, especially at dawn and dusk.

Winter Sports and Activities

Parents and caregivers should inspect equipment and the environment for possible hazards before children engage in winter activities such as sledding, ice skating, and skiing. Remind children not to push, shove, or roughhouse while engaging in sports, and tell them always to wait their turn.

Ice Skating

In 1999, more than 16,000 children ages 5 to 14 were treated in emergency rooms for injuries related to ice skating. But with extra care, even children as young as age 4, as long as they are steady walkers, can enjoy the sport. Allow children to skate only on approved surfaces. Check for signs posted by local police or recreation departments, or call your local police department to find out which areas have been approved. Children should be taught to:

- Skate in the same direction as the crowd.

- Avoid darting across the ice.

- Never skate alone.

- Never go out on ice that an adult has not approved.

- Throw away chewing gum or candy before skating onto the ice.

- If a child falls through the ice, he should stretch his arms over the ice and kick as if swimming, in an attempt to crawl back onto the solid ice.

Sledding

More than 14,000 children ages 5 to 14 were treated in emergency rooms in 1999 for injuries related to sledding. Parents and caregivers should remember the following tips:

- Make sure terrain is free of obstacles and far from traffic. Children should sled on packed snow (not ice) that is free of debris. Check carefully for snow-covered hazards such as rocks, tree limbs, and stumps that could endanger sledders or skiers.

- Use equipment that is sturdy and safely constructed. Avoid equipment with sharp and jagged edges.

- Look for energy absorbing pads on sled seats.

- Examine handholds on sleds to be sure they are secure.

- Ensure sleds and toboggans have easy steering, non-jamming devices.

Parents should remind children to:

- Sled only on terrain that is free of obstacles.

- Make sure the bottom of the slope is far from streets and traffic.

- Always use a sled with a steering mechanism. Avoid makeshift sleds.

- Avoid lying flat on the sled while riding down hill. Always sit up with feet forward—lying flat increases the chance of head and abdominal injuries.

- Never ride in a sled that is being pulled by a motorized vehicle.

- Make sure the number of children riding on the sled does not exceed the manufacturer's recommendations.

Snow Skiing and Snowboarding

According to the National Sporting Goods Association, nearly 10 million persons participate in alpine skiing more than once a year and up to 2.5 million snowboard each year. Skiing, snowboarding, and sledding can be great fun and are terrific ways to exercise. But they can also be risky. The U.S. Consumer Product Safety Commission (CPSC) estimates that 84,200 skiing injuries and 37,600 snowboarding injuries were treated in hospital emergency rooms in the United States in 1997, including approximately 17,500 head injuries. However, the most common skiing-related injuries are knee and ankle sprains and fractures. While most skiing and snowboarding injuries occur among adults, the majority of sledding-related injuries are among children 5-14 years old. More than 14,500 children in this age group were treated for sledding-related injuries in the United States in 1997.

The estimated number of skiing-related injuries declined by more than 25 percent from 1993 to 1997, partly because of improvements in ski equipment, such as redesigned bindings. However, during that same period, snowboarding injuries nearly tripled and the number of head injuries from snowboarding increased five-fold.

A CPSC study found there were 17,500 head injuries associated with skiing and snowboarding in 1997. This study estimated that 7,700 head injuries, including 2,600 head injuries to children, could be prevented or reduced in severity each year by using skiing or snowboarding helmets. The study also showed that helmet use could prevent about 11 skiing- and snowboarding-related deaths annually. As a result of these findings, CPSC recommends skiers and snowboarders wear helmets specifically designed for these activities to prevent head injuries from falls and collisions.

Preparation

- Before you get out on the slopes, be sure you're in shape. You'll enjoy the sports more and have lower risk of injury if you're physically fit.

- Take a lesson (or several) from a qualified instructor. Like anything, you'll improve the most when you receive expert guidance. And be sure to learn how to fall correctly and safely to reduce the risk of injury.

- Don't start jumping maneuvers until you've had proper instruction on how to jump and have some experience. Jumps are the most common cause of spinal injuries among snowboarders.

- Obtain proper equipment. Be sure that your equipment is in good condition and have your ski or snowboard bindings adjusted correctly at a local ski shop. (Extra tip for snowboarders: wrist guards and knee pads can help protect you when you fall.)

- Wear a helmet to prevent head injuries from falls or collisions. (One study showed that helmet use by skiers and snowboarders could prevent or reduce the severity of nearly half of head injuries to adults and more than half of head injuries to children less than 15 years old.) Skiers and snowboarders should wear helmets specifically designed for these sports.

- When buying skiwear, look for fabric that is water and wind-resistant. Look for wind flaps to shield zippers, snug cuffs at wrists and ankles, collars that can be snuggled up to the chin, and drawstrings that can be adjusted for comfort and to keep the wind out.

- Dress in layers. Layering allows you to accommodate your body's constantly changing temperature. For example, dress in polypropylene underwear (top and bottoms), which feels good next to the skin, dries quickly, absorbs sweat, and keeps you warm. Wear a turtleneck, sweater, and jacket.

- Be prepared for changes in the weather. Bring a headband or hat with you to the slopes (60 percent of heat-loss is through the head) and wear gloves or mittens.

- Protect your skin from the sun and wind by using a sun screen or sun block. The sun reflects off the snow and is stronger than you think, even on cloudy days!

- Always use appropriate eye protection. Sunglasses or goggles will help protect your vision from glare, help you to see the terrain better, and help shield your eyes from flying debris.

When You're on the Slopes

- The key to successful skiing and snowboarding is control. To have it, you must be aware of your technique and level of ability, the terrain, and the skiers and snowboarders around you.

- Take a couple of slow ski or snowboard runs to warm up at the start of each day.

- Ski or snowboard with partners and stay within sight of each other, if possible. If one partner loses the other, stop, and wait.

- Stay on marked trails and avoid potential avalanche areas such as steep hillsides with little vegetation. Begin a run slowly. Watch out for rocks and patches of ice on the trails.

- Be aware of the weather and snow conditions and how they can change. Make adjustments for icy conditions, deep snow powder, wet snow, and adverse weather conditions.

- If you find yourself on a slope that exceeds your ability level, always leave your skis or snowboard on and sidestep down the slope.

- If you find yourself skiing or snowboarding out of control, fall down on your rear end or on your side, the softest parts of your body.

- Drink plenty of water to avoid becoming dehydrated.

- Avoid alcohol consumption. Skiing and snowboarding do not mix well with alcohol or drugs. Beware of medicines or drugs that impair the senses or make you drowsy.

- If you're tired, stop, and rest. Fatigue is a risk factor for injuries.

The National Ski Areas Association endorses a responsibility code for skiers. This code can be applied to snowboarders also. The following are the code's seven safety rules of the slopes:

1. Always stay in control and be able to stop or avoid other people or objects.

2. People ahead of you have the right of way. It is your responsibility to avoid them.

3. You must not stop where you obstruct a trail or are not visible from above.

4. Whenever starting downhill or merging into a trail, look uphill, and yield to others.

5. Always use devices to help prevent runaway equipment.

6. Observe all posted signs and warnings.

6. Keep off closed trails and out of closed areas. Prior to using any lift, you must have the knowledge and ability to load, ride, and unload safely.

Snowmobiling

Snowmobiles can weigh up to 600 pounds and travel at speeds in excess of 90 mph. Head injuries are the leading cause of snowmobile-related deaths. In 1999, nearly 1,500 children ages 14 and under were treated in emergency rooms for snowmobile-related injuries. The American Academy of Pediatrics has stated that operating snowmobiles is inappropriate for children under age 16. If a child is riding as a passenger on a snowmobile, be sure he is wearing an approved helmet. Children ages 5 and under should never ride on snowmobiles.

References

American Academy of Orthopaedic Surgeons. *Skiing*. Available at www.aaos.org/wordhtml/pat_educ/skiing.htm. Accessed December 10, 1999.

American Academy of Orthopaedic Surgeons. *Sledding Safety*. Available at www.aaos.org/wordhtml/papers/position/sledding.htm. Accessed December 10, 1999.

Caine D, Caine C, Lindner K, editors. Epidemiology of Sports Injuries. Champaign, IL: *Human Kinetics*, 1996:29-40.

National Ski Areas Association. *Ski and Snowboarding Tips*. Available at www.nsaa.org/MemberUpdate/skitips.htm. Accessed December 13, 1999.

National Ski Areas Association. *Your Responsibility Code*. Available at www.nsaa.org/MemberUpdate/thecode.htm. Accessed December 13, 1999.

SAFE KIDS. *Sports and Recreational Activity Injury*. Available at www.safekids.org/fact99/sports99.html. Accessed December 10, 1999.

U.S. Consumer Product Safety Commission. *CPSC Staff Recommends Use of Helmets for Skiers, Snowboarders to Prevent Head Injuries*. Available at www.cpsc.gov/cpscpub/prerel/prhtm199/99046.html. Accessed December 10, 1999.

Safety Resources

American Academy of Orthopaedic Surgeons
6300 North River Road
Rosemont, IL 60018-4262
Toll-Free: 800-346-AAOS
Tel: 847-823-7186
Fax: 847-823-8125
Fax on Demand: 800-999-2939
Website: www.aaos.org

Through the public information link to patient education on the AAOS home page www.aaos.org, you can access fact sheets on injury prevention for many sports, including skiing and sledding.

American Academy of Pediatrics
141 Northwest Point Boulevard
Elk Grove Village, IL 60007-1098
Tel: 847-434-4000
Fax: 847-434-8000
Website: www.aap.org
E-mail: kidsdocs@aap.org

AAP has safety tips for the winter holidays (including tips on outdoor sports) at www.aap.org/advocacy/releases/novsafe.htm.

National Safety Council
1121 Spring Lake Drive
Itasca, IL 60143-3201
Tel: 630-285-1121
Fax: 630-285-1315
Website: www.nsc.org

National Ski Areas Association
133 S. Van Gordon Street, Suite 300
Lakewood, CO 80228
Tel 303-987-1111
Fax: 303-986-2345
Website: www.nsaa.org
E-mail: nsaa@nsaa.org

NSAA is the trade association for ski area owners and operators. Suggestions for safe skiing and snowboarding can be found on their web site at www.nsaa.org/MemberUpdate/skitips.htm.

National Ski Patrol
133 S. Van Gordon Street
Suite 100
Lakewood, CO 80228
Tel 303-987-1111
Fax: 303-988-3005
Website: www.nsp.org
E-mail: nsp@nsp.org

NSP is a nonprofit membership association providing education services about emergency care and safety to the public and mountain recreation industry.

SAFE KIDS
1301 Pennsylvania Ave., N.W.
Suite 1000
Washington, DC 20004
Tel: 202-662-0600
Fax: 202-393-2072
Website: www.safekids.org
E-mail: info@safekids.org

U.S. Consumer Product Safety Commission
Washington, DC 20207-0001
Toll-Free: 800-638-2772
Toll-Free Teletypewriter: 800-638-8270
TTY: 800-638-8270
Website: www.cpsc.gov
E-mail: info@cpsc.gov

Part Nine

Additional Help and Information

Chapter 61

Glossary of Terms

A

Acute: An illness or injury that lasts for a short time and may be intense.

Audiogram: Graph of hearing threshold level as a function of frequency.

B

Baseline audiogram: The audiogram obtained from an audiometric examination administered before employment or within the first 30 days of employment that is preceded by a period of at least 12 hours of quiet. The baseline audiogram is the audiogram against which subsequent audiograms will be compared for the calculation of significant threshold shift.

This chapter includes glossary information from the following sources: "Q & A about Sprains and Strains," (NIAMS), December 1999; "Occupational Safety and Health Definitions," Bureau of Labor Statistics, 2001; "Census of Fatal Occupational Injuries: Definitions" [Accessibility Information], "Neck (Cervical Spine) Disorders," 2000, and "Repetitive Motion Disorders," 2000, National Institute of Arthritis and Musculoskeletal and Skin Diseases (NIAMS); and excerpts from Chapters 2 and 6 of *Occupational Noise Exposure, Recommendations for a Noise Standard*, National Institute for Occupational Safety and Health (NIOSH), 1998.

Bursitis: Inflammation of the bursa, a small fluid-containing sac that reduces friction where parts of the body move over or against each other, especially around joints.

C

Carpal tunnel syndrome: Pressure on the median nerve as it passes through the wrist; caused by swelling of the tissues around the nerve or by bony injuries to the wrist.

Chronic: An illness or injury that lasts for a long time.

Conductive hearing losses: These are usually traceable to diseases of the outer and middle ear.

Continuous noise: Noise with negligibly small fluctuations of level within the period of observation.

CT scan (computerized tomography scanning): A diagnostic technique in which the combined use of a computer and x-rays passed through the body at different angles produces clear cross-sectional images of the tissue being examined. CT scanning is more sensitive than x-rays, which alone do not permit cross-sectional views.

Cubital tunnel syndrome: Compression or injury of the ulnar nerve at the elbow as it passes through an opening formed by a ligament, muscle, or other tissue. Symptoms may include pain in the elbow and/or forearm, numbness in the ring or little fingers, and weakness of specific muscles in the forearm and hand.

D

Decibel (dB): Unit of level when the base of the logarithm is the 10th root of 10 and the quantities concerned are proportional to power.

Decompression: Relief of pressure, such as that exerted on the spinal cord or nerve roots by a disc or part of the bone of the spine.

Derate: To use a fraction of a hearing protectors noise reduction rating (NRR) to calculate the noise exposure of a worker wearing that hearing protector. (See NRR.)

Discography (diskography): A diagnostic technique in which a dye visible on x-ray films is injected into an intervertebral disc.

E

Epicondylitis: Inflammation of the outer side of the bony projection at the elbow, usually at the origin of one of the muscles that straightens (extends) the wrist. (Sometimes referred to as "tennis elbow.")

Equal-energy hypothesis: A hypothesis stating that equal amounts of sound energy will produce equal amounts of hearing impairment, regardless of how the sound energy is distributed in time.

Event or exposure: Signifies the manner in which the injury or illness was produced or inflicted, for example, overexertion while lifting or fall from ladder.

Excess risk: Percentage with material impairment of hearing in an occupational-noise-exposed population after subtracting the percentage who would normally incur such impairment from other causes in a population not exposed to occupational noise.

F

Femur: The upper leg or thigh bone, which extends into the hip socket at its upper end and down to the knee at its lower end.

Fence: The hearing threshold level above which a material impairment of hearing is considered to have occurred.

Fibula: The thin, outer bone of the leg that forms part of the ankle joint at its lower end.

G

Ganglion cyst: Fluid-filled, closed cavity, or sac that usually occurs in ligaments or other connective tissues in the wrist and hand., caused by repetitive motions or injury.

H

Hearing threshold level (HTL): For a specified signal, amount in decibels by which the hearing threshold for a listener, for one or both ears, exceeds a specified reference equivalent threshold level.

I

Immission level: A descriptor for noise exposure, in decibels, representing the total sound energy incident on the ear over a specified period of time (e.g., months, years).

Inflammation: A characteristic reaction of tissues to disease or injury; it is marked by four signs: swelling, redness, heat, and pain.

Intermittent noise: Noise levels that are interrupted by intervals of relatively low sound levels.

Intervertebral foramina: A normal opening between vertebrae that permits passage of a spinal nerve and blood vessels.

J

Joint: A junction where two bones meet.

L

Laminectomy: Surgical removal of usually a part of the bony arches of the vertebrae that surround the spinal cord to relieve pressure on the cord or nerve roots.

Ligament: A band of tough, fibrous tissue that connects two or more bones at a joint and prevents excessive movement of the joint.

Lost workday cases: Cases which involve days away from work, or days of restricted work activity, or both. Lost workday cases involving days away from work are those cases which result in days away from work, or a combination of days away from work and days of restricted work activity. Lost workday cases involving restricted work activity are those cases which result in restricted work activity only.

M

Medullary vessels: Blood vessels that run along the spinal cord.

MRI (magnetic resonance imaging): Diagnostic technique that provides high-quality cross-sectional images without x-rays or other radiation. The patient lies inside a massive, hollow, cylindrical magnet and is exposed to short bursts of powerful magnetic fields and radio waves. The bursts stimulate hydrogen atoms in the tissues to emit signals that are detected and analyzed by computer to create an image of a slice of the tissue. "Open" MRI units are available for patients who feel claustrophobic in common MRI units.

Muscle: Tissue composed of bundles of specialized cells that contract and produce movement when stimulated by nerve impulses.

Myelography (myelogram): Injection of an opaque substance into the spinal column that shows up on x-ray, permitting visualization of pathology. This technique is being replaced by the newer CT scan and MRI techniques.

Myelopathy: Nervous system problems caused by pressure on the spinal cord.

N

Nature of injury or illness: Names the principal physical characteristic of a disabling condition, such as sprain/strain, cut/laceration, or carpal tunnel syndrome.

Noise: (1) Undesired sound. By extension, noise is any unwarranted disturbance within a useful frequency band, such as undesired electric waves in a transmission channel or device. (2) Erratic, intermittent, or statistically random oscillation.

Noise reduction rating (NRR): The NRR, which indicates a hearing protectors noise reduction capabilities, is a single-number rating that is required by law to be shown on the label of each hearing protector sold in the United States.

O

Occupational injury: Any injury such as a cut, fracture, sprain, amputation, etc., which results from a work-related event or from a single instantaneous exposure in the work environment.

Occupational illness: Any abnormal condition or disorder, other than one resulting from an occupational injury, produced in the work environment over a period longer than one workday or shift, caused by exposure to factors associated with employment. It includes acute and chronic illnesses or disease which may be caused by inhalation, absorption, ingestion, or direct contact.

Oseous protrusion: A bony projection.

Osteophyte: A bony outgrowth.

P

Part of body affected: The body part directly linked to the nature of injury or illness cited, for example, back sprain, finger cut, or wrist and carpal tunnel syndrome.

Permanent threshold shift (PTS): Permanent increase in the threshold of audibility for an ear.

Presbycusis: The sensorineural hearing loss that occurs naturally because of aging.

Pulse range: Difference in decibels between the peak level of an impulsive signal and the root-mean-square level of a continuous noise.

R

Radiculopathy: Pressure on a nerve root as it branches off the spinal cord, causing symptoms in the area stimulated by the nerve root.

Range of motion: The arc of movement of a joint from one extreme position to the other; range-of-motion exercises help increase or maintain flexibility and movement in muscles, tendons, ligaments, and joints.

Recordable injuries: Recordable injuries and illnesses are:

1. Occupational deaths, regardless of the time between injury and death, or the length of the illness; or

2. Nonfatal occupational illnesses; or

3. Nonfatal occupational injuries which involve one or more of the following: Loss of consciousness, restriction of work or motion, transfer to another job, or medical treatment (other than first aid).

S

Significant threshold shift: A shift in hearing threshold, outside the range of audiometric testing variability (5 dB), that warrants follow-up action to prevent further hearing loss. NIOSH defines significant threshold shift as an increase in the HTL of 15 dB or more at any frequency (500, 1000, 2000, 3000, 4000, or 6000 Hz) in either ear that is confirmed for the same ear and frequency by a second test within 30 days of the first test.

Sociocusis: Hearing loss caused by exposure to nonoccupational noise is collectively called sociocusis.

Source of injury or illness: The object, substance, exposure, or bodily motion that directly produced or inflicted the disabling condition cited. Examples are a heavy box, a toxic substance, fire/flame, and bodily motion of injured/ill worker.

Spondylosis: An osteoarthritic condition of the spine.

Sprain: An injury to a ligament—a stretching or a tearing. One or more ligaments can be injured during a sprain. The severity of the injury will depend on the extent of injury to a single ligament (whether the tear is partial or complete) and the number of ligaments involved.

Stenosis: A narrowing of the spinal canal or intervertebral foramen.

Strain: An injury to either a muscle or a tendon. Depending on the severity of the injury, a strain may be a simple overstretch of the muscle or tendon, or it can result in a partial or complete tear.

Subluxation: Slippage or a partial dislocation of a vertebra.

T

Temporary threshold shift: Temporary increase in the threshold of audibility for an ear caused by exposure to high-intensity acoustic stimuli. Such a shift may be caused by other means such as use of aspirin or other drugs.

Tendinitis: Inflammation of a tendon.

Tendons: Tough, fibrous cords of tissue that connect muscle to bone.

Tenosynovitis: Inflammation of tissue that covers tendons to permit them to move without friction.

Thoracic outlet syndrome: A series of symptoms involving pain in the arms and shoulders, tingling in the fingers, and a weak grip caused by pressure on the brachial plexus (nerves that pass into the arms from the neck).

Tibia: The thick, long bone of the lower leg (also called the shin) that forms part of the knee joint at its upper end and the ankle joint at its lower end.

Traumatic injury: A traumatic injury is any unintentional or intentional wound or damage to the body resulting from acute exposure to energy—such as heat or electricity or kinetic energy from a crash—or from the absence of such essentials as heat or oxygen caused by a specific event, incident, or series of events within a single workday or shift.

Trigger finger: Pain and inability to extend (straighten) a finger, resulting either from a thickening of the flexor tendon or its surrounding membrane. Occasionally the involved finger will momentarily lock in a bent (flexed) position.

V

Varying noise: Noise, with or without audible tones, for which the level varies substantially during the period of observation.

W

Work relationship criteria: A work relationship exists if an event or exposure results in the fatal injury or illness of a person: (1) ON the employer's premises and the person was there to work; or (2) OFF the employer's premises and the person was there to work, or the event or exposure was related to the person's work or status as an employee. The employer's premises include buildings, grounds, parking lots, and other facilities and property used in the conduct of business. Work is defined as duties, activities, or tasks that produce a product or result; that are done in exchange for money, goods, services, profit, or benefit; and, that are legal activities in the United States. The following are clarifications of the CFOI work relationship criteria.

- **Volunteer workers:** Fatalities to volunteer workers who are exposed to the same work hazards and perform the same duties or functions as paid employees and that meet the CFOI work relationship criteria are IN scope.

- **Institutionalized persons:** Fatalities to institutionalized persons, including inmates of penal and mental institutions, sanitariums, and homes for the aged, infirm and needy, are OUT of scope unless they are employed off the premises of their institutions.

- **Suicides and homicides** that meet the CFOI work relationship criteria are IN scope.

- **Fatal heart attacks and strokes** are IN scope if they occurred ON or OFF the employer's premises and the person was there to work. Those fatal heart attacks and strokes that occurred under other circumstances are OUT of scope, unless work relationship is verified.

- **Recreational activities:** Fatal events or exposures that occurred during a person's recreational activities, that were not required by the person's employer, are OUT of scope.

- **Travel status:** Fatal events or exposures that occurred when a person was in travel status are IN scope if the travel was for work purposes or was a condition of employment.

- **Commuting:** Fatal events or exposures that occurred during a person's commute to or from work are OUT of scope.

Chapter 62

Directory of Resources

Note: All listed prices are subject to change.

Injury Resources

National Center for Injury Prevention and Control
Office of Communications Resources
Mailstop K65
4770 Buford Highway NE
Atlanta, GA 30341
Tel: 770-488-1506
Fax: 770-488-1667
Website: www.cdc.gov/ncipc
E-mail: OHCINFO@cdc.gov

A national agency to reduce injury, disability, death, and costs associated with injuries outside the workplace; established in 1992 by the Centers for Disease Control and Prevention.

This chapter includes information from "National Poison Prevention Week—List of Materials," Consumer Product Safety Commission, Document 385; a resource list from "Traumatic Brain Injury: Cognitive and Communication Disorders," National Institute on Deafness and Other Communication Disorders (NIDCD), 1998; and the "Trauma, Burn, and Injury: Resources," Fact Sheet, National Institute of General Medical Sciences (NIGMS), updated March 13, 2001.

American Academy of Orthopaedic Surgeons
6300 North River Road
Rosemont, IL 60018-4262
Toll-Free: 800-346-AAOS
Tel: 847-823-7186
Fax: 847-823-8125
Fax on Demand: 800-999-2939
Website: www.aaos.org

The orthopaedist's scope of practice includes disorders of the body's bones, joints, ligaments, muscles, and tendons.

American Academy of Pediatrics
141 Northwest Point Boulevard
Elk Grove Village, IL 60007-1098
Tel: 847-434-4000
Fax: 847-434-8000
Website: www.aap.org
E-mail: kidsdocs@aap.org

The American Academy of Pediatrics (AAP) and its member pediatricians dedicate their efforts and resources to the health, safety, and well-being of infants, children, adolescents, and young adults. Activities of the AAP include advocacy for children and youth, public education, research, professional education, and membership service and advocacy for pediatricians.

American Chronic Pain Association (ACPA)
P.O. Box 850
Rocklin, CA 95677-0850
Tel: 916-632-0922
Fax: 916-632-3208
Website: www.theacpa.org
E-mail: ACPA@pacbell.net

American College of Rheumatology
1800 Century Place, Suite 250
Atlanta, GA 30329
Tel: 404-633-3777
Fax: 404-633-1870
Website: www.rheumatology.org
E-mail: acr@rheumatology.org

This national professional organization can provide referrals to rheumatologists and allied health professionals, such as physical therapists. One-page fact sheets are available on various forms of arthritis. Lists of specialists by geographic area and fact sheets are also available on this website.

American College of Surgeons
633 North St. Clair Street
Chicago, IL 60611-3211
Tel: 312-202-5155
Website: www.facs.org

American Physical Therapy Association
1111 N. Fairfax Street
Alexandria, VA 22314
Toll-Free: 800-999-APTA (2782)
Tel: 703-684-2783
Fax: 703-683-6748
TDD: 703-683-6748
Website: www.apta.org

American Podiatric Medical Association
9312 Old Georgetown Road
Bethesda, MD 20814
Tel: 301-571-9200
Fax: 301-530-2725
Website: www.apma.org
E-mail: aaskapma@apma.org

Arthritis Foundation
1330 West Peachtree Street
Atlanta, GA 30309
Toll-Free: 800-283-7800
Tel: 404-872-7100 or call your local chapter (listed in the local telephone directory)
Website: www.arthritis.org

The foundation has several free brochures about coping with arthritis, taking nonsteroid and steroid medicines, and exercise. A free brochure on protecting your joints is titled "Using Your Joints Wisely." The foundation also can provide addresses and phone numbers for local chapters and physician and clinic referrals.

National Arthritis and Musculoskeletal and Skin Diseases Information Clearinghouse (NAMSIC)
National Institutes of Health
1 AMS Circle
Bethesda, MD 20892-3675
Toll-Free: 877-22-NIAMS
Tel: 301-495-4484
Fax: 301-718-6366
TTY: 301-565-2966
Website: www.nih.gov/niams
E-mail: niamsinfo@mail.nih.gov

National Chronic Pain Outreach Association (NCPOA)
7979 Old Georgetown Road, Suite 100
Bethesda, MD 20814-2429
Tel: 301-652-4948
Fax: 301-907-0745
E-mail: ncpoa@cfw.com

National Headache Foundation
428 W. St. James Pl., 2nd Floor
Chicago IL 60614-2750
Toll-Free: 888-NHF-5552 (643-5552)
Tel: 773-388-6399
Fax: 773-525-7357
Website: www.headaches.org
E-mail: info@headaches.org

National Institute of General Medical Sciences, NIH
45 Center Drive MSC 6200
Bethesda, MD 20892-6200
Tel: 301-496-7301
Website: www.nigms.nih.gov
E-mail: pub_info@nigms.nih.gov

Spinal Cord Injury and Traumatic Brain Injury Resources

ABLEDATA
8630 Fenton Street
Suite 930
Silver Spring, MD 20910
Toll-Free: 800-227-0216
TTY: 301-608-8912
Website: www.abledata.com
E-mail: abledata@macroint.com

Provides computerized searches for assistive devices, products, and equipment. Searches include distributor information and product descriptions. Fact sheets and information on catalogs are also available. The database can be searched from the ABLEDATA website.

American Academy of Neurology
1080 Montreal Avenue
St. Paul, MN 55116
Toll-Free: 800-879-1960
Tel: 612-695-1940
Website: www.aan.com
E-mail: web@aan.com

American Speech-Language-Hearing Association
10801 Rockville Pike
Rockville, MD 20852
Toll-Free: 800-638-8255
Tel: 301-987-5700 Voice/TTY
Fax: 301-571-0457
Website: www.asha.org
E-mail: actioncenter@asha.org

Brain Injury Association, Inc.
105 North Alfred Street
Alexandria, VA 22314
Toll-Free: 800-444-6443
Tel: 703-236-6000
Fax: 703-236-6001
Website: www.biausa.org
E-mail: familyhelpline@biausa.org

Christopher Reeve Paralysis Foundation

500 Morris Avenue
Springfield, NJ 07081
Toll-Free: 800-225-0292
Tel: 973-379-2690
Fax: 973-912-9433
Website: www.paralysis.org
E-mail: info@crpf.org

Kent Waldrep National Paralysis Foundation

16415 Addison Road, Suite 550
Addison, TX 75001
Toll-Free: 800-SCI-CURE (925-2873)
Tel: 972-248-7100
Fax: 972-248-7313
Website: www.spinalvictory.org
E-mail: kwaldrep@spinalvictory.org

Marketing Health Promotion, Wellness, and Risk Information to Spinal Cord Injury Survivors in the Community

Craig Hospital
3425 South Clarkson Street
Englewood, CO 80110
Tel: 303-789-8417
Website: www.craig-hospital.org

Project offers information to assist SCI survivors, caregivers, and researchers in the areas of health maintenance, lifestyle choices, and improving quality of life. Website features the "Wellness and Risk Assessment Profile," which can be completed online.

Miami Project to Cure Paralysis/Buoniconti Fund

P.O. Box 016960 R-48
Miami, FL 33101-6960
Toll-Free: 800-STANDUP (782-6387)
Tel: 305-243-6001
Fax: 305-243-6017
Website: www.miamiproject.miami.edu
E-mail: mpinfo@miamiproject.med.miami.edu

A science and clinical research effort dedicated to finding new treatments and ultimately, a cure for paralysis. Project offers research and rehabilitation information packets. Website includes project overview, newsletter, and latest research findings.

National Center for Medical Rehabilitation Research (NCMRR)
National Institutes of Health
Executive Building, Room 2A03
6100 Executive Blvd., MSC 7510
Bethesda, MD 20892-7510
Tel: 301-402-2242
Website: www.nichd.nih.gov/about/ncmrr/ncmrr.htm

National Center for Neurogenic Communication Disorders
Speech and Hearing Sciences
P.O. Box 210071
1131 E. 2nd Street
Tucson, AZ 85721-0071
Tel: 520-621-1644
Website: http://w3.arizona.edu/~sphweb
E-mail: sphweb@w3.arizona.edu

National Institute of Child Health and Human Development (NICHD)
31 Center Drive
National Institutes of Health
Bldg. 31, Rm. 2A32, MSC 2425
Bethesda, MD 20892-2425
Toll-Free: 800-370-2943
Fax: 301-984-1473
Website: www.nichd.nih.gov
E-mail: NICHDClearinghouse@mail.nih.gov

National Institute of Mental Health (NIMH)
National Institutes of Health
6001 Executive Boulevard, Rm. 8184, MSC 9663
Bethesda, MD 20892
Tel: 301-443-4513
TTY: 301-443-8431
Fax: 301-443-4279
Website: www.nimh.nih.gov
E-mail: nimhinfo@nih.gov

National Institute of Neurological Disorders and Stroke (NINDS)
National Institutes of Health
P.O. Box 5801
Bethesda, MD 20892
Toll-Free: 800-352-9424
Tel: 301-496-5751
Fax: 301-402-2186
Website: www.ninds.nih.gov

National Institute on Aging (NIA)
National Institutes of Health
NIA Information Office
P.O. Box 8057
Gaithersburg, MD 20898-8057
Toll-Free: 800-222-2225 (Voice)
Toll-Free: 800-222-4225 (TTY)
Website: www.nih.gov/nia

National Institute of Neurological Disorders and Stroke
National Institutes of Health
P.O. Box 5801
Bethesda, MD 20894
Toll-Free: 800-352-9424
Website: www.ninds.nih.gov

Provides scientific documents, research reports, and publications. Website includes up-to-date research findings, health information, and a publications guide.

National Rehabilitation Information Center (NARIC)
1010 Wayne Avenue Suite 800
Silver Spring, MD 20910-5633
Toll-Free: 800-346-2742
Tel: 301-562-2400
Fax: 301-562-2401
TTY: 301-495-5626
Website: www.naric.com
E-mail: naricinfo@kra.com

National Spinal Cord Injury Association
6701 Democracy Blvd. #300-9
Bethesda, MD 20817
Toll-Free: 800-962-9629
Tel: 301-588-6959
Fax: 301-588-9414
Website: www.spinalcord.org
E-mail: NSCIA2@aol.com

Serves as a comprehensive information source for anyone effected by spinal cord injury. Referrals and consultations are available through the national office or one of the many state chapters. Web site includes fact sheets, rehabilitation centers by state, and state chapter information.

National Spinal Cord Injury Hotline
2200 Kernan Drive
Baltimore, MD 21207
Toll-Free: 800-526-3456
Website: www.paralinks.net/national_sci_injury_hotline.html
E-mail: scihotline@aol.com

The 24-hour hotline serves as a network for peer support and offers assistance in locating physicians, services, and equipment. Information on accessing resources in one's community is also available. Website explains the hotline's objectives.

Paralyzed Veterans of America (PVA)
801 18th Street NW
Washington, DC 20006-3517
Toll-Free: 800-424-8200
Tel: 202-USA-1300 (872-1300)
Fax: 202-785-4452
Website: www.pva.org
E-mail: info@pva.org

Advocacy and information association with brochures covering such topics as accessibility, legislation, assistive technology, and sports. Website includes SCI related news, research and treatment guides, chapter information, and Internet links.

Rehabilitation Research and Training Center on Secondary Conditions of Spinal Cord Injury
University of Alabama/Birmingham
Department of Physical Medicine and Rehabilitation
619 19th St. South
SRC 529
Birmingham, AL 35249-7330
Tel: 205-975-4691
TTY: 205-934-4642
Website: www.spinalcord.uab.edu
E-mail: rtc@uab.edu

Spinal Cord Society
19051 County Highway 1
Fergus Falls, MN 56537-7609
Website: members.aol.com/scsweb
Tel: 218-739-5252 or 218-739-5261
Fax: 218-739-5262

Center disseminates information based on research activities surrounding the prevention and treatment of secondary complications of SCI. Topics include urology, respiratory health, and treatments for pain and depression. Website contains an extensive variety of reports and fact sheets.

Psychological Effects of Trauma Resources

American Psychiatric Association
1400 K Street, N.W.
Washington, DC 20005
Toll-Free: 888-357-7924
Tel: 202-682-6000
Fax: 202-682-6850
Website: www.psych.org
E-mail: apa@psych.org

Anxiety Disorders Association of America, Inc.
11900 Parklawn Drive, Suite 100
Rockville, MD 20852-2624
Tel: 301-231-9350
Website: www.adaa.org

International Society for Traumatic Stress Studies
60 Revere Drive, Suite 500
Northbrook, IL 60062
Tel: 847-480-9028
Fax: 847-480-9282
Website: www.istss.org
E-mail: istss@istss.org

National Center for PTSD
VA Medical Center (116D)
White River Junction, VT 05009
Tel: 802-296-5132
Fax: 802-296-5135
Website: www.ncptsd.org
E-mail: ptsd@dartmouth.edu

National Institute of Mental Health Public Inquiries
6001 Executive Blvd., Room 8184 MSC 9663
Bethesda, MD 20892-9663
Tel: 301-443-4513
TTY: 301-443-8431
Fax: 301-443-4279
Facts on Demand: 301-443-5158
Website: www.nimh.nih.gov
E-mail: nimhinfo@nih.gov

National Organization for Victim Assistance
1730 Park Road, N.W.
Washington, DC 20010
Tel: 202-232-6682
Fax: 202-462-2255
Website: www.try-nova.org

U.S. Veterans Administration
Mental Health and Behavioral Sciences Services
Room 990
810 Vermont Avenue, N.W.
Washington, DC 20410
Tel: 202-273-8431
Website: www.va.gov

Trauma, Burn, and Injury Resources

Alisa Ann Ruch Burn Foundation
3600 Ocean View Boulevard, #1
Glendale, CA 91208
Toll-Free: 800-242-2876
Tel: 818-249-2230
Fax: 818-249-2488
Website: www.aarbf.org
E-mail: aarbf@aarbf.org

A nonprofit health organization dedicated to burn prevention and survivor assistance.

American Burn Association
625 N. Michigan Avenue
Suite 1530
Chicago, IL 60611
Toll-Free: 800-548-2876
Tel: 312-642-9260
Fax: 312-642-9260
Website: www.ameriburn.org
E-mail: info@ameriburn.org

Nonprofit health association dedicated to addressing the problems of burn injuries and burn survivors throughout the United States, Canada, and other countries.

American Trauma Society
8903 Presidential Parkway
Suite 512
Upper Marlboro, MD 20772
Toll-Free: 800-556-7890
Tel: 301-420-4189
Website: www.amtrauma.org
E-mail: atstrauma@aol.com

A nonprofit health association dedicated to the prevention of trauma and the improvement of trauma care.

Burn Survivors Online Inc.

28997 Nicholas Road
Norwalk, WI 54648
Tel: 608-337-4272
Website: www.BurnSurvivorsOnline.com
E-mail: info@burnsurvivorsonline.com

An online resource providing information and support for burn survivors and family members.

MEDLINEplus Health Topics: Burns

National Library of Medicine
8600 Rockville Pike
Bethesda, MD 20894
Toll-Free: 888-346-3656
Website: www.nlm.nih.gov/medlineplus/burns.html

A variety of online resources maintained by the National Library of Medicine.

The Phoenix Society for Burn Survivors, Inc.

2153 Wealthy Street SE, Suite 215
East Grand Rapids, MI 49506
Toll-Free: 800-888-2876
Tel: 616-458-2773
Fax: 616-458-2831
Website: www.phoenix-society.org
E-mail: info@phoenix-society.org

An international, nonprofit organization helping burn survivors and their families.

Shriners Hospitals for Children

International Shrine Headquarters
2900 Rocky Point Drive
Tampa, FL 33607
Toll-Free: 800-237-5055
Tel: 813-281-0300
Website: www.shrinershq.org

A nationwide network of 22 hospitals that provide no-cost orthopedic and burn care to children under 18 years of age, regardless of financial need.

The Shock Society
1021 15th Street, Suite 9
Augusta, GA 30901
Tel: 706-722-7511
Website: www2.musc.edu/shock.html
E-mail: maps@csranet.com

A Society whose purpose is to facilitate the integration of basic and clinical disciplines in the study of the causes of, and treatments for, traumatic injury and shock.

Society of Critical Care Medicine
701 Lee Street Suite 200
Des Plaines, IL 60016
Tel: 847-827-6869
Fax: 847-827-6886
Website: www.sccm.org
E-mail: info@sccm.org

A nonprofit international, multidisciplinary, scientific, and educational organization whose mission is to secure the highest quality care for all critically ill and injured patients.

International Shrine Headquarters
2900 Rocky Point Dr.
Tampa, FL 33607-1460
Tel: 813-281-0300
Website: www.shrinershq.org

Poison Prevention Information

Brochures, Flyers, and Pamphlets

Closure Manufacturers Association (CMA)
1627 K St., N.W., Suite 800
Washington, DC 20006
Tel: 202-223-9050
Website: www.cmadc.org
E-mail: cmadc@erols.com

Tips on Child Safety contains facts on proper use and life-saving effectiveness of safety caps, advice on how to instill safety consciousness in preschoolers, and general home safety tips. Send stamped, self-addressed, business-size envelope to Safety Tips.

The Soap and Detergent Association
1500 K Street NW, Suite 300
Washington, DC 20005
Tel: 202-347-2900
Fax: 202-347-4110
Website: www.sdahq.org

- *Home Safe Home* has tips for parents on how to protect young children in the home environment. Spanish versions available. Up to 100 copies free. Ask for information on larger orders.

- *Clean and Safe* is a four-page guide to safe use and storage of household cleaning products that explains the information given on package labels, procedures for safe storage and use of cleaning products, and what to do in case of emergency involving accidental exposure. Up to 30 copies free. Ask for information on larger orders.

- *Managing Allergies and Asthma: A Consumer Cleaning Guide* a 14-page booklet recommending lifestyle strategies and cleaning practices that can help bring allergies and asthma under control. Focuses on using cleaning products safely and effectively to control allergens in the home. Up to 10 copies free. Larger orders, 50¢ per copy.

Council on Family Health
1155 Connecticut Avenue, N.W., Suite 400
Washington, DC 20036
Tel: 202-429-6600
Website: www.cfhinfo.org

- *Ten Guides to Proper Medicine Use* is a brochure describing steps for consumers to follow when buying and taking prescription and nonprescription medicines. Available in English and Spanish. Up to 50 copies free; 10¢ per brochure for requests over 50.

- *Medicines and You: A Guide for Older Americans* is a brochure to help older adults in taking their medicines. Includes a sample medicine chart. Up to 50 copies free; 10¢ per brochure for requests over 50.

- *How to Prevent Drug Interactions* is a brochure highlighting the three types of potential drug interactions and how to prevent them, the drug interaction warning signs to note, and specific questions people should ask their physicians in order to avoid possible problems. Up to 50 copies free; 10¢ per brochure for requests over 50.

- *The Medicine Label...Your Road Map to Good Health* is a brochure that maps out what to look for on the medicine label and where to find it. Explains the importance of reading the medicine label every time you take or administer medicine. Up to 50 copies free; 10¢ per brochure for requests over 50.

The Consumer Healthcare Products Association
Office of Public Affairs
1150 Connecticut Ave., N.W. 12th Floor
Washington, DC 20036-4193.
Tel: 202-429-9260
Fax: 202-223-6835
Website: www.chpa-info.org

Nonprescription Medicines: What's Right For You? Offers consumers tips on reading the nonprescription, over-the-counter (OTC) medicine label, avoiding drug interactions, using OTCs when pregnant or nursing, dosing children, child-resistant and tamper-resistant packaging, and more. Up to 100 copies free.

Bronson Hospital Poison Prevention
601 John St.
Kalamazoo, Ml 49007
Tel: 616-341-7654
Website: www.bronsonhealth.com

Plants That Poison is an illustrated chart of common poisonous plants indicating size, toxic parts, and symptoms of poisoning. Contains information on preventing plant poisoning and emergency measures. Single copy free. Must send self addressed, stamped, business envelope.

Consumer Product Safety Commission
Washington, DC 20207
Toll-Free: 800-638-2772
Fax: 800-809-0924
Website: www.cpsc.gov
E-mail: info@cpsc.gov

Protect Your Family From Lead in Your Home is a booklet about the dangers of lead-based paint, how you can test the paint in your home for lead, and ways to reduce your exposure. Prepared by the U.S. Consumer Product Safety Commission and the Environmental Protection Agency. Single copy free.

The Art and Creative Materials Institute, Inc.
P.O. Box 479
Hanson, MA 02341-0479
Tel: 781-293-4100
Fax: 781-294-0808
Website: www.acminet.org

What You Need to Know About the Safety of Art & Craft Materials is a twelve page booklet that answers commonly asked questions about the safe use of materials. Single copies free: quantities upon request.

American Academy of Pediatrics
141 Northwest Point Blvd.
Elk Grove Village, IL 60007-1098
Toll-Free: 847-434-4000
Fax: 847-434-8000
Website: www.aap.org.

- *Injury Prevention Program Sheets–TIPP* a specific age-related safety sheet for each of eight age groups, providing focused information to parents about common childhood injuries. Some also available in Spanish. Each questionnaire is $19.95 for 100 copies plus $5.50 shipping and handling. Prepaid orders only.

- *Injury Prevention Program Safety Surveys–TIPP* are five questionnaires, in checklist format, concerning poisons, burns, falls, and other hazards are available. Some also available in Spanish. Each questionnaire is $19.95 for 100 copies plus $5.50 shipping and handling. Prepaid orders only.

- *Injury Prevention Program Economy Pack–TIPP* includes 8 age-related sheets with safety information on poisons, burns, falls, and other hazards and five color-coded safety questionnaires. $185.00 for 100 copies of each of the 13 components plus $18.50 shipping and handling. Prepaid orders only.

- *Choking Prevention and First Aid for Infants and Children* is a brochure that includes clear, concise text with helpful diagrams and instructions outlining what parents should do in an actual emergency. Includes a list of dangerous foods and prevention tips. $34.95 for 100 copies plus $7.50 shipping and handling. Prepaid orders only.

- *Child Safety Slips and Bicycle Safety Sheet—TIPP* Each of the eleven *Child Safety Slips* provides guidelines for the prevention of injury hazards. These handouts for parents highlight some of the frequent causes of childhood accidents. Topics are:

  - Infant Furniture: Cribs
  - Baby Sitting Reminders
  - Safety Tips for Home Playground Equipment
  - Safe Driving: A Parental Responsibility
  - Protect Your Child—Prevent Poisoning
  - Protect Your Home Against Fire—Planning Saves Lives
  - Water Safety for Your School-Aged Child
  - Lawn Mower Safety
  - Home Water Hazards for Infants and Toddlers
  - Pool Safety for Toddlers
  - Life Jackets and Life Preservers

- *Bicycle Safety Sheets*

  - About Bicycle Helmets
  - Bicycle Safety: Myths and Facts
  - Tips for Getting Your Kids to Wear Helmets
  - Choosing the Right Size Bicycle For Your Child
  - The Child as Passenger on an Adult's Bicycle
  - Safe Bicycling Starts Early

Each topic is available in packages of 100 for $19.95 plus $5.50 shipping and handling. Prepaid orders only.

- *First Aid Chart* an 11" x 17" chart with first aid instructions for poisoning and for several other types of injury. Single copies $2.95, $55 for 100 copies plus $9.50 shipping and handling charge. Prepaid orders only.

Chemical Specialties Manufacturers Association
1913 Eye Street, N.W.
Washington, DC 20006
Tel: 202-872-8110
Fax: 202-872-8114
Website: www.pressroom.com/~csma/home.htm
E-mail: CSMA@juno.com

- *Fighting Back: Helping Young People Kick the Sniffing Habit* a 12-page illustrated booklet. Discusses the nature of inhalation abuse, identifies substances typically misused by adolescents, and gives practical guidelines for adults on how to deal with the problem before seeking outside help. Single copy free with self-addressed stamped #10 envelope. For bulk quantities, request in writing for bulk price information. Orders under $100.00 must be pre-paid.

- *En Pie de Lucha: Ayudando a Los Jovenas a Combatir el Habito de Aspirar Substancias Nocivas* is a Spanish version of *Fighting Back: Helping Young People Kick the Sniffing Habit*.

- *Sniffing Abuse: It Can Kill* is an 8-1/2" x 11", 12 page, two-color booklet. Speaks to young people about the hard facts of inhalant abuse. Explains that sniffing is a drug problem; discusses the right and wrong use of breathing and inhaling; includes news bulletins of sniffing incidents and deaths; shows a diagram of body organs damaged by sniffing; describes how a youngster might be deprived of the joys of normal living. Single copy free with self-addressed stamped (55 cents) 9" x 12" envelope. Request in writing for price information on bulk quantities. Orders under $100.00 must be prepaid.

- *Don't Sniff to Get High — You May Die* a 4-color, 8-1/2" x 11" poster that folds-out to 11" x 17" poster for young people. Front of poster features warning that death could result from sniffing; back presents key messages on the dangers of inhalation abuse. Single copy free with self-addressed stamped (55 cents) 9" x 12" envelope. For bulk quantities, request in writing for price information. Orders under $100.00 must be pre-paid.

National Service Center for Environmental Publications
P.O. Box 42419
Cincinnati, OH 45242-2419
Toll-Free: 800-490-9198
Website: www.epa.gov/ncepihom/index.htm

* *Pesticides and Child Safety* (EPA #735-R-95-050R) Contains tips on safeguarding children from accidental pesticide poisonings or exposures and important contact phone numbers on who to call if an accident occurs. Also available in Spanish. Free.

* *Read the Label First! Protect Your Kids* (EPA #740-F-00-001) A brochure about protecting children from exposure to household cleaners and pesticides. Free

* *Ten Tips to Protect Children from Pesticide* and *Lead Poisoning Around the Home* (EPA #735-F-97-001) Free

Films, Slides, Talks, and Media Aids

National Technical Information Service
National Audiovisual Center
5285 Port Royal Road
Springfield, VA 22161
Toll-Free: 800-553-6847
Tel: 703-605-6000
Website: www.ntis.gov

The Travels of Timothy Trent explains that safety packaging is a valuable tool that offers an additional margin of safety from accidental poisoning of children. Demonstrates this point through the character of Timothy Trent, a young fellow who can't resist putting everything he can reach in his mouth. Order no.: AVA03690VNB1, $50.00, 10 min., 1976. U.S. Consumer Product Safety Commission.

YES Technologies
320 S. Willson Ave.
Bozeman, MT 59715
Tel: 406-586-2002
Fax: 406-586-8818
Website: www.yestech.com
E-mail: yes@yestech.com

Child-Resistant Packaging Videos includes three short segments emphasizing the need to use child-resistant packaging. The first two video segments (each 3:45 in length) are narrated by grandparents. The third (4:15 in length) is a simulated TV news story about a child who swallowed his grandparent's heart medicine. To order a 1/2" VHS videocassette of all three video segments, send a check for $25.

American Academy of Pediatrics
Publications Department
P.O. Box 747
Elk Grove Village, IL 60009-0747
Toll-Free: 888-227-1770
Website: www.aap.org

Childhood Injury: It's No Accident is a speaker's kit containing narrative and slides on the prevention of childhood injury. Also includes a home safety checklist. Prices, $35.00, prepaid orders only.

Hyper.Active Media and Content Inc.
1240 Bay Street
Suite 500
Toronto, Ontario, Canada M5R2A7
Tel: 416-324-1771
E-mail: dyorke@hypn.com

Poison Proof Your Home is a 30-minute interactive video which shows parents how to prevent child poisonings. Presents a room-by-room and step-by-step outline of what hazardous substances are available in a typical household. Cost: $6.95

Miscellaneous Poison Prevention Information

Poison Prevention Week Council
P.O. Box 1543
Washington, DC 20013
Tel: 301-504-0580 x1184
Fax: 301-504-0862
Website: www.poisonprevention.org

- *National Poison Prevention Week Packet* is a folder containing lists of available materials, fact sheets, and other promotional materials for the National Poison Prevention Week Observance.

- Annual Report for NPPW-2000. Single free copies available.

- Presidential Proclamation. Single copies of the President's proclamation are available.

- *Locked Up Poisons* is an 8-1/2" x 11" pamphlet with safety recommendations for poison prevention. 100 copies of this pamphlet are available. You may add your own name and address when you reprint this pamphlet. Also available in Spanish.

Cooperative Extension System Resources
Selection of programs/publications varies from state to state

Educational programs and materials are available from the Cooperative Extension Service in each state. Information on parent education, childcare provider training, food safety, farm and pesticide safety, and health/wellness issues can meet your needs for poison prevention education. Information in the form of publications, courses/workshops, and speakers/consultation are usually available. County Cooperative Extension Service offices are listed under county government in the telephone directory. Cooperative Extension resources are made available by a partnership between USDA, State Land-Grant Universities, and county government.

National Council on Patient Information and Education (NCPIE)
4915 Saint Elmo Ave., Suite 505
Bethesda, MD 20814-6082
Tel: 301-656-8565
Fax: 301-656-4464
Website: www.talkaboutrx.org
E-mail: ncpie@erols.com

The National Council on Patient Information and Education provides prescription medicine information and education resources. These items are designed to help consumers and their health care providers better communicate about prescription medicines.

National SAFE KIDS Campaign
1301 Pennsylvania Ave., N.W., Suite 1000
Washington, DC 20004
Tel: 202-662-0600
Fax: 202-393-2072
E-mail: info@safekids.org
Website: www.safekids.org

The National SAFE KIDS Campaign has developed several poison prevention resources including a poison injury fact sheet, an informational brochure for adults, and an educational children's booklet, "Filbert Prevents a Poison."

Council on Family Health
1155 Connecticut Avenue, N.W., Suite 400
Washington, DC 20036
Tel: 202-429-6600
Website: www.cfhinfo.org

Emergency Telephone Stickers for your telephone with spaces to include doctor, pharmacy and poison control numbers. Up to 50 copies free; 10¢ per sticker for requests over 50.

American Academy of Pediatrics
Publications Department
P.O. Box 747
Elk Grove Village, IL 60009-0747
Toll-Free: 888-227-1770
Website: www.aap.org

Handbook of Common Poisonings in Children, 3rd edition. Provides the practitioner with essential information needed to assess poisoning exposures and initiate a course of action. Cost is $44.95 per copy plus $7.50 shipping and handling. Prepaid orders only. The 3rd edition of *the Handbook of Common Poisonings in Children* contains many areas of interest:

- Poison Prevention
- General Management of Acute Poisonings
- Drugs Used in Poisoned Patients
- Toxicity Calculations
- Specific Poisons (Drugs, Abuse Drugs, Chemicals, and Biological Toxins) and much more.

Children's Hospital of Pittsburgh
Attn: Marketing Department
3705 Fifth Avenue
Pittsburgh, PA 15213
Tel: 412-692-5325
Website: www.chp.edu
E-mail: petrast@chplink.chp.edu

Understanding Cards and Mr. Yuk Stickers. These 4" x 8-3/4" cards are a new approach to teach poison prevention. Six flash cards in brilliant, attractive colors explain the four forms of poison. The instructions on back of each card make this prevention effort ideal for school, home, or presentations. One set of cards costs $2.00.

Mr. Yuk Means No! Stay Away! Use this sticker to teach your children about poisonous products. Mr. Yuk stickers can be customized for orders of 5,000 or more. $85.00 per 1,000. Shipping costs:

- $1.00 for orders under $5.00
- Orders under $50.00 = $5.50
- Orders $50.01 to $100.00 = $8.50
- Orders over $101.00
- "Order total" x .07 = shipping charges

The U.S. Consumer Product Safety Commission
Toll-Free Hotline:800-638-2772
Teletypewriter: 800-638-8270
E-mail: info@cpsc.gov
Website: www.cpsc.gov

The CPSC protects the public from the unreasonable risk of injury or death from 15,000 types of consumer products under the agency's jurisdiction. To report a dangerous product or a product-related injury, you can go to CPSC's forms page and use the first on-line form on that page. Or, you can call CPSC's hotline or teletypewriter, or E-Mail the information.

Safety and Prevention Resources

American Gas Association
400 N. Capitol Street, NW
Washington, DC 20001
Tel: 202-824-7000
Fax: 202-842-7115
Website: www.aga.org

The Chemosensory Disorders Group
The Smell and Taste Disorders Clinic
SUNY Health Science Center
750 East Adams Street
Syracuse, NY 13210
Tel: 315-464-5588
Fax: 315-464-7712
Website: www.upstate.edu/ent/smelltaste.shtml

Indoor Air Quality Information Clearinghouse (IAQ INFO)
P.O. Box 37133
Washington, DC 20013-7133
Toll-Free: 800-438-4318
Tel: 703-356-4020
Website: www.epa.gov/iaq/iaqinfo.html
E-mail: iaqinfo@aol.com

National Audiovisual Center
U.S. Department of Commerce Technology Administration
National Technical Information Service
5285 Port Royal Road
Springfield, VA 22161
Tel: 703-605-6000
Website: www.ntis.gov

National Institute for Occupational Safety and Health (NIOSH)
Occupational Safety and Health Administration (OSHA)
U.S. Department of Labor
200 Constitution Avenue, N.W.
Washington, DC 20210
Toll-Free: 800-356-4674
Fax: 513-533-8573
Fax-on-Demand: 888-232-3299
Website: www.cdc.gov/niosh
E-mail: eidtechinfo@cdc.gov

NIDCD Information Clearinghouse
1 Communication Avenue
Bethesda, MD 20892-3456
Toll-Free: 800-241-1044
TTY: 800-241-1055
Website: www.nidcd.nih.gov
E-mail: nidcdinfo@nidcd.nih.gov

National Institute on Deafness and Other Communication Disorders
National Institutes of Health
31 Center Drive, MSC 2320
Bethesda, MD 20892-2320
Tel: 301-496-7243
TTY: 301-402-0252
Website: www.nidcd.nih.gov

National Program for Playground Safety
School of Health, Physical Education & Leisure Services
WRC 205, University of Northern Iowa
Cedar Falls, IA 50614-0618
Toll-Free: 800-554-PLAY
Tel: 319-273-7308
Fax: 319-273-7308
Website: www.uni.edu/playground
E-mail: playground-safety@uni.edu

National Safety Council
1121 Spring Lake Drive
Itasca, IL 60143-3201
Tel: 630-285-1121
Fax: 630-285-1315
Website: www.nsc.org

National Ski Areas Association
133 S. Van Gordon Street, Suite 300
Lakewood, CO 80228
Tel: 303-987-1111
Fax: 303-986-2345
Website: www.nsaa.org
E-mail: nsaa@nsaa.org

National Ski Patrol
133 South Van Gordon Street
Suite 100
Lakewood, Colorado 80228
Tel: 303-988-1111
Fax: 303-988-3005
Website: www.nsp.org
E-mail: nsp@nsp.org

SafeUSA
P.O. Box 8189
Silver Springs, MD 20907-9189
Toll-Free: 888-252-7751
Website: www.cdc.gov/safeusa
E-mail: sainfo@cdc.gov

Chapter 63

Injury-Related Websites

Inclusion on this list does not constitute an endorsement of these organizations or their programs by the Centers for Disease Control Prevention (CDC), the National Center for Injury Prevention and Control (NCIPC), or the Federal government, and none should be inferred. CDC and NCIPC are not responsible for the content of the individual organizations' web pages found at these links.

A

ABLEDATA
Website: www.abledata.com/index.htm

Adults and Children Together Against Violence-ACT
Website: www.actagainstviolence.org/homepage.html

Alcohol-Related Injury & Violence (ARIV) Project
Website: www.tf.org/tf/alcohol/ariv

American Academy of Family Physicians
Website: www.aafp.org

American Academy of Neurology
Website: www.aan.com

"Injury Related Web Sites," National Center for Injury Prevention and Control, available at www.cdc.gov/ncipc/injweb/websites.htm, reviewed April 18, 2001.

American Academy of Pediatrics
Website: www.aap.org

American Association of Poison Control Centers
Website: www.aapcc.org

American Association of Spinal Cord Injury Nurses
Website: www.aascin.org/default.html

American Association of Suicidology
Website: www.suicidology.org

American Burn Association
Website: www.ameriburn.org

American College of Physicians
Website: www.acponline.org

American Foundation for Suicide Prevention
Website: www.afsp.org

American Hospital Association
Website: www.aha.org

American Medical Association
Website: www.ama-assn.org/home.htm

American Paralysis Association
Website: www.apacure.com

American Paraplegia Society
Website: www.apssci.org/default.html

American Psychological Association
Website: www.apa.org

American Public Health Association Injury Control and Emergency Services (APHA ICEHS)
Website: www.injurycontrol.com/ICEHS/welcome.htm

American Spinal Injury Association
Website: www.asia-spinalinjury.org

American Trauma Society
Website: www.amtrauma.org

Arizona Rape Prevention Education Project
Website: www.u.arizona.edu/~sexasslt/arpep

Ask NOAH About: Spinal Cord and Head Injuries
Website: www.noah.cuny.edu/illness/neuro/spinal.html

Association for the Advancement of Automotive Medicine
Website: www.carcrash.org

Association of American Medical Colleges
Website: www.aamc.org

Australian Institute of Criminology
Website: www.aic.gov.au/index.html

B

Bike Helmet Safety Institute
Website: www.bhsi.org

A comprehensive site for bicycle helmet information of all kinds.

Brain Injury Association
Website: www.biausa.org

Brain Injury Law Office
Website: www.tbilaw.com

Brain Train Software
Website: www.brain-train.com

British Columbia Injury Research and Prevention Unit
Website: www.injuryresearch.bc.ca

Building Safe Communities
Website: www.edc.org/HHD/csn/bsc

Bureau of Justice Statistics
Website: www.ojp.usdoj.gov/bjs

Bureau of Transportation Statistics
Website: www.bts.gov/contents.html

Burn and Shock Trauma Institute - Injury Prevention
Website: www.meddean.luc.edu/lumen/DeptWebs/brnshock/
preventi.htm

C

California Department of Health Services
Website: www.dhs.ca.gov/cdic/epic

Canadian Hospitals Injury Reporting and Prevention Program, Child Injury Division
Website: www.hc-sc.gc.ca/main/1cdc/web/brch/injury.html

Center for the Advanced Study of Public Safety and Injury Prevention
Website: www.albany.edu/sph/injury_3.html

Center for Rural Emergency Medicine at West Virginia University
Website: www.hsc.wvu.edu/som/crem

Center for the Study and Prevention of Violence
Website: www.colorado.edu/cspv

Center for Violence Prevention and Control—University of Minnesota
Website: www.umn.edu/cvpc

Child and Adolescent Emergency Department Visit Databook
Website: www.pgh.auhs.edu/childed

Child Maltreatment 1995: Reports from the States to the National Child Abuse and Neglect Data System
Website: www.acf.dhhs.gov/programs/cb/stats/ncands

Children's Safety Network
Website: www.edc.org/HHD/csn

Colorado Injury Control Research Center
Website: www.ColoState.EDU/Orgs/CICRC

The Connecticut Childhood Injury Prevention Center
Website: www.ccmckids.org/departments/ccipc.htm

Consumer Product Safety Commission
Website: www.cpsc.gov

County of San Diego Office of Violence & Injury Prevention
Website: www.sdvip.org

Craig Hospital
Website: www.craighospital.org

Crash Analysis and Reporting Environment (CARE)
Website: http://care.cs.ua.edu

Creative Partnerships for Prevention - A Drug and Violence Prevention Resource
Website: www.CPPrev.org

Crossroads from the National Safety Council
Website: www.crossroads.nsc.org/index.cfm

D

Drunk Busters of America
Website: www.drunkbusters.com

E

Emergency Medical Services for Children
Website: www.ems-c.org

Emory Center for Injury Control
Website: www.sph.emory.edu/CIC

EuroSafetyNet
Website: www.ecosa.org/csi/ecosa.nsf/orhome/home

F

Fact Sheets on Trauma and Burn Injury Statistics, Research, and Resources—National Institute of General Medical Sciences
Website: www.nih.gov/nigms/news/facts

Family Caregiver Alliance
Website: www.caregiver.org

Family Health and Safety (Safe Ride News)
Website: www.twbc.com

Family Violence Prevention Fund
Website: www.igc.apc.org/fund

Family Violence & Sexual Assault Institute (FVSAI)
Website: www.fvsai.org/index.htm

Family and Youth Services (FYSB)
Website: www.acf.dhhs.gov/programs/fysb

FBI's Supplementary Homicide Reports, 1980-1995
Website: www.ncjrs.org/ojjdp/html/ezaccess.htm.#SHR

Foundation for Spinal Cord Injury Prevention, Care & Cure
Website: www.fscip.org

FSU Juvenile Justice Clearinghouse
Website: www.fxu.edu/~crimdo/jjclearinghouse/jjclearinghouse.html

G

Great Lakes Area Regional Resource Center (GLARRC) Early Prevention of Violence Database
Website: www.csnp.ohio-state.edu/glarrc/vpdb.htm

H

Harborview Injury Prevention and Research Center
Website: http://depts.washington.edu/hiprc

Harvard Injury Control Research Center
Website: www.hsph.harvard.edu/hicrc

Health Canada
Website: www.hc-sc.gc.ca/english

Health Resources and Services Administration (HRSA)
Website: www.hrsa.dhhs.gov

Healthy People 2010 Objectives Injury Prevention
Website: www.injuryprevention.org/hp2010/hp2010.htm

I

International Collaborative Effort (ICE) on Injury Statistics
Website: www.cdc.gov/nchswww/about/otheract/ice/ice.htm

In Remembrance Project
Website: www.inremembrance.org

Injury Control Resource Information Network
Website: www.injurycontrol.com/icrin

Injury Facts for New York State
Website: www.health.state.ny.us/nysdoh/research/injury/injury.htm

Injury Free Coalition for Kids
Website: www.injuryfree.org

Injury Prevention Centre, Alberta, Canada
Website: www.inj-prev.ab.ca

Injury Prevention Web
Website: www.InjuryPreventionWeb.org

Institute for Global Communications-Violence Against Women
Website: www.egc.org/igc/issues/violencewn

Institute for Preventative Sports Medicine
Website: http://www.ipsm.org

Institute of Transportation Engineers
Website: www.ite.org

Insurance Institute for Highway Safety
Website: www.highwaysafety.org

Integrated Network of Disability Information and Education (Indie)
Website: http://laurence.canlearn.ca/English/learn/accessibility2001/indie

International Society for Child and Adolescent Injury Prevention (ISCAIP)
Website: www.iscaip.org

J

Johns Hopkins Center for Injury Research and Policy
Website: www.jhsph.edu/Research/enters/CIRP

K

Kentucky Injury Prevention and Research Center
Website: www.kiprc.uky.edu

L

Loyola University Medical Center
Website: www.meddean.luc.edu/lumen/DeptWebs/brnshock/preventi.htm

M

Maternal and Child Health Bureau
Website: www.os.dhhs.gov/hrsa/mchb

Publications on child passenger safety for out-of-home child care settings.

Mild Traumatic Brain Injury Task Force
Website: www.med.ualberta.ca/PHS/staff/Cassidy's%20Website/MTBI2/MTBI%20website

Missouri Model Spinal Cord Injury System
Website: www.hsc.missouri.edu/~momscis/momscis.htm

Model Spinal Cord Injury Care System at the University of Michigan
Website: www.med.umich.edu/pmr/model_sci

N

NAICRC Member Research Project DataBank
Website: www.quickbase.com/db/6tejwf5t

National Association of EMS Physicians
Website: www.naemsp.org

National Association of Governors' Highway Safety Representatives (NAGHSR)
Website: www.magjsr/prg

National Center for Health Statistics
Website: www.cdc.gov/nchswww/releases/98facts/98sheets/injury.htm

National Association of Injury Control Research Centers
Website: www.naicrc.org

National Center on Physical Activity and Disability
Website: http://ncpad.cc.uic.edu/home.htm

National Children's Center for Rural and Agricultural Health and Safety
Website: http://research.marshfieldclinic.org/children

National Clearinghouse for Justice Information and Statistics
Website: www.ch.search.org

National Clearinghouse on Families and Youth (NCFY)
Website: www.ncfy.com

National Clearinghouse of Rehabilitation Training Materials
Website: www.nchrtm.okstate.edu/forms/mainquery.html

National Committee to Prevent Child Abuse
Website: www.childabuse.org

The National Consortium on Violence Research (NCOVR)
Website: www.ncovr.heinz.cmu.edu

National Crash Outcome Data Evaluation System (CODES)
Website: www.upmc.edu/codes

National Criminal Justice Reference Service
Website: http://aspensys.com:81/new2/homepage.html

National Data Archive on Child Abuse and Neglect
Website: www.ndacan.cornell.edu

National Fire Protection Association
Website: www.nfpa.org

National Group Rides and Designated Drivers (National GRADD)
Website: www.ntlgradd.w1.com/htmlcode.html

National Highway Traffic Safety Administration
Website: www.nhtsa.dot.gov

National Highway Traffic Safety Administration Kid's Page
Website: www.nhtsa.dot.gov/kids

National Injury Surveillance Unit (NISU) Web Site
Website: www.nisu.flinders.edu.au/welcome.html

National Institute of Justice (NIJ)
Website: www.ojp.usdoj.gov/nij

National Institute on Disability & Rehabilitation Research (NIDRR)
Website: www.ed.gov/offices/OSERS/NIDRR

National Organizations for Youth Safety
Website: www.noys.com

National Pediatric Trauma Registry
Website: www.nemc.org/rehab/nptrhome.htm

National Program for Playground Safety
Website: www.uni.edu/playground

National Rehabilitation Information Center Home Page (NARIC)
Website: www.cais.net/naric

National Resource Center on Aging and Injury
Website: www.olderadultinjury.org

National SafeKids Campaign
Website: www.safekids.org

National Safety Council
Website: www.nsc.org

National Suicide Prevention Strategy
Website: www.sg.gov/library/calltoaction/strategymain.htm

National Spinal Cord Injury Association
Website: www.erols.com/nscia

National Youth Violence Resource Center
Website: www.safeyouth.org

National Women's Health Information Center
Website: www.4women.org

The NeuroScience Center
Website: www.neruoscience.cnter.com

Northwest Regional Spinal Cord Injury System
Website: http://weber.u.washington.edu/~rehab/sci

O

Oklahoma State Department of Health Injury Control Division
Website: www.health.state.ok.us/program/injury/index.html

Operation LifeSaver
Website: www.oli.org

Preventing deaths and injuries at places where the roadway crosses the railroad tracks and on railroad rights-of-way.

P

Pacific Center for Violence Prevention
Website: www.pcvp.org

Paralyzed Veterans of America
Website: www.pva.org

PAVNET
Website: www.pavnet.org

PERIL Project Earth Risk Identification Lifeline
Website: www.uoguelph.ca/cntc/educat/peril/index.html

The Perspectives Network
Website: www.tbi.org

PoinTIS (Point of Care, Team Information System)
Website: http://calder.med.miami.edu/pointis/index.html

Preventing falls among the elderly:
"Preventing Falls among Seniors"
Website: www.cdc.gov/ncipc/duip/spotlite/falls.htm
"Preventing Falls in the Elderly"
Website: www.healthatoz.com/atoz/Lifestyles/Home/homefalls.html
"Preventing Falls in the Elderly"
Website: www.ext.colostate.edu/pubs/consumer/10242.html

R

Rehabilitation Institute of Chicago
Website: www.rehabchicago.org

Rehabilitation Learning Center
Website: http://weber.u.washington.edu/~rlc

Rehabilitation Research & Training Center in Secondary Complications in SCI
Website: www.spinalcord.uab.edu

Rehabilitation Services Administration
Website: www.ed.gov/offices/OSERS/RSA/rsa.html

Reproductive Health and Violence
Website: www.cdc.gov/nccdphp/drh/wh_violence.htm

Research and Training Center in Rehabilitation and Childhood Trauma
Website: www.nemc.org/rehab/homepg.htm

Resources for Youth, California Wellness Foundation
Website: www.preventviolence.org/home.html

Rocky Mountain Model Spinal Cord Injury System
Website: www.csn.net/~gale

S

Safe Start, USA, Inc.—Drowning Prevention
Website: http://safestart.org

SafetyBeltSafe USA
Website: www.carseat.org

Safe Communities Foundation
Website: www.safecommunities.ca

Safe Communities Service Center
Website: www.nhtsa.dot.gov/safecommunities

SafeUSA
Website: www.cdc.gov/safeusa

The Samaritans of Boston
Website: http://vcc.mit.edu/comm/samaritans

San Francisco Injury Center
Website: http://itsa.ucsf.edu/~sfic/INDEX.html

The Science and Practice of Injury Control
Website: www.circl.pitt.edu/home/seminar%20archive.htm

Society for Public Health Education (SOPHE)
Website: www.sophe.org/Unintentional-Injury/index.html

Southern California Injury Prevention Research Center
Website: www.ph.ucla.edu/sciprc/sciprc1.htm

Southside Teens About Respect (STAR)
Website: www.uic.edu/~schewepa

South Texas Injury Prevention and Research Center
Website: http://sthrc.uthscsa.edu/stiprc

Spinal Cord Injury Information Network
Website: www.sci.rehabm.uab.edu

Spinal Cord Injury Resources
Website: www.eskimo.com/~jlubin/disabled/sci.htm

Spokane Domestic Violence Consortium
Website: www.domesticviolence.net

State and Territorial Injury Prevention Directors Association
Website: www.stipda.org

Suicide Awareness: Voices of Education (SA\VE)
Website: www.save.org

Suicide Information and Education Centre
Website: www.siec.ca/siec/information.html

Suicide Prevention Advocacy Network (SPAN)
Website: http://spanusa.org

Systematic Reviews of Childhood Injury Prevention/ Interventions
Website: http://weber.u.washington.edu/d02/hiprc/childinjury

T

Temple University Fall Prevention Project
Website: www.temple.edu/older_adult

Texas Department of Health, Bureau of Emergency Management
Website: www.tdh.state.tx.us/hcqs/ems/emshome.htm

Texas Department of Health, Injury Epidemiology and Surveillance Program
Website: www.tdh.state.tx.us/injury

THINK FIRST Foundation
Website: www.thinkfirst.org

THINK FIRST—Oregon injury prevention website
Website: www.ohsu.edu/hosp-thinkfirst

Trauma & Emergency Surgery Unit Web Site
Website: www.trauma.org.tr/en/index.html

Traumatic Brain and Spinal Cord Injury Projects
Website: www.tbi-sci.org/index.html

TraumLink: The Interdisciplinary Pediatric Injury Control Research Center
Website: www.med.upenn.edu/trauma

Trauma Foundation at San Francisco General Hospital
Website: www.tf.org

U

Unintentional Injury: A Resource for Health Education and Health Promotion
Website: www.sophe.org/Unintentional-Injury/index.html

United Tribes Technical College Injury Prevention Program
Website: www.injuryprevention.cc

University of Alabama Injury Control Research Center
Website: www.uab.edu/icrc

University of Iowa Injury Prevention Research Center
Website: www.pmeh.uiowa.edu/iprc

University of Michigan Transportation Research Institute
Website: www.umtri.umich.edu

University of North Carolina Injury Prevention Research Center
Website: www.sph.unc.edu/iprc

University of Otago Injury Prevention and Research Unit
Website: www.otago.ac.nz/Web_menus/Dept_Homepages/IPRU/home.html

University of Pittsburgh Center for Injury Research and Control
Website: www.circl.pitt.edu

University of Texas Health Science Center at San Antonio's Trauma
Website: http://rmstewart.uthscsa.edu

U.S. Fire Administration Kid's Pages
Website: www.usfa.fema.gov/kids

U.S. Department of Health and Human Services Kid's Pages
Website: www.hhs.gov/kids

U.S. Department of Justice
Website: www.ojp.usdoj.gov

U.S Department of Justice Kid's Pages
Website: www.usdoj.gov/kidspage

U.S. Department of Labor Kid's Pages
Website: www.dol.gov/dol/asp/public/fibre/main.htm

V

VincentWeb
Website: www.sph.unc.edu/vincentweb

Violence and Injury Prevention-WHO
Website: www.who.int/violence_injury_prevention/index.html

Violence Against Women Office (VAWO)
Website: www.usdoj.gov/vawo

Violence Against Women—IGC
Website: www.igc.org/igc/issues/violencewn

Violence and Injury Control Education through Networking and Training (VINCENT)
Website: www.sph.unc.edu/iprc/vincent.htm

Violence and Injury Prevention (VIP) Program— University of South Florida
Website: www.fmhi.usf.edu/amh/homicide-suicide

W

Washington State Drowning Prevention Project
Website: www. chmc.org/DP

WHO Helmet Initiative
Website: www.sph.emory.edu/Helmets

WHO Violence and Injury Prevention
Website: www.who.int/violence_injury_prevention/index.html

Whole Brain Atlas
Website: www.med.harvard.edu/AANLIB/home.html

William Lehman Injury Research Center, University of Miami
Website: http://trauma.med.miami.edu

Wisconsin Chapter of the American College of Emergency Physicians
Website: www.pmihwy.com/~wacep

Y

Youth and Violence: Education/Intervention Resources
Website: www.humanitarian.net

Index

Index

Page numbers followed by 'n' indicate a footnote. Page numbers in *italics* indicate a table or illustration.

A

AAP *see* American Academy of Pediatrics
abandonment, elders 205
"The ABC's of Safe and Healthy Child Care" (DHQP) 188n
"The ABC's of Safe and Healthy Child Care" (NCIPC) 297n
abdomninal pain treatment 297
ABEM *see* American Board of Emergency Medicine
ABLEDATA
  contact information 607
  Web site address 631
abrasions, treatment 75–76, 297–99
abuse
  alcohol use 210–15
  statistics *208*
  see also child abuse; dating violence; elder abuse; family violence; intimate partner violence
ACEP *see* American College of Emergency Physicians

ACPA *see* American Chronic Pain Association
acromioclavicular joint 149
acromion 149
Actonel (risedronate) 97
acute, defined 593
acute stress disorder (ASD) 266
A.D.A.M. Inc., neck injuries publication 143n
ADEAR *see* Alzheimer's Disease Education & Referral Center
adhesive capsulitis *see* frozen shoulder
Administration on Aging (AoA), elder abuse publication 201n
"Adolescent Health Chartbook" (NCHS) 33n
adolescents
  alcohol-related accidents 470
  antisocial personality disorder 213
  firearms 240
  growth plate injuries 99
  injury statistics 33–48
  motor vehicle accidents 461–63
  spinal cord injury 245
  tramatic brain injury 254
  workplace injuries 431–38
  see also children
adult protective services (APS), elder abuse 209–10

651

American College of Emergency Physicians (ACEP), continued
  household accidents 321n
  medical emergencies 281n
  serious cuts 305n
American College of Physicians, Web site address 632
American College of Rheumatology, contact information 141, 160, 604
American College of Surgeons, contact information 605
American Federation of State, County, and Municipal Employees, Web site address 450
American Foundation for Suicide Prevention, Web site address 632
American Gas Association, contact information 368, 626
American Hospital Association, Web site address 632
American Medical Association, Web site address 632
American Orthopaedic Society for Sports Medicine, contact information 107
American Paralysis Association, Web site address 632
American Paraplegia Society, Web site address 632
American Physical Therapy Association, contact information 141–42, 161, 605
American Podiatric Medical Association (APMA)
  contact information 86, 605
  foot injuries publication 83n
American Psychiatric Association
  contact information 271, 612
  post-traumatic stress disorder publication 265n
American Public Health Association Injury Control and Emergency Services, Web site address 632
American Red Cross, contact information 343
American Speech-Language-Hearing Association, contact information 607
American Spinal Injury Association, Web site address 632

American Trauma Society
  contact information 614
  Web site address 633
amputations 73
amusement ride injuries 533–43
"Amusement Ride-Related Injuries and Deaths in the United States: 1987-1999" (Morris) 533n
animal bites
  prevention 377–79
  treatment 67–69, 298, 306
ankle
  injuries 83–86
  sprains *164*, 164–65, 585
"Annual Report: All-Terrain Vehicle (ATV)-Related Deaths and Injuries" (CPSC) 497n
anterior cruciate ligament
  described 128
  injuries 133–35
anticoagulant medications, head injuries 110
antidepressant medications, post-traumatic stress syndrome 271
antisocial personality disorder (ASPD) 213
Anxiety Disorders Association of America, Inc., contact information 271, 612
AoA *see* Administration on Aging
APMA *see* American Podiatric Medical Association
APS agencies *see* adult protective services
"Are You a Working Teen?" (NIOSH) 431n
Arizona Rape Prevention Education Project, Web site address 633
The Art and Creative Materials Institues, Inc., contact information 619
arthritis
  elbow 82
  knees 129–30
  shoulders 158–59
  see also osteoarthritis; rheumatoid arthritis
Arthritis Foundation, contact information 142, 161, 605

I

National Institute of Mental Health,
contact information 609
National Institute of Mental Health
Public Inquiries, contact information 272, 613
National Institute of Neurological
Disorders and Stroke (NINDS)
contact information 610
publications
spinal cord injury 243n
whiplash injury 143n
National Institute on Aging (NIA)
contact information 610
head injury publication 109n
National Institute on Alcohol and Alcoholism (NIAAA), publications
injury risks 315n
transportation safety 469n
violence 210n
National Institute on Deafness and
Other Communications Disorders
(NIDCD)
Clearinghouse contact information
367, 628
contact information 368, 628
publications
gas detectors 361n
traumatic brain injury 603n
National Institute on Disability and
Rehabilitation Research, Web site
address 640
National Institutes of Justice, Web
site address 640
National Organization for Victim Assistance, contact information 272,
613
National Organizations for Youth
Safety, Web site address 640
National Pediatric Trauma Registry,
Web site address 641
"National Poison Prevention Week -
List of Materials" (CPSC) 603
*National Poison Prevention Week
Packet* (Poison Prevention Week
Council) 623
National Program for Playground
Safety
contact information 385, 628
Web site address 641

National Rehabilitation Information
Center
contact information 610
Web site address 641
National Resource Center on Aging
and Injury, Web site address 641
National SAFE KIDS Campaign
contact information 579, 624
publications
childhood injury seasonality 28n
hidden hazards 25n
scooter injuries 545n
winter sports safety 581n
National SafeKids Campaign, Web
site address 641
National Safety Council
contact information 628
Web site address 641
National Service Center for Environmental Publications, contact information 622
National Ski Areas Association, contact information 589, 628
National Ski Patrol, contact information 589, 629
National Spinal Cord Injury Association
contact information 611
Web site address 641
National Spinal Cord Injury Hotline,
contact information 611
National Spinal Cord Injury Statistical Center, publication 243n
National Suicide Prevention Strategy,
Web site address 641
National Technical Information Service, contact information 622
National Violent Death Reporting
System 6
National Women's Health Information Center, Web site address 641
National Youth Sports Safety Foundation, contact information 579
National Youth Violence Resource
Center, Web site address 641
natural gas detectors 364–67
nature of illness, defined 597
nature of injury, defined 597
NCEA *see* National Center on Elder
Abuse

Health Reference Series
COMPLETE CATALOG

Adolescent Health Sourcebook

Basic Consumer Health Information about Common Medical, Mental, and Emotional Concerns in Adolescents, Including Facts about Acne, Body Piercing, Mononucleosis, Nutrition, Eating Disorders, Stress, Depression, Behavior Problems, Peer Pressure, Violence, Gangs, Drug Use, Puberty, Sexuality, Pregnancy, Learning Disabilities, and More

Along with a Glossary of Terms and Other Resources for Further Help and Information

Edited by Chad T. Kimball. 700 pages. 2002. 0-7808-0248-9. $78.

■

AIDS Sourcebook, 1st Edition

Basic Information about AIDS and HIV Infection, Featuring Historical and Statistical Data, Current Research, Prevention, and Other Special Topics of Interest for Persons Living with AIDS

Along with Source Listings for Further Assistance

Edited by Karen Bellenir and Peter D. Dresser. 831 pages. 1995. 0-7808-0031-1. $78.

"One strength of this book is its practical emphasis. The intended audience is the lay reader . . . useful as an educational tool for health care providers who work with AIDS patients. Recommended for public libraries as well as hospital or academic libraries that collect consumer materials."
— *Bulletin of the Medical Library Association, Jan '96*

"This is the most comprehensive volume of its kind on an important medical topic. Highly recommended for all libraries."　— *Reference Book Review, '96*

"Very useful reference for all libraries."
— *Choice, Association of College and Research Libraries, Oct '95*

"There is a wealth of information here that can provide much educational assistance. It is a must book for all libraries and should be on the desk of each and every congressional leader. Highly recommended."
— *AIDS Book Review Journal, Aug '95*

"Recommended for most collections."
— *Library Journal, Jul '95*

■

AIDS Sourcebook, 2nd Edition

Basic Consumer Health Information about Acquired Immune Deficiency Syndrome (AIDS) and Human Immunodeficiency Virus (HIV) Infection, Featuring Updated Statistical Data, Reports on Recent Research and Prevention Initiatives, and Other Special Topics of Interest for Persons Living with AIDS, Including New Antiretroviral Treatment Options, Strategies for Combating Opportunistic Infections, Information about Clinical Trials, and More

Along with a Glossary of Important Terms and Resource Listings for Further Help and Information

Edited by Karen Bellenir. 751 pages. 1999. 0-7808-0225-X. $78.

"Highly recommended."
— *American Reference Books Annual, 2000*

"Excellent sourcebook. This continues to be a highly recommended book. There is no other book that provides as much information as this book provides."
— *AIDS Book Review Journal, Dec-Jan 2000*

"Recommended reference source."
— *Booklist, American Library Association, Dec '99*

"A solid text for college-level health libraries."
— *The Bookwatch, Aug '99*

Cited in *Reference Sources for Small and Medium-Sized Libraries, American Library Association, 1999*

■

Alcoholism Sourcebook

Basic Consumer Health Information about the Physical and Mental Consequences of Alcohol Abuse, Including Liver Disease, Pancreatitis, Wernicke-Korsakoff Syndrome (Alcoholic Dementia), Fetal Alcohol Syndrome, Heart Disease, Kidney Disorders, Gastrointestinal Problems, and Immune System Compromise and Featuring Facts about Addiction, Detoxification, Alcohol Withdrawal, Recovery, and the Maintenance of Sobriety

Along with a Glossary and Directories of Resources for Further Help and Information

Edited by Karen Bellenir. 613 pages. 2000. 0-7808-0325-6. $78.

"This title is one of the few reference works on alcoholism for general readers. For some readers this will be a welcome complement to the many self-help books on the market. Recommended for collections serving general readers and consumer health collections."
— *E-Streams, Mar '01*

"This book is an excellent choice for public and academic libraries."
— *American Reference Books Annual, 2001*

"Recommended reference source."
— *Booklist, American Library Association, Dec '00*

"Presents a wealth of information on alcohol use and abuse and its effects on the body and mind, treatment, and prevention." — *SciTech Book News, Dec '00*

"Important new health guide which packs in the latest consumer information about the problems of alcoholism." — *Reviewer's Bookwatch, Nov '00*

SEE ALSO *Drug Abuse Sourcebook, Substance Abuse Sourcebook*

Allergies Sourcebook, 1st Edition

Basic Information about Major Forms and Mechanisms of Common Allergic Reactions, Sensitivities, and Intolerances, Including Anaphylaxis, Asthma, Hives and Other Dermatologic Symptoms, Rhinitis, and Sinusitis

Along with Their Usual Triggers Like Animal Fur, Chemicals, Drugs, Dust, Foods, Insects, Latex, Pollen, and Poison Ivy, Oak, and Sumac; Plus Information on Prevention, Identification, and Treatment

Edited by Allan R. Cook. 611 pages. 1997. 0-7808-0036-2. $78.

■

Allergies Sourcebook, 2nd Edition

Basic Consumer Health Information about Allergic Disorders, Triggers, Reactions, and Related Symptoms, Including Anaphylaxis, Rhinitis, Sinusitis, Asthma, Dermatitis, Conjunctivitis, and Multiple Chemical Sensitivity

Along with Tips on Diagnosis, Prevention, and Treatment, Statistical Data, a Glossary, and a Directory of Sources for Further Help and Information

Edited by Annemarie S. Muth. 598 pages. 2002. 0-7808-0376-0. $78.

■

Alternative Medicine Sourcebook

Basic Consumer Health Information about Alternatives to Conventional Medicine, Including Acupressure, Acupuncture, Aromatherapy, Ayurveda, Bioelectromagnetics, Environmental Medicine, Essence Therapy, Food and Nutrition Therapy, Herbal Therapy, Homeopathy, Imaging, Massage, Naturopathy, Reflexology, Relaxation and Meditation, Sound Therapy, Vitamin and Mineral Therapy, and Yoga, and More

Edited by Allan R. Cook. 737 pages. 1999. 0-7808-0200-4. $78.

"Recommended reference source."
—*Booklist, American Library Association, Feb '00*

"A great addition to the reference collection of every type of library." —*American Reference Books Annual, 2000*

■

Alzheimer's, Stroke & 29 Other Neurological Disorders Sourcebook, 1st Edition

Basic Information for the Layperson on 31 Diseases or Disorders Affecting the Brain and Nervous System, First Describing the Illness, Then Listing Symptoms, Diagnostic Methods, and Treatment Options, and Including Statistics on Incidences and Causes

Edited by Frank E. Bair. 579 pages. 1993. 1-55888-748-2. $78.

"Nontechnical reference book that provides reader-friendly information."
—*Family Caregiver Alliance Update, Winter '96*

"Should be included in any library's patient education section." —*American Reference Books Annual, 1994*

"Written in an approachable and accessible style. Recommended for patient education and consumer health collections in health science center and public libraries." —*Academic Library Book Review, Dec '93*

"It is very handy to have information on more than thirty neurological disorders under one cover, and there is no recent source like it." —*Reference Quarterly, American Library Association, Fall '93*

SEE ALSO Brain Disorders Sourcebook

■

Alzheimer's Disease Sourcebook, 2nd Edition

Basic Consumer Health Information about Alzheimer's Disease, Related Disorders, and Other Dementias, Including Multi-Infarct Dementia, AIDS-Related Dementia, Alcoholic Dementia, Huntington's Disease, Delirium, and Confusional States

Along with Reports Detailing Current Research Efforts in Prevention and Treatment, Long-Term Care Issues, and Listings of Sources for Additional Help and Information

Edited by Karen Bellenir. 524 pages. 1999. 0-7808-0223-3. $78.

"Provides a wealth of useful information not otherwise available in one place. This resource is recommended for all types of libraries."
—*American Reference Books Annual, 2000*

"Recommended reference source."
—*Booklist, American Library Association, Oct '99*

■

Arthritis Sourcebook

Basic Consumer Health Information about Specific Forms of Arthritis and Related Disorders, Including Rheumatoid Arthritis, Osteoarthritis, Gout, Polymyalgia Rheumatica, Psoriatic Arthritis, Spondyloarthropathies, Juvenile Rheumatoid Arthritis, and Juvenile Ankylosing Spondylitis

Along with Information about Medical, Surgical, and Alternative Treatment Options, and Including Strategies for Coping with Pain, Fatigue, and Stress

Edited by Allan R. Cook. 550 pages. 1998. 0-7808-0201-2. $78.

". . . accessible to the layperson."
—*Reference and Research Book News, Feb '99*

■

Asthma Sourcebook

Basic Consumer Health Information about Asthma, Including Symptoms, Traditional and Nontraditional Remedies, Treatment Advances, Quality-of-Life Aids, Medical Research Updates, and the Role of Allergies, Exercise, Age, the Environment, and Genetics in the Development of Asthma

Along with Statistical Data, a Glossary, and Directories of Support Groups, and Other Resources for Further Information

Edited by Annemarie S. Muth. 628 pages. 2000. 0-7808-0381-7. $78.

"A worthwhile reference acquisition for public libraries and academic medical libraries whose readers desire a quick introduction to the wide range of asthma information." — *Choice, Association of College & esearch Libraries, Jun '01*

"Recommended reference source." — *Booklist, American Library Association, Feb '01*

"Highly recommended." — *The Bookwatch, Jan '01*

"There is much good information for patients and their families who deal with asthma daily." — *American Medical Writers Association Journal, Winter '01*

"This informative text is recommended for consumer health collections in public, secondary school, and community college libraries and the libraries of universities with a large undergraduate population." — *American Reference Books Annual, 2001*

■

Back & Neck Disorders Sourcebook

Basic Information about Disorders and Injuries of the Spinal Cord and Vertebrae, Including Facts on Chiropractic Treatment, Surgical Interventions, Paralysis, and Rehabilitation

Along with Advice for Preventing Back Trouble

Edited by Karen Bellenir. 548 pages. 1997. 0-7808-0202-0. $78.

"The strength of this work is its basic, easy-to-read format. Recommended." — *Reference and User Services Quarterly, American Library Association, Winter '97*

■

Blood & Circulatory Disorders Sourcebook

Basic Information about Blood and Its Components, Anemias, Leukemias, Bleeding Disorders, and Circulatory Disorders, Including Aplastic Anemia, Thalassemia, Sickle-Cell Disease, Hemochromatosis, Hemophilia, Von Willebrand Disease, and Vascular Diseases

Along with a Special Section on Blood Transfusions and Blood Supply Safety, a Glossary, and Source Listings for Further Help and Information

Edited by Karen Bellenir and Linda M. Shin. 554 pages. 1998. 0-7808-0203-9. $78.

"Recommended reference source." — *Booklist, American Library Association, Feb '99*

"An important reference sourcebook written in simple language for everyday, non-technical users." — *Reviewer's Bookwatch, Jan '99*

Brain Disorders Sourcebook

Basic Consumer Health Information about Strokes, Epilepsy, Amyotrophic Lateral Sclerosis (ALS/Lou Gehrig's Disease), Parkinson's Disease, Brain Tumors, Cerebral Palsy, Headache, Tourette Syndrome, and More

Along with Statistical Data, Treatment and Rehabilitation Options, Coping Strategies, Reports on Current Research Initiatives, a Glossary, and Resource Listings for Additional Help and Information

Edited by Karen Bellenir. 481 pages. 1999. 0-7808-0229-2. $78.

"Belongs on the shelves of any library with a consumer health collection." — *E-Streams, Mar '00*

"Recommended reference source." — *Booklist, American Library Association, Oct '99*

SEE ALSO *Alzheimer's, Stroke & 29 Other Neurological Disorders Sourcebook, 1st Edition*

■

Breast Cancer Sourcebook

Basic Consumer Health Information about Breast Cancer, Including Diagnostic Methods, Treatment Options, Alternative Therapies, Self-Help Information, Related Health Concerns, Statistical and Demographic Data, and Facts for Men with Breast Cancer

Along with Reports on Current Research Initiatives, a Glossary of Related Medical Terms, and a Directory of Sources for Further Help and Information

Edited by Edward J. Prucha and Karen Bellenir. 580 pages. 2001. 0-7808-0244-6. $78.

"Recommended reference source." — *Booklist, American Library Association, Jan '02*

"This reference source is highly recommended. It is quite informative, comprehensive and detailed in nature, and yet it offers practical advice in easy-to-read language. It could be thought of as the 'bible' of breast cancer for the consumer." — *E-Streams, Jan '02*

"From the pros and cons of different screening methods and results to treatment options, *Breast Cancer Sourcebook* provides the latest information on the subject." — *Library Bookwatch, Dec '01*

"This thoroughgoing, very readable reference covers all aspects of breast health and cancer. . . . Readers will find much to consider here. Recommended for all public and patient health collections." — *Library Journal, Sep '01*

SEE ALSO *Cancer Sourcebook for Women, 1st and 2nd Editions, Women's Health Concerns Sourcebook*

Breastfeeding Sourcebook

Basic Consumer Health Information about the Benefits of Breastmilk, Preparing to Breastfeed, Breastfeeding as a Baby Grows, Nutrition, and More, Including Information on Special Situations and Concerns Such as Mastitis, Illness, Medications, Allergies, Multiple Births, Prematurity, Special Needs, and Adoption

Along with a Glossary and Resources for Additional Help and Information

Edited by Jenni Lynn Colson. 350 pages. 2002. 0-7808-0332-9. $78.

SEE ALSO Pregnancy & Birth Sourcebook

■

Burns Sourcebook

Basic Consumer Health Information about Various Types of Burns and Scalds, Including Flame, Heat, Cold, Electrical, Chemical, and Sun Burns

Along with Information on Short-Term and Long-Term Treatments, Tissue Reconstruction, Plastic Surgery, Prevention Suggestions, and First Aid

Edited by Allan R. Cook. 604 pages. 1999. 0-7808-0204-7. $78.

"This is an exceptional addition to the series and is highly recommended for all consumer health collections, hospital libraries, and academic medical centers."
—*E-Streams, Mar '00*

"This key reference guide is an invaluable addition to all health care and public libraries in confronting this ongoing health issue."
—*American Reference Books Annual, 2000*

"Recommended reference source."
—*Booklist, American Library Association, Dec '99*

SEE ALSO Skin Disorders Sourcebook

■

Cancer Sourcebook, 1st Edition

Basic Information on Cancer Types, Symptoms, Diagnostic Methods, and Treatments, Including Statistics on Cancer Occurrences Worldwide and the Risks Associated with Known Carcinogens and Activities

Edited by Frank E. Bair. 932 pages. 1990. 1-55888-888-8. $78.

Cited in *Reference Sources for Small and Medium-Sized Libraries, American Library Association, 1999*

"Written in nontechnical language. Useful for patients, their families, medical professionals, and librarians."
—*Guide to Reference Books, 1996*

"Designed with the non-medical professional in mind. Libraries and medical facilities interested in patient education should certainly consider adding the *Cancer Sourcebook* to their holdings. This compact collection of reliable information . . . is an invaluable tool for helping patients and patients' families and friends to take the first steps in coping with the many difficulties of cancer."
—*Medical Reference Services Quarterly, Winter '91*

"Specifically created for the nontechnical reader . . . an important resource for the general reader trying to understand the complexities of cancer."
—*American Reference Books Annual, 1991*

"This publication's nontechnical nature and very comprehensive format make it useful for both the general public and undergraduate students."
—*Choice, Association of College and Research Libraries, Oct '90*

■

New Cancer Sourcebook, 2nd Edition

Basic Information about Major Forms and Stages of Cancer, Featuring Facts about Primary and Secondary Tumors of the Respiratory, Nervous, Lymphatic, Circulatory, Skeletal, and Gastrointestinal Systems, and Specific Organs; Statistical and Demographic Data; Treatment Options; and Strategies for Coping

Edited by Allan R. Cook. 1,313 pages. 1996. 0-7808-0041-9. $78.

"An excellent resource for patients with newly diagnosed cancer and their families. The dialogue is simple, direct, and comprehensive. Highly recommended for patients and families to aid in their understanding of cancer and its treatment."
—*Booklist Health Sciences Supplement, American Library Association, Oct '97*

"The amount of factual and useful information is extensive. The writing is very clear, geared to general readers. Recommended for all levels."
—*Choice, Association of College and Research Libraries, Jan '97*

■

Cancer Sourcebook, 3rd Edition

Basic Consumer Health Information about Major Forms and Stages of Cancer, Featuring Facts about Primary and Secondary Tumors of the Respiratory, Nervous, Lymphatic, Circulatory, Skeletal, and Gastrointestinal Systems, and Specific Organs

Along with Statistical and Demographic Data, Treatment Options, Strategies for Coping, a Glossary, and a Directory of Sources for Additional Help and Information

Edited by Edward J. Prucha. 1,069 pages. 2000. 0-7808-0227-6. $78.

"This title is recommended for health sciences and public libraries with consumer health collections."
—*E-Streams, Feb '01*

". . . can be effectively used by cancer patients and their families who are looking for answers in a language they can understand. Public and hospital libraries should have it on their shelves."
—*American Reference Books Annual, 2001*

"Recommended reference source."
—*Booklist, American Library Association, Dec '00*

Cancer Sourcebook for Women, 1st Edition

Basic Information about Specific Forms of Cancer That Affect Women, Featuring Facts about Breast Cancer, Cervical Cancer, Ovarian Cancer, Cancer of the Uterus and Uterine Sarcoma, Cancer of the Vagina, and Cancer of the Vulva; Statistical and Demographic Data; Treatments, Self-Help Management Suggestions, and Current Research Initiatives

Edited by Allan R. Cook and Peter D. Dresser. 524 pages. 1996. 0-7808-0076-1. $78.

". . . written in easily understandable, non-technical language. Recommended for public libraries or hospital and academic libraries that collect patient education or consumer health materials."
— *Medical Reference Services Quarterly, Spring '97*

"Would be of value in a consumer health library. . . . written with the health care consumer in mind. Medical jargon is at a minimum, and medical terms are explained in clear, understandable sentences."
— *Bulletin of the Medical Library Association, Oct '96*

"The availability under one cover of all these pertinent publications, grouped under cohesive headings, makes this certainly a most useful sourcebook."
— *Choice, Association of College and Research Libraries, Jun '96*

"Presents a comprehensive knowledge base for general readers. Men and women both benefit from the gold mine of information nestled between the two covers of this book. Recommended."
— *Academic Library Book Review, Summer '96*

"This timely book is highly recommended for consumer health and patient education collections in all libraries."
— *Library Journal, Apr '96*

SEE ALSO *Breast Cancer Sourcebook, Women's Health Concerns Sourcebook*

Cancer Sourcebook for Women, 2nd Edition

Basic Consumer Health Information about Gynecologic Cancers and Related Concerns, Including Cervical Cancer, Endometrial Cancer, Gestational Trophoblastic Tumor, Ovarian Cancer, Uterine Cancer, Vaginal Cancer, Vulvar Cancer, Breast Cancer, and Common Non-Cancerous Uterine Conditions, with Facts about Cancer Risk Factors, Screening and Prevention, Treatment Options, and Reports on Current Research Initiatives

Along with a Glossary of Cancer Terms and a Directory of Resources for Additional Help and Information

Edited by Karen Bellenir. 604 pages. 2002. 0-7808-0226-8. $78.

SEE ALSO *Breast Cancer Sourcebook, Women's Health Concerns Sourcebook*

Cardiovascular Diseases & Disorders Sourcebook, 1st Edition

Basic Information about Cardiovascular Diseases and Disorders, Featuring Facts about the Cardiovascular System, Demographic and Statistical Data, Descriptions of Pharmacological and Surgical Interventions, Lifestyle Modifications, and a Special Section Focusing on Heart Disorders in Children

Edited by Karen Bellenir and Peter D. Dresser. 683 pages. 1995. 0-7808-0032-X. $78.

". . . comprehensive format provides an extensive overview on this subject." — *Choice, Association of College & Research Libraries, Jun '96*

". . . an easily understood, complete, up-to-date resource. This well executed public health tool will make valuable information available to those that need it most, patients and their families. The typeface, sturdy non-reflective paper, and library binding add a feel of quality found wanting in other publications. Highly recommended for academic and general libraries. "
— *Academic Library Book Review, Summer '96*

SEE ALSO *Healthy Heart Sourcebook for Women, Heart Diseases & Disorders Sourcebook, 2nd Edition*

Caregiving Sourcebook

Basic Consumer Health Information for Caregivers, Including a Profile of Caregivers, Caregiving Responsibilities and Concerns, Tips for Specific Conditions, Care Environments, and the Effects of Caregiving

Along with Facts about Legal Issues, Financial Information, and Future Planning, a Glossary, and a Listing of Additional Resources

Edited by Joyce Brennfleck Shannon. 600 pages. 2001. 0-7808-0331-0. $78.

"An ideal addition to the reference collection of any public library. Health sciences information professionals may also want to acquire the *Caregiving Sourcebook* for their hospital or academic library for use as a ready reference tool by health care workers interested in aging and caregiving." — *E-Streams, Jan '02*

"Recommended reference source."
— *Booklist, American Library Association, Oct '01*

Colds, Flu & Other Common Ailments Sourcebook

Basic Consumer Health Information about Common Ailments and Injuries, Including Colds, Coughs, the Flu, Sinus Problems, Headaches, Fever, Nausea and Vomiting, Menstrual Cramps, Diarrhea, Constipation, Hemorrhoids, Back Pain, Dandruff, Dry and Itchy Skin, Cuts, Scrapes, Sprains, Bruises, and More

Along with Information about Prevention, Self-Care, Choosing a Doctor, Over-the-Counter Medications, Folk Remedies, and Alternative Therapies, and Including a Glossary of Important Terms and a Directory of Resources for Further Help and Information

Edited by Chad T. Kimball. 638 pages. 2001. 0-7808-0435-X. $78.

"Will prove valuable to any library seeking to maintain a current, comprehensive reference collection of health resources. . . . Excellent reference."
— *The Bookwatch, Aug '01*

"Recommended reference source."
— *Booklist, American Library Association, July '01*

■

Communication Disorders Sourcebook

Basic Information about Deafness and Hearing Loss, Speech and Language Disorders, Voice Disorders, Balance and Vestibular Disorders, and Disorders of Smell, Taste, and Touch

Edited by Linda M. Ross. 533 pages. 1996. 0-7808-0077-X. $78.

"This is skillfully edited and is a welcome resource for the layperson. It should be found in every public and medical library." — *Booklist Health Sciences Supplement, American Library Association, Oct '97*

■

Congenital Disorders Sourcebook

Basic Information about Disorders Acquired during Gestation, Including Spina Bifida, Hydrocephalus, Cerebral Palsy, Heart Defects, Craniofacial Abnormalities, Fetal Alcohol Syndrome, and More

Along with Current Treatment Options and Statistical Data

Edited by Karen Bellenir. 607 pages. 1997. 0-7808-0205-5. $78.

"Recommended reference source."
— *Booklist, American Library Association, Oct '97*

SEE ALSO Pregnancy & Birth Sourcebook

■

Consumer Issues in Health Care Sourcebook

Basic Information about Health Care Fundamentals and Related Consumer Issues, Including Exams and Screening Tests, Physician Specialties, Choosing a Doctor, Using Prescription and Over-the-Counter Medications Safely, Avoiding Health Scams, Managing Common Health Risks in the Home, Care Options for Chronically or Terminally Ill Patients, and a List of Resources for Obtaining Help and Further Information

Edited by Karen Bellenir. 618 pages. 1998. 0-7808-0221-7. $78.

"Both public and academic libraries will want to have a copy in their collection for readers who are interested in self-education on health issues."
— *American Reference Books Annual, 2000*

"The editor has researched the literature from government agencies and others, saving readers the time and effort of having to do the research themselves. Recommended for public libraries."
— *Reference and User Services Quarterly, American Library Association, Spring '99*

"Recommended reference source."
— *Booklist, American Library Association, Dec '98*

■

Contagious & Non-Contagious Infectious Diseases Sourcebook

Basic Information about Contagious Diseases like Measles, Polio, Hepatitis B, and Infectious Mononucleosis, and Non-Contagious Infectious Diseases like Tetanus and Toxic Shock Syndrome, and Diseases Occurring as Secondary Infections Such as Shingles and Reye Syndrome

Along with Vaccination, Prevention, and Treatment Information, and a Section Describing Emerging Infectious Disease Threats

Edited by Karen Bellenir and Peter D. Dresser. 566 pages. 1996. 0-7808-0075-3. $78.

■

Death & Dying Sourcebook

Basic Consumer Health Information for the Layperson about End-of-Life Care and Related Ethical and Legal Issues, Including Chief Causes of Death, Autopsies, Pain Management for the Terminally Ill, Life Support Systems, Insurance, Euthanasia, Assisted Suicide, Hospice Programs, Living Wills, Funeral Planning, Counseling, Mourning, Organ Donation, and Physician Training

Along with Statistical Data, a Glossary, and Listings of Sources for Further Help and Information

Edited by Annemarie S. Muth. 641 pages. 1999. 0-7808-0230-6. $78.

"Public libraries, medical libraries, and academic libraries will all find this sourcebook a useful addition to their collections."
— *American Reference Books Annual, 2001*

"An extremely useful resource for those concerned with death and dying in the United States."
— *Respiratory Care, Nov '00*

"Recommended reference source."
— *Booklist, American Library Association, Aug '00*

"This book is a definite must for all those involved in end-of-life care." — *Doody's Review Service, 2000*

■

Diabetes Sourcebook, 1st Edition

Basic Information about Insulin-Dependent and Non-insulin-Dependent Diabetes Mellitus, Gestational Diabetes, and Diabetic Complications, Symptoms, Treatment, and Research Results, Including Statistics on Prevalence, Morbidity, and Mortality

Along with Source Listings for Further Help and Information

Edited by Karen Bellenir and Peter D. Dresser. 827 pages. 1994. 1-55888-751-2. $78.

". . . very informative and understandable for the layperson without being simplistic. It provides a comprehensive overview for laypersons who want a general understanding of the disease or who want to focus on various aspects of the disease."
— *Bulletin of the Medical Library Association, Jan '96*

■

Diabetes Sourcebook, 2nd Edition

Basic Consumer Health Information about Type 1 Diabetes (Insulin-Dependent or Juvenile-Onset Diabetes), Type 2 (Noninsulin-Dependent or Adult-Onset Diabetes), Gestational Diabetes, and Related Disorders, Including Diabetes Prevalence Data, Management Issues, the Role of Diet and Exercise in Controlling Diabetes, Insulin and Other Diabetes Medicines, and Complications of Diabetes Such as Eye Diseases, Periodontal Disease, Amputation, and End-Stage Renal Disease

Along with Reports on Current Research Initiatives, a Glossary, and Resource Listings for Further Help and Information

Edited by Karen Bellenir. 688 pages. 1998. 0-7808-0224-1. $78.

"An invaluable reference." — *Library Journal, May '00*

Selected as one of the 250 "Best Health Sciences Books of 1999." — *Doody's Rating Service, Mar-Apr 2000*

"This comprehensive book is an excellent addition for high school, academic, medical, and public libraries. This volume is highly recommended."
— *American Reference Books Annual, 2000*

"Provides useful information for the general public."
— *Healthlines, University of Michigan Health Management Research Center, Sep/Oct '99*

". . . provides reliable mainstream medical information . . . belongs on the shelves of any library with a consumer health collection." — *E-Streams, Sep '99*

"Recommended reference source."
— *Booklist, American Library Association, Feb '99*

■

Diet & Nutrition Sourcebook, 1st Edition

Basic Information about Nutrition, Including the Dietary Guidelines for Americans, the Food Guide Pyramid, and Their Applications in Daily Diet, Nutritional Advice for Specific Age Groups, Current Nutritional Issues and Controversies, the New Food Label and How to Use It to Promote Healthy Eating, and Recent Developments in Nutritional Research

Edited by Dan R. Harris. 662 pages. 1996. 0-7808-0084-2. $78.

"Useful reference as a food and nutrition sourcebook for the general consumer." — *Booklist Health Sciences Supplement, American Library Association, Oct '97*

"Recommended for public libraries and medical libraries that receive general information requests on nutrition. It is readable and will appeal to those interested in learning more about healthy dietary practices."
— *Medical Reference Services Quarterly, Fall '97*

"An abundance of medical and social statistics is translated into readable information geared toward the general reader." — *Bookwatch, Mar '97*

"With dozens of questionable diet books on the market, it is so refreshing to find a reliable and factual reference book. Recommended to aspiring professionals, librarians, and others seeking and giving reliable dietary advice. An excellent compilation." — *Choice, Association of College and Research Libraries, Feb '97*

SEE ALSO Digestive Diseases & Disorders Sourcebook, Gastrointestinal Diseases & Disorders Sourcebook

■

Diet & Nutrition Sourcebook, 2nd Edition

Basic Consumer Health Information about Dietary Guidelines, Recommended Daily Intake Values, Vitamins, Minerals, Fiber, Fat, Weight Control, Dietary Supplements, and Food Additives

Along with Special Sections on Nutrition Needs throughout Life and Nutrition for People with Such Specific Medical Concerns as Allergies, High Blood Cholesterol, Hypertension, Diabetes, Celiac Disease, Seizure Disorders, Phenylketonuria (PKU), Cancer, and Eating Disorders, and Including Reports on Current Nutrition Research and Source Listings for Additional Help and Information

Edited by Karen Bellenir. 650 pages. 1999. 0-7808-0228-4. $78.

"This book is an excellent source of basic diet and nutrition information." — *Booklist Health Sciences Supplement, American Library Association, Dec '00*

"This reference document should be in any public library, but it would be a very good guide for beginning students in the health sciences. If the other books in this publisher's series are as good as this, they should all be in the health sciences collections."
— *American Reference Books Annual, 2000*

"This book is an excellent general nutrition reference for consumers who desire to take an active role in their health care for prevention. Consumers of all ages who select this book can feel confident they are receiving current and accurate information." — *Journal of Nutrition for the Elderly, Vol. 19, No. 4, '00*

"Recommended reference source."
— *Booklist, American Library Association, Dec '99*

SEE ALSO Digestive Diseases & Disorders Sourcebook, Gastrointestinal Diseases & Disorders Sourcebook

Digestive Diseases & Disorders Sourcebook

Basic Consumer Health Information about Diseases and Disorders that Impact the Upper and Lower Digestive System, Including Celiac Disease, Constipation, Crohn's Disease, Cyclic Vomiting Syndrome, Diarrhea, Diverticulosis and Diverticulitis, Gallstones, Heartburn, Hemorrhoids, Hernias, Indigestion (Dyspepsia), Irritable Bowel Syndrome, Lactose Intolerance, Ulcers, and More

Along with Information about Medications and Other Treatments, Tips for Maintaining a Healthy Digestive Tract, a Glossary, and Directory of Digestive Diseases Organizations

Edited by Karen Bellenir. 335 pages. 2000. 0-7808-0327-2. $78.

"This title would be an excellent addition to all public or patient-research libraries."
—American Reference Books Annual, 2001

"This title is recommended for public, hospital, and health sciences libraries with consumer health collections." *—E-Streams, Jul-Aug '00*

"Recommended reference source."
—Booklist, American Library Association, May '00

SEE ALSO Diet & Nutrition Sourcebook, 1st and 2nd Editions, Gastrointestinal Diseases & Disorders Sourcebook

■

Disabilities Sourcebook

Basic Consumer Health Information about Physical and Psychiatric Disabilities, Including Descriptions of Major Causes of Disability, Assistive and Adaptive Aids, Workplace Issues, and Accessibility Concerns

Along with Information about the Americans with Disabilities Act, a Glossary, and Resources for Additional Help and Information

Edited by Dawn D. Matthews. 616 pages. 2000. 0-7808-0389-2. $78.

"A much needed addition to the Omnigraphics *Health Reference Series*. A current reference work to provide people with disabilities, their families, caregivers or those who work with them, a broad range of information in one volume, has not been available until now. . . . It is recommended for all public and academic library reference collections." *—E-Streams, May '01*

"An excellent source book in easy-to-read format covering many current topics; highly recommended for all libraries." *— Choice, Association of College and Research Libraries, Jan '01*

"Recommended reference source."
—Booklist, American Library Association, Jul '00

"An involving, invaluable handbook."
— The Bookwatch, May '00

Domestic Violence & Child Abuse Sourcebook

Basic Consumer Health Information about Spousal/ Partner, Child, Sibling, Parent, and Elder Abuse, Covering Physical, Emotional, and Sexual Abuse, Teen Dating Violence, and Stalking; Includes Information about Hotlines, Safe Houses, Safety Plans, and Other Resources for Support and Assistance, Community Initiatives, and Reports on Current Directions in Research and Treatment

Along with a Glossary, Sources for Further Reading, and Governmental and Non-Governmental Organizations Contact Information

Edited by Helene Henderson. 1,064 pages. 2001. 0-7808-0235-7. $78.

"This is important information. The Web has many resources but this sourcebook fills an important societal need. I am not aware of any other resources of this type." *—Doody's Review Service, Sep '01*

"Recommended for all libraries, scholars, and practitioners." *—Choice, Association of College & Research Libraries, Jul '01*

"Recommended reference source."
—Booklist, American Library Association, Apr '01

"Important pick for college-level health reference libraries." *— The Bookwatch, Mar '01*

"Because this problem is so widespread and because this book includes a lot of issues within one volume, this work is recommended for all public libraries."
—American Reference Books Annual, 2001

■

Drug Abuse Sourcebook

Basic Consumer Health Information about Illicit Substances of Abuse and the Diversion of Prescription Medications, Including Depressants, Hallucinogens, Inhalants, Marijuana, Narcotics, Stimulants, and Anabolic Steroids

Along with Facts about Related Health Risks, Treatment Issues, and Substance Abuse Prevention Programs, a Glossary of Terms, Statistical Data, and Directories of Hotline Services, Self-Help Groups, and Organizations Able to Provide Further Information

Edited by Karen Bellenir. 629 pages. 2000. 0-7808-0242-X. $78.

"Containing a wealth of information, this book will be useful to the college student just beginning to explore the topic of substance abuse. This resource belongs in libraries that serve a lower-division undergraduate or community college clientele as well as the general public." *— Choice, Association of College and Research Libraries, Jun '01*

"Recommended reference source."
— Booklist, American Library Association, Feb '01

"Highly recommended." *— The Bookwatch, Jan '01*

"Even though there is a plethora of books on drug abuse, this volume is recommended for school, public, and college libraries."
—American Reference Books Annual, 2001

SEE ALSO Alcoholism Sourcebook, Substance Abuse Sourcebook

■

Ear, Nose & Throat Disorders Sourcebook

Basic Information about Disorders of the Ears, Nose, Sinus Cavities, Pharynx, and Larynx, Including Ear Infections, Tinnitus, Vestibular Disorders, Allergic and Non-Allergic Rhinitis, Sore Throats, Tonsillitis, and Cancers That Affect the Ears, Nose, Sinuses, and Throat

Along with Reports on Current Research Initiatives, a Glossary of Related Medical Terms, and a Directory of Sources for Further Help and Information

Edited by Karen Bellenir and Linda M. Shin. 576 pages. 1998. 0-7808-0206-3. $78.

"Overall, this sourcebook is helpful for the consumer seeking information on ENT issues. It is recommended for public libraries."
—American Reference Books Annual, 1999

"Recommended reference source."
—Booklist, American Library Association, Dec '98

■

Eating Disorders Sourcebook

Basic Consumer Health Information about Eating Disorders, Including Information about Anorexia Nervosa, Bulimia Nervosa, Binge Eating, Body Dysmorphic Disorder, Pica, Laxative Abuse, and Night Eating Syndrome

Along with Information about Causes, Adverse Effects, and Treatment and Prevention Issues, and Featuring a Section on Concerns Specific to Children and Adolescents, a Glossary, and Resources for Further Help and Information

Edited by Dawn D. Matthews. 322 pages. 2001. 0-7808-0335-3. $78.

"This volume is another convenient collection of excerpted articles. Recommended for school and public library patrons; lower-division undergraduates; and two-year technical program students."
—Choice, Association of College & Research Libraries, Jan '02

"Recommended reference source." —Booklist, American Library Association, Oct '01

■

Endocrine & Metabolic Disorders Sourcebook

Basic Information for the Layperson about Pancreatic and Insulin-Related Disorders Such as Pancreatitis, Diabetes, and Hypoglycemia; Adrenal Gland Disorders Such as Cushing's Syndrome, Addison's Disease, and Congenital Adrenal Hyperplasia; Pituitary Gland Disorders Such as Growth Hormone Deficiency, Acromegaly, and Pituitary Tumors; Thyroid Disorders Such as Hypothyroidism, Graves' Disease, Hashimoto's Disease, and Goiter; Hyperparathyroidism; and Other Diseases and Syndromes of Hormone Imbalance or Metabolic Dysfunction

Along with Reports on Current Research Initiatives

Edited by Linda M. Shin. 574 pages. 1998. 0-7808-0207-1. $78.

"Omnigraphics has produced another needed resource for health information consumers."
—American Reference Books Annual, 2000

"Recommended reference source."
—Booklist, American Library Association, Dec '98

■

Environmentally Induced Disorders Sourcebook

Basic Information about Diseases and Syndromes Linked to Exposure to Pollutants and Other Substances in Outdoor and Indoor Environments Such as Lead, Asbestos, Formaldehyde, Mercury, Emissions, Noise, and More

Edited by Allan R. Cook. 620 pages. 1997. 0-7808-0083-4. $78.

"Recommended reference source."
—Booklist, American Library Association, Sep '98

"This book will be a useful addition to anyone's library." —Choice Health Sciences Supplement, Association of College and Research Libraries, May '98

". . . a good survey of numerous environmentally induced physical disorders . . . a useful addition to anyone's library."
—Doody's Health Sciences Book Reviews, Jan '98

". . . provide[s] introductory information from the best authorities around. Since this volume covers topics that potentially affect everyone, it will surely be one of the most frequently consulted volumes in the Health Reference Series." —Rettig on Reference, Nov '97

■

Ethnic Diseases Sourcebook

Basic Consumer Health Information for Ethnic and Racial Minority Groups in the United States, Including General Health Indicators and Behaviors, Ethnic Diseases, Genetic Testing, the Impact of Chronic Diseases, Women's Health, Mental Health Issues, and Preventive Health Care Services

Along with a Glossary and a Listing of Additional Resources

Edited by Joyce Brennfleck Shannon. 664 pages. 2001. 0-7808-0336-1. $78.

"Recommended for health sciences libraries where public health programs are a priority."
—E-Streams, Jan '02

"Recommended reference source."
—Booklist, American Library Association, Oct '01

"Will prove valuable to any library seeking to maintain

a current, comprehensive reference collection of health resources. . . . An excellent source of health information about genetic disorders which affect particular ethnic and racial minorities in the U.S."

—*The Bookwatch, Aug '01*

Family Planning Sourcebook

Basic Consumer Health Information about Planning for Pregnancy and Contraception, Including Traditional Methods, Barrier Methods, Hormonal Methods, Permanent Methods, Future Methods, Emergency Contraception, and Birth Control Choices for Women at Each Stage of Life

Along with Statistics, a Glossary, and Sources of Additional Information

Edited by Amy Marcaccio Keyzer. 520 pages. 2001. 0-7808-0379-5. $78.

"Recommended reference source."

—*Booklist, American Library Association, Oct '01*

"Will prove valuable to any library seeking to maintain a current, comprehensive reference collection of health resources. . . . Excellent reference."

—*The Bookwatch, Aug '01*

SEE ALSO Pregnancy & Birth Sourcebook

Fitness & Exercise Sourcebook, 1st Edition

Basic Information on Fitness and Exercise, Including Fitness Activities for Specific Age Groups, Exercise for People with Specific Medical Conditions, How to Begin a Fitness Program in Running, Walking, Swimming, Cycling, and Other Athletic Activities, and Recent Research in Fitness and Exercise

Edited by Dan R. Harris. 663 pages. 1996. 0-7808-0186-5. $78.

"A good resource for general readers." —*Choice, Association of College and Research Libraries, Nov '97*

"The perennial popularity of the topic . . . make this an appealing selection for public libraries."

—*Rettig on Reference, Jun/Jul '97*

Fitness & Exercise Sourcebook, 2nd Edition

Basic Consumer Health Information about the Fundamentals of Fitness and Exercise, Including How to Begin and Maintain a Fitness Program, Fitness as a Lifestyle, the Link between Fitness and Diet, Advice for Specific Groups of People, Exercise as It Relates to Specific Medical Conditions, and Recent Research in Fitness and Exercise

Along with a Glossary of Important Terms and Resources for Additional Help and Information

Edited by Kristen M. Gledhill. 646 pages. 2001. 0-7808-0334-5. $78.

"Highly recommended for public, consumer, and school grades fourth through college."

—*E-Streams, Nov '01*

"Recommended reference source." —*Booklist, American Library Association, Oct '01*

"The information appears quite comprehensive and is considered reliable. . . . This second edition is a welcomed addition to the series."

—*Doody's Review Service, Sep '01*

"This reference is a valuable choice for those who desire a broad source of information on exercise, fitness, and chronic-disease prevention through a healthy lifestyle." —*American Medical Writers Association Journal, Fall '01*

"Will prove valuable to any library seeking to maintain a current, comprehensive reference collection of health resources. . . . Excellent reference."

—*The Bookwatch, Aug '01*

Food & Animal Borne Diseases Sourcebook

Basic Information about Diseases That Can Be Spread to Humans through the Ingestion of Contaminated Food or Water or by Contact with Infected Animals and Insects, Such as Botulism, E. Coli, Hepatitis A, Trichinosis, Lyme Disease, and Rabies

Along with Information Regarding Prevention and Treatment Methods, and Including a Special Section for International Travelers Describing Diseases Such as Cholera, Malaria, Travelers' Diarrhea, and Yellow Fever, and Offering Recommendations for Avoiding Illness

Edited by Karen Bellenir and Peter D. Dresser. 535 pages. 1995. 0-7808-0033-8. $78.

"Targeting general readers and providing them with a single, comprehensive source of information on selected topics, this book continues, with the excellent caliber of its predecessors, to catalog topical information on health matters of general interest. Readable and thorough, this valuable resource is highly recommended for all libraries."

—*Academic Library Book Review, Summer '96*

"A comprehensive collection of authoritative information." —*Emergency Medical Services, Oct '95*

Food Safety Sourcebook

Basic Consumer Health Information about the Safe Handling of Meat, Poultry, Seafood, Eggs, Fruit Juices, and Other Food Items, and Facts about Pesticides, Drinking Water, Food Safety Overseas, and the Onset, Duration, and Symptoms of Foodborne Illnesses, Including Types of Pathogenic Bacteria, Parasitic Protozoa, Worms, Viruses, and Natural Toxins

Along with the Role of the Consumer, the Food Handler, and the Government in Food Safety; a Glossary, and Resources for Additional Help and Information

Edited by Dawn D. Matthews. 339 pages. 1999. 0-7808-0326-4. $78.

"This book is recommended for public libraries and universities with home economic and food science programs." —E-Streams, Nov '00

"Recommended reference source."
—Booklist, American Library Association, May '00

"This book takes the complex issues of food safety and foodborne pathogens and presents them in an easily understood manner. [It does] an excellent job of covering a large and often confusing topic."
—American Reference Books Annual, 2000

■

Forensic Medicine Sourcebook

Basic Consumer Information for the Layperson about Forensic Medicine, Including Crime Scene Investigation, Evidence Collection and Analysis, Expert Testimony, Computer-Aided Criminal Identification, Digital Imaging in the Courtroom, DNA Profiling, Accident Reconstruction, Autopsies, Ballistics, Drugs and Explosives Detection, Latent Fingerprints, Product Tampering, and Questioned Document Examination

Along with Statistical Data, a Glossary of Forensics Terminology, and Listings of Sources for Further Help and Information

Edited by Annemarie S. Muth. 574 pages. 1999. 0-7808-0232-2. $78.

"Given the expected widespread interest in its content and its easy to read style, this book is recommended for most public and all college and university libraries."
—E-Streams, Feb '01

"Recommended for public libraries."
—Reference & User Services Quarterly, American Library Association, Spring 2000

"Recommended reference source."
—Booklist, American Library Association, Feb '00

"A wealth of information, useful statistics, references are up-to-date and extremely complete. This wonderful collection of data will help students who are interested in a career in any type of forensic field. It is a great resource for attorneys who need information about types of expert witnesses needed in a particular case. It also offers useful information for fiction and nonfiction writers whose work involves a crime. A fascinating compilation. All levels." —Choice, Association of College and Research Libraries, Jan 2000

"There are several items that make this book attractive to consumers who are seeking certain forensic data. . . . This is a useful current source for those seeking general forensic medical answers."
—American Reference Books Annual, 2000

■

Gastrointestinal Diseases & Disorders Sourcebook

Basic Information about Gastroesophageal Reflux Disease (Heartburn), Ulcers, Diverticulosis, Irritable Bowel Syndrome, Crohn's Disease, Ulcerative Colitis, Diarrhea, Constipation, Lactose Intolerance, Hemorrhoids, Hepatitis, Cirrhosis, and Other Digestive Problems, Featuring Statistics, Descriptions of Symptoms,

and Current Treatment Methods of Interest for Persons Living with Upper and Lower Gastrointestinal Maladies

Edited by Linda M. Ross. 413 pages. 1996. 0-7808-0078-8. $78.

". . . very readable form. The successful editorial work that brought this material together into a useful and understandable reference makes accessible to all readers information that can help them more effectively understand and obtain help for digestive tract problems."
—Choice, Association of College and Research Libraries, Feb '97

SEE ALSO Diet & Nutrition Sourcebook, 1st and 2nd Editions, Digestive Diseases & Disorders

■

Genetic Disorders Sourcebook, 1st Edition

Basic Information about Heritable Diseases and Disorders Such as Down Syndrome, PKU, Hemophilia, Von Willebrand Disease, Gaucher Disease, Tay-Sachs Disease, and Sickle-Cell Disease, Along with Information about Genetic Screening, Gene Therapy, Home Care, and Including Source Listings for Further Help and Information on More Than 300 Disorders

Edited by Karen Bellenir. 642 pages. 1996. 0-7808-0034-6. $78.

"Recommended for undergraduate libraries or libraries that serve the public."
—Science & Technology Libraries, Vol. 18, No. 1, '99

"Provides essential medical information to both the general public and those diagnosed with a serious or fatal genetic disease or disorder." —Choice, Association of College and Research Libraries, Jan '97

"Geared toward the lay public. It would be well placed in all public libraries and in those hospital and medical libraries in which access to genetic references is limited." —Doody's Health Sciences Book Review, Oct '96

■

Genetic Disorders Sourcebook, 2nd Edition

Basic Consumer Health Information about Hereditary Diseases and Disorders, Including Cystic Fibrosis, Down Syndrome, Hemophilia, Huntington's Disease, Sickle Cell Anemia, and More; Facts about Genes, Gene Research and Therapy, Genetic Screening, Ethics of Gene Testing, Genetic Counseling, and Advice on Coping and Caring

Along with a Glossary of Genetic Terminology and a Resource List for Help, Support, and Further Information

Edited by Kathy Massimini. 768 pages. 2001. 0-7808-0241-1. $78.

"Recommended for public libraries and medical and hospital libraries with consumer health collections."
—E-Streams, May '01

"Recommended reference source."
—Booklist, American Library Association, Apr '01

■

Head Trauma Sourcebook

Basic Information for the Layperson about Open-Head and Closed-Head Injuries, Treatment Advances, Recovery, and Rehabilitation

Along with Reports on Current Research Initiatives

Edited by Karen Bellenir. 414 pages. 1997. 0-7808-0208-X. $78.

■

Headache Sourcebook

Basic Consumer Health Information about Migraine, Tension, Cluster, Rebound and Other Types of Headaches, with Facts about the Cause and Prevention of Headaches, the Effects of Stress and the Environment, Headaches during Pregnancy and Menopause, and Childhood Headaches

Along with a Glossary and Other Resources for Additional Help and Information

Edited by Dawn D. Matthews. 362 pages. 2002. 0-7808-0337-X. $78.

■

Health Insurance Sourcebook

Basic Information about Managed Care Organizations, Traditional Fee-for-Service Insurance, Insurance Portability and Pre-Existing Conditions Clauses, Medicare, Medicaid, Social Security, and Military Health Care

Along with Information about Insurance Fraud

Edited by Wendy Wilcox. 530 pages. 1997. 0-7808-0222-5. $78.

■

Health Reference Series Cumulative Index 1999

A Comprehensive Index to the Individual Volumes of the Health Reference Series, Including a Subject Index, Name Index, Organization Index, and Publication Index

Along with a Master List of Acronyms and Abbreviations

Edited by Edward J. Prucha, Anne Holmes, and Robert Rudnick. 990 pages. 2000. 0-7808-0382-5. $78.

■

Healthy Aging Sourcebook

Basic Consumer Health Information about Maintaining Health through the Aging Process, Including Advice on Nutrition, Exercise, and Sleep, Help in Making Decisions about Midlife Issues and Retirement, and Guidance Concerning Practical and Informed Choices in Health Consumerism

Along with Data Concerning the Theories of Aging, Different Experiences in Aging by Minority Groups, and Facts about Aging Now and Aging in the Future; and Featuring a Glossary, a Guide to Consumer Help, Additional Suggested Reading, and Practical Resource Directory

Edited by Jenifer Swanson. 536 pages. 1999. 0-7808-0390-6. $78.

SEE ALSO Physical & Mental Issues in Aging Sourcebook

■

Healthy Heart Sourcebook for Women

Basic Consumer Health Information about Cardiac Issues Specific to Women, Including Facts about Major Risk Factors and Prevention, Treatment and Control Strategies, and Important Dietary Issues

Along with a Special Section Regarding the Pros and Cons of Hormone Replacement Therapy and Its Impact on Heart Health, and Additional Help, Including Recipes, a Glossary, and a Directory of Resources

Edited by Dawn D. Matthews. 336 pages. 2000. 0-7808-0329-9. $78.

SEE ALSO *Cardiovascular Diseases & Disorders Sourcebook, 1st Edition, Heart Diseases & Disorders Sourcebook, 2nd Edition, Women's Health Concerns Sourcebook*

■

Heart Diseases & Disorders Sourcebook, 2nd Edition

Basic Consumer Health Information about Heart Attacks, Angina, Rhythm Disorders, Heart Failure, Valve Disease, Congenital Heart Disorders, and More, Including Descriptions of Surgical Procedures and Other Interventions, Medications, Cardiac Rehabilitation, Risk Identification, and Prevention Tips

Along with Statistical Data, Reports on Current Research Initiatives, a Glossary of Cardiovascular Terms, and Resource Directory

Edited by Karen Bellenir. 612 pages. 2000. 0-7808-0238-1. $78.

SEE ALSO *Cardiovascular Diseases & Disorders Sourcebook, 1st Edition; Healthy Heart Sourcebook for Women*

■

Household Safety Sourcebook

Basic Consumer Health Information about Household Safety, Including Information about Poisons, Chemicals, Fire, and Water Hazards in the Home

Along with Advice about the Safe Use of Home Maintenance Equipment, Choosing Toys and Nursery Furniture, Holiday and Recreation Safety, a Glossary, and Resources for Further Help and Information

Edited by Dawn D. Matthews. 606 pages. 2002. 0-7808-0338-8. $78.

■

Immune System Disorders Sourcebook

Basic Information about Lupus, Multiple Sclerosis, Guillain-Barré Syndrome, Chronic Granulomatous Disease, and More

Along with Statistical and Demographic Data and Reports on Current Research Initiatives

Edited by Allan R. Cook. 608 pages. 1997. 0-7808-0209-8. $78.

Infant & Toddler Health Sourcebook

Basic Consumer Health Information about the Physical and Mental Development of Newborns, Infants, and Toddlers, Including Neonatal Concerns, Nutrition Recommendations, Immunization Schedules, Common Pediatric Disorders, Assessments and Milestones, Safety Tips, and Advice for Parents and Other Caregivers

Along with a Glossary of Terms and Resource Listings for Additional Help

Edited by Jenifer Swanson. 585 pages. 2000. 0-7808-0246-2. $78.

■

Injury & Trauma Sourcebook

Basic Consumer Health Information about the Impact of Injury, the Diagnosis and Treatment of Common and Traumatic Injuries, Emergency Care, and Specific Injuries Related to Home, Community, Workplace, Transportation, and Recreation

Along with Guidelines for Injury Prevention, a Glossary, and a Directory of Additional Resources

Edited by Joyce Brennfleck Shannon. 696 pages. 2002. 0-7808-0421-X. $78.

■

Kidney & Urinary Tract Diseases & Disorders Sourcebook

Basic Information about Kidney Stones, Urinary Incontinence, Bladder Disease, End Stage Renal Disease, Dialysis, and More

Along with Statistical and Demographic Data and Reports on Current Research Initiatives

Edited by Linda M. Ross. 602 pages. 1997. 0-7808-0079-6. $78.

■

Learning Disabilities Sourcebook

Basic Information about Disorders Such as Dyslexia, Visual and Auditory Processing Deficits, Attention Deficit/Hyperactivity Disorder, and Autism

Along with Statistical and Demographic Data, Reports on Current Research Initiatives, an Explanation of the Assessment Process, and a Special Section for Adults with Learning Disabilities

Edited by Linda M. Shin. 579 pages. 1998. 0-7808-0210-1. $78.

Liver Disorders Sourcebook

Basic Consumer Health Information about the Liver and How It Works; Liver Diseases, Including Cancer, Cirrhosis, Hepatitis, and Toxic and Drug Related Diseases; Tips for Maintaining a Healthy Liver; Laboratory Tests, Radiology Tests, and Facts about Liver Transplantation

Along with a Section on Support Groups, a Glossary, and Resource Listings

Edited by Joyce Brennfleck Shannon. 591 pages. 2000. 0-7808-0383-3. $78.

Lung Disorders Sourcebook

Basic Consumer Health Information about Emphysema, Pneumonia, Tuberculosis, Asthma, Cystic Fibrosis, and Other Lung Disorders, Including Facts about Diagnostic Procedures, Treatment Strategies, Disease Prevention Efforts, and Such Risk Factors as Smoking, Air Pollution, and Exposure to Asbestos, Radon, and Other Agents

Along with a Glossary and Resources for Additional Help and Information

Edited by Dawn D. Matthews. 678 pages. 2002. 0-7808-0339-6. $78.

Medical Tests Sourcebook

Basic Consumer Health Information about Medical Tests, Including Periodic Health Exams, General Screening Tests, Tests You Can Do at Home, Findings of the U.S. Preventive Services Task Force, X-ray and Radiology Tests, Electrical Tests, Tests of Blood and Other Body Fluids and Tissues, Scope Tests, Lung Tests, Genetic Tests, Pregnancy Tests, Newborn Screening Tests, Sexually Transmitted Disease Tests, and Computer Aided Diagnoses

Along with a Section on Paying for Medical Tests, a Glossary, and Resource Listings

Edited by Joyce Brennfleck Shannon. 691 pages. 1999. 0-7808-0243-8. $78.

Men's Health Concerns Sourcebook

Basic Information about Health Issues That Affect Men, Featuring Facts about the Top Causes of Death in Men, Including Heart Disease, Stroke, Cancers, Prostate Disorders, Chronic Obstructive Pulmonary Disease, Pneumonia and Influenza, Human Immunodeficiency Virus and Acquired Immune Deficiency Syndrome, Diabetes Mellitus, Stress, Suicide, Accidents and Homicides; and Facts about Common Concerns for Men, Including Impotence, Contraception, Circumcision, Sleep Disorders, Snoring, Hair Loss, Diet, Nutrition, Exercise, Kidney and Urological Disorders, and Backaches

Edited by Allan R. Cook. 738 pages. 1998. 0-7808-0212-8. $78.

Mental Health Disorders Sourcebook, 1st Edition

Basic Information about Schizophrenia, Depression, Bipolar Disorder, Panic Disorder, Obsessive-Compulsive Disorder, Phobias and Other Anxiety Disorders, Paranoia and Other Personality Disorders, Eating Disorders, and Sleep Disorders

Along with Information about Treatment and Therapies

Edited by Karen Bellenir. 548 pages. 1995. 0-7808-0040-0. $78.

"This is an excellent new book . . . written in easy-to-understand language."
—*Booklist Health Sciences Supplement, American Library Association, Oct '97*

". . . useful for public and academic libraries and consumer health collections."
—*Medical Reference Services Quarterly, Spring '97*

"The great strengths of the book are its readability and its inclusion of places to find more information. Especially recommended." —*Reference Quarterly, American Library Association, Winter '96*

". . . a good resource for a consumer health library."
—*Bulletin of the Medical Library Association, Oct '96*

"The information is data-based and couched in brief, concise language that avoids jargon. . . . a useful reference source." —*Readings, Sep '96*

"The text is well organized and adequately written for its target audience." —*Choice, Association of College and Research Libraries, Jun '96*

". . . provides information on a wide range of mental disorders, presented in nontechnical language."
—*Exceptional Child Education Resources, Spring '96*

"Recommended for public and academic libraries."
—*Reference Book Review, 1996*

■

Mental Health Disorders Sourcebook, 2nd Edition

Basic Consumer Health Information about Anxiety Disorders, Depression and Other Mood Disorders, Eating Disorders, Personality Disorders, Schizophrenia, and More, Including Disease Descriptions, Treatment Options, and Reports on Current Research Initiatives

Along with Statistical Data, Tips for Maintaining Mental Health, a Glossary, and Directory of Sources for Additional Help and Information

Edited by Karen Bellenir. 605 pages. 2000. 0-7808-0240-3. $78.

"Well organized and well written."
—*American Reference Books Annual, 2001*

"Recommended reference source."
—*Booklist, American Library Association, Jun '00*

■

Mental Retardation Sourcebook

Basic Consumer Health Information about Mental Retardation and Its Causes, Including Down Syndrome, Fetal Alcohol Syndrome, Fragile X Syndrome, Genetic Conditions, Injury, and Environmental Sources

Along with Preventive Strategies, Parenting Issues, Educational Implications, Health Care Needs, Employment and Economic Matters, Legal Issues, a Glossary, and a Resource Listing for Additional Help and Information

Edited by Joyce Brennfleck Shannon. 642 pages. 2000. 0-7808-0377-9. $78.

"Public libraries will find the book useful for reference and as a beginning research point for students, parents, and caregivers."
—*American Reference Books Annual, 2001*

"The strength of this work is that it compiles many basic fact sheets and addresses for further information in one volume. It is intended and suitable for the general public. This sourcebook is relevant to any collection providing health information to the general public."
—*E-Streams, Nov '00*

"From preventing retardation to parenting and family challenges, this covers health, social and legal issues and will prove an invaluable overview."
—*Reviewer's Bookwatch, Jul '00*

■

Obesity Sourcebook

Basic Consumer Health Information about Diseases and Other Problems Associated with Obesity, and Including Facts about Risk Factors, Prevention Issues, and Management Approaches

Along with Statistical and Demographic Data, Information about Special Populations, Research Updates, a Glossary, and Source Listings for Further Help and Information

Edited by Wilma Caldwell and Chad T. Kimball. 376 pages. 2001. 0-7808-0333-7. $78.

"This is a very useful resource book for the lay public."
—*Doody's Review Service, Nov '01*

"Well suited for the health reference collection of a public library or an academic health science library that serves the general population." —*E-Streams, Sep '01*

"Recommended reference source."
—*Booklist, American Library Association, Apr '01*

" Recommended pick both for specialty health library collections and any general consumer health reference collection." —*The Bookwatch, Apr '01*

■

Ophthalmic Disorders Sourcebook

Basic Information about Glaucoma, Cataracts, Macular Degeneration, Strabismus, Refractive Disorders, and More

Along with Statistical and Demographic Data and Reports on Current Research Initiatives

Edited by Linda M. Ross. 631 pages. 1996. 0-7808-0081-8. $78.

■

Oral Health Sourcebook

Basic Information about Diseases and Conditions Affecting Oral Health, Including Cavities, Gum Disease, Dry Mouth, Oral Cancers, Fever Blisters, Canker Sores, Oral Thrush, Bad Breath, Temporomandibular Disorders, and other Craniofacial Syndromes

Along with Statistical Data on the Oral Health of Americans, Oral Hygiene, Emergency First Aid, In-

formation on *Treatment Procedures and Methods of Replacing Lost Teeth*

Edited by Allan R. Cook. 558 pages. 1997. 0-7808-0082-6. $78.

"Unique source which will fill a gap in dental sources for patients and the lay public. A valuable reference tool even in a library with thousands of books on dentistry. Comprehensive, clear, inexpensive, and easy to read and use. It fills an enormous gap in the health care literature." — *Reference and User Services Quarterly, American Library Association, Summer '98*

"Recommended reference source."
— *Booklist, American Library Association, Dec '97*

■

Osteoporosis Sourcebook

Basic Consumer Health Information about Primary and Secondary Osteoporosis and Juvenile Osteoporosis and Related Conditions, Including Fibrous Dysplasia, Gaucher Disease, Hyperthyroidism, Hypophosphatasia, Myeloma, Osteopetrosis, Osteogenesis Imperfecta, and Paget's Disease

Along with Information about Risk Factors, Treatments, Traditional and Non-Traditional Pain Management, a Glossary of Related Terms, and a Directory of Resources

Edited by Allan R. Cook. 584 pages. 2001. 0-7808-0239-X. $78.

"This would be a book to be kept in a staff or patient library. The targeted audience is the layperson, but the therapist who needs a quick bit of information on a particular topic will also find the book useful."
— *Physical Therapy, Jan '02*

"Recommended for all public libraries and general health collections, especially those supporting patient education or consumer health programs."
— *E-Streams, Nov '01*

"Will prove valuable to any library seeking to maintain a current, comprehensive reference collection of health resources. . . . From prevention to treatment and associated conditions, this provides an excellent survey."
— *The Bookwatch, Aug '01*

"Recommended reference source."
— *Booklist, American Library Association, July '01*

SEE ALSO *Women's Health Concerns Sourcebook*

■

Pain Sourcebook, 1st Edition

Basic Information about Specific Forms of Acute and Chronic Pain, Including Headaches, Back Pain, Muscular Pain, Neuralgia, Surgical Pain, and Cancer Pain

Along with Pain Relief Options Such as Analgesics, Narcotics, Nerve Blocks, Transcutaneous Nerve Stimulation, and Alternative Forms of Pain Control, Including Biofeedback, Imaging, Behavior Modification, and Relaxation Techniques

Edited by Allan R. Cook. 667 pages. 1997. 0-7808-0213-6. $78.

"The text is readable, easily understood, and well indexed. This excellent volume belongs in all patient education libraries, consumer health sections of public libraries, and many personal collections."
— *American Reference Books Annual, 1999*

"A beneficial reference." — *Booklist Health Sciences Supplement, American Library Association, Oct '98*

"The information is basic in terms of scholarship and is appropriate for general readers. Written in journalistic style . . . intended for non-professionals. Quite thorough in its coverage of different pain conditions and summarizes the latest clinical information regarding pain treatment." — *Choice, Association of College and Research Libraries, Jun '98*

"Recommended reference source."
— *Booklist, American Library Association, Mar '98*

■

Pain Sourcebook, 2nd Edition

Basic Consumer Health Information about Specific Forms of Acute and Chronic Pain, Including Muscle and Skeletal Pain, Nerve Pain, Cancer Pain, and Disorders Characterized by Pain, Such as Fibromyalgia, Shingles, Angina, Arthritis, and Headaches

Along with Information about Pain Medications and Management Techniques, Complementary and Alternative Pain Relief Options, Tips for People Living with Chronic Pain, a Glossary, and a Directory of Sources for Further Information

Edited by Karen Bellenir. 650 pages. 2002. 0-7808-0612-3. $78.

■

Pediatric Cancer Sourcebook

Basic Consumer Health Information about Leukemias, Brain Tumors, Sarcomas, Lymphomas, and Other Cancers in Infants, Children, and Adolescents, Including Descriptions of Cancers, Treatments, and Coping Strategies

Along with Suggestions for Parents, Caregivers, and Concerned Relatives, a Glossary of Cancer Terms, and Resource Listings

Edited by Edward J. Prucha. 587 pages. 1999. 0-7808-0245-4. $78.

"An excellent source of information. Recommended for public, hospital, and health science libraries with consumer health collections." — *E-Streams, Jun '00*

"Recommended reference source."
— *Booklist, American Library Association, Feb '00*

"A valuable addition to all libraries specializing in health services and many public libraries."
— *American Reference Books Annual, 2000*

Physical & Mental Issues in Aging Sourcebook

Basic Consumer Health Information on Physical and Mental Disorders Associated with the Aging Process, Including Concerns about Cardiovascular Disease, Pulmonary Disease, Oral Health, Digestive Disorders, Musculoskeletal and Skin Disorders, Metabolic Changes, Sexual and Reproductive Issues, and Changes in Vision, Hearing, and Other Senses

Along with Data about Longevity and Causes of Death, Information on Acute and Chronic Pain, Descriptions of Mental Concerns, a Glossary of Terms, and Resource Listings for Additional Help

Edited by Jenifer Swanson. 660 pages. 1999. 0-7808-0233-0. $78.

"This is a treasure of health information for the layperson." — Choice Health Sciences Supplement, Association of College & Research Libraries, May 2000

"Recommended for public libraries." —American Reference Books Annual, 2000

"Recommended reference source." — Booklist, American Library Association, Oct '99

SEE ALSO Healthy Aging Sourcebook

■

Podiatry Sourcebook

Basic Consumer Health Information about Foot Conditions, Diseases, and Injuries, Including Bunions, Corns, Calluses, Athlete's Foot, Plantar Warts, Hammertoes and Clawtoes, Clubfoot, Heel Pain, Gout, and More

Along with Facts about Foot Care, Disease Prevention, Foot Safety, Choosing a Foot Care Specialist, a Glossary of Terms, and Resource Listings for Additional Information

Edited by M. Lisa Weatherford. 380 pages. 2001. 0-7808-0215-2. $78.

■

Pregnancy & Birth Sourcebook

Basic Information about Planning for Pregnancy, Maternal Health, Fetal Growth and Development, Labor and Delivery, Postpartum and Perinatal Care, Pregnancy in Mothers with Special Concerns, and Disorders of Pregnancy, Including Genetic Counseling, Nutrition and Exercise, Obstetrical Tests, Pregnancy Discomfort, Multiple Births, Cesarean Sections, Medical Testing of Newborns, Breastfeeding, Gestational Diabetes, and Ectopic Pregnancy

Edited by Heather E. Aldred. 737 pages. 1997. 0-7808-0216-0. $78.

"A well-organized handbook. Recommended." — Choice, Association of College and Research Libraries, Apr '98

"Recommended reference source." — Booklist, American Library Association, Mar '98

"Recommended for public libraries." —American Reference Books Annual, 1998

SEE ALSO Congenital Disorders Sourcebook, Family Planning Sourcebook

■

Prostate Cancer Sourcebook

Basic Consumer Health Information about Prostate Cancer, Including Information about the Associated Risk Factors, Detection, Diagnosis, and Treatment of Prostate Cancer

Along with Information on Non-Malignant Prostate Conditions, and Featuring a Section Listing Support and Treatment Centers and a Glossary of Related Terms

Edited by Dawn D. Matthews. 358 pages. 2001. 0-7808-0324-8. $78.

"Recommended reference source." —Booklist, American Library Association, Jan '02

Public Health Sourcebook

Basic Information about Government Health Agencies, Including National Health Statistics and Trends, Healthy People 2000 Program Goals and Objectives, the Centers for Disease Control and Prevention, the Food and Drug Administration, and the National Institutes of Health

Along with Full Contact Information for Each Agency

Edited by Wendy Wilcox. 698 pages. 1998. 0-7808-0220-9. $78.

"Recommended reference source." — Booklist, American Library Association, Sep '98

"This consumer guide provides welcome assistance in navigating the maze of federal health agencies and their data on public health concerns." — SciTech Book News, Sep '98

■

Reconstructive & Cosmetic Surgery Sourcebook

Basic Consumer Health Information on Cosmetic and Reconstructive Plastic Surgery, Including Statistical Information about Different Surgical Procedures, Things to Consider Prior to Surgery, Plastic Surgery Techniques and Tools, Emotional and Psychological Considerations, and Procedure-Specific Information

Along with a Glossary of Terms and a Listing of Resources for Additional Help and Information

Edited by M. Lisa Weatherford. 374 pages. 2001. 0-7808-0214-4. $78.

"Recommended for health science libraries that are open to the public, as well as hospital libraries that are open to the patients. This book is a good resource for the consumer interested in plastic surgery." —E-Streams, Dec '01

"Recommended reference source." —Booklist, American Library Association, July '01

Rehabilitation Sourcebook

Basic Consumer Health Information about Rehabilitation for People Recovering from Heart Surgery, Spinal Cord Injury, Stroke, Orthopedic Impairments, Amputation, Pulmonary Impairments, Traumatic Injury, and More, Including Physical Therapy, Occupational Therapy, Speech/ Language Therapy, Massage Therapy, Dance Therapy, Art Therapy, and Recreational Therapy

Along with Information on Assistive and Adaptive Devices, a Glossary, and Resources for Additional Help and Information

Edited by Dawn D. Matthews. 531 pages. 1999. 0-7808-0236-5. $78.

"This is an excellent resource for public library reference and health collections."
—American Reference Books Annual, 2001

"Recommended reference source."
—Booklist, American Library Association, May '00

■

Respiratory Diseases & Disorders Sourcebook

Basic Information about Respiratory Diseases and Disorders, Including Asthma, Cystic Fibrosis, Pneumonia, the Common Cold, Influenza, and Others, Featuring Facts about the Respiratory System, Statistical and Demographic Data, Treatments, Self-Help Management Suggestions, and Current Research Initiatives

Edited by Allan R. Cook and Peter D. Dresser. 771 pages. 1995. 0-7808-0037-0. $78.

"Designed for the layperson and for patients and their families coping with respiratory illness. . . . an extensive array of information on diagnosis, treatment, management, and prevention of respiratory illnesses for the general reader." *— Choice, Association of College and Research Libraries, Jun '96*

"A highly recommended text for all collections. It is a comforting reminder of the power of knowledge that good books carry between their covers."
— Academic Library Book Review, Spring '96

"A comprehensive collection of authoritative information presented in a nontechnical, humanitarian style for patients, families, and caregivers."
—Association of Operating Room Nurses, Sep/Oct '95

■

Sexually Transmitted Diseases Sourcebook, 1st Edition

Basic Information about Herpes, Chlamydia, Gonorrhea, Hepatitis, Nongonoccocal Urethritis, Pelvic Inflammatory Disease, Syphilis, AIDS, and More

Along with Current Data on Treatments and Preventions

Edited by Linda M. Ross. 550 pages. 1997. 0-7808-0217-9. $78.

Sexually Transmitted Diseases Sourcebook, 2nd Edition

Basic Consumer Health Information about Sexually Transmitted Diseases, Including Information on the Diagnosis and Treatment of Chlamydia, Gonorrhea, Hepatitis, Herpes, HIV, Mononucleosis, Syphilis, and Others

Along with Information on Prevention, Such as Condom Use, Vaccines, and STD Education; And Featuring a Section on Issues Related to Youth and Adolescents, a Glossary, and Resources for Additional Help and Information

Edited by Dawn D. Matthews. 538 pages. 2001. 0-7808-0249-7. $78.

"Every school and public library should have a copy of this comprehensive and user-friendly reference book."
—Choice, Association of College & Research Libraries, Sep '01

"This is a highly recommended book. This is an especially important book for all school and public libraries." *—AIDS Book Review Journal, Jul-Aug '01*

"Recommended reference source."
— Booklist, American Library Association, Apr '01

"Recommended pick both for specialty health library collections and any general consumer health reference collection." *— The Bookwatch, Apr '01*

■

Skin Disorders Sourcebook

Basic Information about Common Skin and Scalp Conditions Caused by Aging, Allergies, Immune Reactions, Sun Exposure, Infectious Organisms, Parasites, Cosmetics, and Skin Traumas, Including Abrasions, Cuts, and Pressure Sores

Along with Information on Prevention and Treatment

Edited by Allan R. Cook. 647 pages. 1997. 0-7808-0080-X. $78.

". . . comprehensive, easily read reference book."
—Doody's Health Sciences Book Reviews, Oct '97

SEE ALSO Burns Sourcebook

■

Sleep Disorders Sourcebook

Basic Consumer Health Information about Sleep and Its Disorders, Including Insomnia, Sleepwalking, Sleep Apnea, Restless Leg Syndrome, and Narcolepsy

Along with Data about Shiftwork and Its Effects, Information on the Societal Costs of Sleep Deprivation, Descriptions of Treatment Options, a Glossary of Terms, and Resource Listings for Additional Help

Edited by Jenifer Swanson. 439 pages. 1998. 0-7808-0234-9. $78.

"This text will complement any home or medical library. It is user-friendly and ideal for the adult reader."
—American Reference Books Annual, 2000

"A useful resource that provides accurate, relevant, and accessible information on sleep to the general public. Health care providers who deal with sleep disorders patients may also find it helpful in being prepared to answer some of the questions patients ask."
— *Respiratory Care, Jul '99*

"Recommended reference source."
— *Booklist, American Library Association, Feb '99*

■

Sports Injuries Sourcebook

Basic Consumer Health Information about Common Sports Injuries, Prevention of Injury in Specific Sports, Tips for Training, and Rehabilitation from Injury

Along with Information about Special Concerns for Children, Young Girls in Athletic Training Programs, Senior Athletes, and Women Athletes, and a Directory of Resources for Further Help and Information

Edited by Heather E. Aldred. 624 pages. 1999. 0-7808-0218-7. $78.

"While this easy-to-read book is recommended for all libraries, it should prove to be especially useful for public, high school, and academic libraries; certainly it should be on the bookshelf of every school gymnasium." — *E-Streams, Mar '00*

"Public libraries and undergraduate academic libraries will find this book useful for its nontechnical language." — *American Reference Books Annual, 2000*

■

Substance Abuse Sourcebook

Basic Health-Related Information about the Abuse of Legal and Illegal Substances Such as Alcohol, Tobacco, Prescription Drugs, Marijuana, Cocaine, and Heroin; and Including Facts about Substance Abuse Prevention Strategies, Intervention Methods, Treatment and Recovery Programs, and a Section Addressing the Special Problems Related to Substance Abuse during Pregnancy

Edited by Karen Bellenir. 573 pages. 1996. 0-7808-0038-9. $78.

"A valuable addition to any health reference section. Highly recommended."
— *The Book Report, Mar/Apr '97*

". . . a comprehensive collection of substance abuse information that's both highly readable and compact. Families and caregivers of substance abusers will find the information enlightening and helpful, while teachers, social workers and journalists should benefit from the concise format. Recommended."
— *Drug Abuse Update, Winter '96/'97*

SEE ALSO *Alcoholism Sourcebook, Drug Abuse Sourcebook*

Transplantation Sourcebook

Basic Consumer Health Information about Organ and Tissue Transplantation, Including Physical and Financial Preparations, Procedures and Issues Relating to Specific Solid Organ and Tissue Transplants, Rehabilitation, Pediatric Transplant Information, the Future of Transplantation, and Organ and Tissue Donation

Along with a Glossary and Listings of Additional Resources

Edited by Joyce Brennfleck Shannon. 628 pages. 2002. 0-7808-0322-1. $78.

■

Traveler's Health Sourcebook

Basic Consumer Health Information for Travelers, Including Physical and Medical Preparations, Transportation Health and Safety, Essential Information about Food and Water, Sun Exposure, Insect and Snake Bites, Camping and Wilderness Medicine, and Travel with Physical or Medical Disabilities

Along with International Travel Tips, Vaccination Recommendations, Geographical Health Issues, Disease Risks, a Glossary, and a Listing of Additional Resources

Edited by Joyce Brennfleck Shannon. 613 pages. 2000. 0-7808-0384-1. $78.

"Recommended reference source."
— *Booklist, American Library Association, Feb '01*

"This book is recommended for any public library, any travel collection, and especially any collection for the physically disabled."
— *American Reference Books Annual, 2001*

■

Women's Health Concerns Sourcebook

Basic Information about Health Issues That Affect Women, Featuring Facts about Menstruation and Other Gynecological Concerns, Including Endometriosis, Fibroids, Menopause, and Vaginitis; Reproductive Concerns, Including Birth Control, Infertility, and Abortion; and Facts about Additional Physical, Emotional, and Mental Health Concerns Prevalent among Women Such as Osteoporosis, Urinary Tract Disorders, Eating Disorders, and Depression

Along with Tips for Maintaining a Healthy Lifestyle

Edited by Heather E. Aldred. 567 pages. 1997. 0-7808-0219-5. $78.

"Handy compilation. There is an impressive range of diseases, devices, disorders, procedures, and other physical and emotional issues covered . . . well organized, illustrated, and indexed." — *Choice, Association of College and Research Libraries, Jan '98*

SEE ALSO *Breast Cancer Sourcebook, Cancer Sourcebook for Women, 1st and 2nd Editions, Healthy Heart Sourcebook for Women, Osteoporosis Sourcebook*

Workplace Health & Safety Sourcebook

Basic Consumer Health Information about Workplace Health and Safety, Including the Effect of Workplace Hazards on the Lungs, Skin, Heart, Ears, Eyes, Brain, Reproductive Organs, Musculoskeletal System, and Other Organs and Body Parts

Along with Information about Occupational Cancer, Personal Protective Equipment, Toxic and Hazardous Chemicals, Child Labor, Stress, and Workplace Violence

Edited by Chad T. Kimball. 626 pages. 2000. 0-7808-0231-4. $78.

"As a reference for the general public, this would be useful in any library." *—E-Streams, Jun '01*

"Provides helpful information for primary care physicians and other caregivers interested in occupational medicine. . . . General readers; professionals."
— Choice, Association of College & Research Libraries, May '01

"Recommended reference source."
—Booklist, American Library Association, Feb '01

"Highly recommended." *— The Bookwatch, Jan '01*

∎

Worldwide Health Sourcebook

Basic Information about Global Health Issues, Including Malnutrition, Reproductive Health, Disease Dispersion and Prevention, Emerging Diseases, Risky Health Behaviors, and the Leading Causes of Death

Along with Global Health Concerns for Children, Women, and the Elderly, Mental Health Issues, Research and Technology Advancements, and Economic, Environmental, and Political Health Implications, a Glossary, and a Resource Listing for Additional Help and Information

Edited by Joyce Brennfleck Shannon. 614 pages. 2001. 0-7808-0330-2. $78.

"Named an Outstanding Academic Title."
—Choice, Association of College & Research Libraries, Jan '02

"Yet another handy but also unique compilation in the extensive Health Reference Series, this is a useful work because many of the international publications reprinted or excerpted are not readily available. Highly recommended."
—Choice, Association of College & Research Libraries, Nov '01

"Recommended reference source."
—Booklist, American Library Association, Oct '01

Health Reference Series

Adolescent Health Sourcebook

AIDS Sourcebook, 1st Edition

AIDS Sourcebook, 2nd Edition

Alcoholism Sourcebook

Allergies Sourcebook, 1st Edition

Allergies Sourcebook, 2nd Edition

Alternative Medicine Sourcebook, 1st Edition

Alternative Medicine Sourcebook, 2nd Edition

Alzheimer's, Stroke & 29 Other Neurological Disorders Sourcebook, 1st Edition

Alzheimer's Disease Sourcebook, 2nd Edition

Arthritis Sourcebook

Asthma Sourcebook

Attention Deficit Disorder Sourcebook

Back & Neck Disorders Sourcebook

Blood & Circulatory Disorders Sourcebook

Brain Disorders Sourcebook

Breast Cancer Sourcebook

Breastfeeding Sourcebook

Burns Sourcebook

Cancer Sourcebook, 1st Edition

Cancer Sourcebook (New), 2nd Edition

Cancer Sourcebook, 3rd Edition

Cancer Sourcebook for Women, 1st Edition

Cancer Sourcebook for Women, 2nd Edition

Cardiovascular Diseases & Disorders Sourcebook, 1st Edition

Caregiving Sourcebook

Colds, Flu & Other Common Ailments Sourcebook

Communication Disorders Sourcebook

Congenital Disorders Sourcebook

Consumer Issues in Health Care Sourcebook

Contagious & Non-Contagious Infectious Diseases Sourcebook

Death & Dying Sourcebook

Diabetes Sourcebook, 1st Edition

Diabetes Sourcebook, 2nd Edition

Diet & Nutrition Sourcebook, 1st Edition

Diet & Nutrition Sourcebook, 2nd Edition

Digestive Diseases & Disorder Sourcebook

Disabilities Sourcebook

Domestic Violence & Child Abuse Sourcebook

Drug Abuse Sourcebook

Ear, Nose & Throat Disorders Sourcebook

Eating Disorders Sourcebook

Emergency Medical Services Sourcebook

Endocrine & Metabolic Disorders Sourcebook

Environmentally Induced Disorders Sourcebook

Ethnic Diseases Sourcebook

Family Planning Sourcebook

Fitness & Exercise Sourcebook, 1st Edition

Fitness & Exercise Sourcebook, 2nd Edition

Food & Animal Borne Diseases Sourcebook

Food Safety Sourcebook

Forensic Medicine Sourcebook

Gastrointestinal Diseases & Disorders Sourcebook